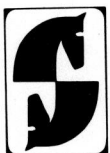

Manual of
Internal Fixation

Technique Recommended by the AO-Group

Swiss Association for the Study of Internal Fixation: ASIF

By M. E. Müller
M. Allgöwer · H. Willenegger

In Collaboration with
W. Bandi · H. R. Bloch · A. Mumenthaler
R. Schneider · B. G. Weber and S. Weller

Translated by J. Schatzker

With 306 Figures

Springer-Verlag
New York · Heidelberg · Berlin 1970

ISBN 0-387-05219-4 Springer-Verlag New York Heidelberg Berlin
ISBN 3-540-05219-4 Springer-Verlag Berlin Heidelberg New York

Translation of MÜLLER / ALLGÖWER / WILLENEGGER, Manual der Osteosynthese (1969)
ISBN 0-387-04663-1 Springer-Verlag New York Heidelberg Berlin
ISBN 3-540-04663-1 Springer-Verlag Berlin Heidelberg New York

Universitätsdruckerei H. Stürtz AG Würzburg

Preface

The German edition of our book entitled *"Operative Frakturen-behandlung"* by M. E. MÜLLER, M. ALLGÖWER and H. WILLENEGGER (Springer, Berlin · Göttingen · Heidelberg, 1963) has been out of print now for more than three years. We are planning a new edition which will deal with the collective experience of 14,000 new cases, all treated by internal fixation, and will include the newest developments in the field of internal fixation. However, it will be some time before this new edition can be published. Increasing demands for a description of the AO technique of internal fixation has stimulated us to publish this manual. In it we shall describe in a comprehensive but somewhat apodictic manner the principles and techniques of the AO methods of fracture treatment and reconstructive surgery, which in our hands, have stood the test of time.

The book is written in a somewhat abbreviated style. It corresponds in subject matter to the teaching given at the AO courses in Davos, but deals with each subject more thoroughly.

We have dispensed with pictures of the instruments, as these may be found in the Synthes Catalogue*.

This manual should be regarded as the product of collective experience, containing new thoughts and new discoveries from basic research.

In considering the risks of mistakes and dangers, we can only reiterate what we have already stated in "Technique of Internal Fixation of Fractures": "Open treatment of fractures is a valuable but difficult method which involves much responsibility. We cannot advise too strongly against internal fixation if it is carried out by an inadequately trained surgeon, and in the absence of full equipment and sterile operating room conditions. Using our methods, enthusiasts who lack self criticism are much more dangerous than skeptics or outright opponents. We hope therefore that readers will understand our efforts in this direction and that they will pass on any constructive criticism to us".

---

* Catalogues can be obtained from distributors all over the world, or from the manufacturers, Synthes, CH-4437 Waldenburg (Switzerland).

We must record our deep appreciation to our publishers as well as to our collaborators. Our gratitude is also due to the artist, Mr. OBERLI, who drew most of the illustrations and to Miss DAXWANGER, who prepared them for publication.

Berne, October, 1970

M. E. MÜLLER
M. ALLGÖWER
H. WILLENEGGER

VI

Table of Contents

VII

Special Part

Internal Fixation of Fresh Fractures

Supplement

Reconstructive Bone Surgery. By M. E. MÜLLER

Authors:
M. E. MÜLLER,
M.D., Professor of Orthopaedic Surgery,
University of Berne Medical School,
Director of the Dept. of Orthopaedics,
University of Berne, Inselspital, CH-3008 Bern

M. ALLGÖWER,
M.D., Professor of Surgery,
University of Basle Medical School,
Director of the Dept. of Surgery,
University of Basle, Bürgerspital, CH-4000 Basel

H. WILLENEGGER,
M.D., Associate Professor of Surgery,
University of Basle Medical School,
Surgeon-in-Chief, Dept. of Surgery,
Kantonsspital, CH-4410 Liestal

Contributors:
W. BANDI,
M.D., Surgeon-in-Chief,
Dept. of Surgery, Bezirksspital,
CH-3800 Interlaken

H. R. BLOCH,
M.D., Surgeon-in-Chief,
Dept. of Surgery, Kantonsspital,
CH-8750 Glarus

A. MUMENTHALER,
M.D., Bezirksspital, CH-4900 Langenthal

R. SCHNEIDER,
M.D., Surgeon-in-Chief,
Dept. of Surgery, Bezirksspital,
CH-3506 Großhöchstetten

B. G. WEBER,
M.D., Surgeon-in-Chief,
Dept. of Orthopaedics and Traumatology,
Kantonsspital, CH-9000 St. Gallen

S. WELLER,
M.D., Professor of Surgery, Surgeon-in-Chief of
Berufsgenossenschaftliche Unfallklinik
D-7400 Tübingen

Translator:
JOSEPH SCHATZKER, M.D., B.Sc. (Med.), F.R.C.S.(C),
University of Toronto, Ontario, Canada

General Considerations

1. The Aims and the Fundamental Principles of the AO Method

The chief aim in fracture treatment is the return of the injured limb to full activity. In order to prevent malunion, joint stiffness and soft tissue damage resulting from circulatory disturbances which have become known as "fracture disease," we aim to achieve such *rigid internal fixation* that a long period in plaster is no longer necessary, and early active joint movement is possible. These principles also apply in elective bone surgery, as the threat of pseudarthrosis has been overcome. It is also possible to shorten the period of time in hospital, and to facilitate earlier weight bearing and a rapid return to work. Our experience has taught us that really rigid internal fixation is best obtained by using *compression techniques* and *intramedullary nailing*.

The value of compression in obtaining rigid internal fixation was recognized by LAMBOTTE, DANIS, KROMPECHER, EGGER, CHARNLEY and many others, long before the foundation of our association (AO). The work of these investigators are the pillars on which we have built the AO method. Clinical experience, histological studies and biomechanical experiments in animals, the development of standard instrument sets, and the founding of a documentation center, have all contributed in enabling us to assess the results of cases operated upon, using compression techniques.

In the next few pages we will show by means of two examples how early mobilization can be achieved. Later we will describe briefly the six basic principles of the AO method.

A. The Aims of the AO Method

The chief aim of the AO method is the *early return to full function* of the injured limb

This is achieved by:

Accurate anatomical reduction. This is of particular importance in intra-articular fractures.	*Rigid internal fixation.*
Atraumatic operative technique preserving the *vitality* of bone and soft tissues.	*Avoidance of soft tissue damage* and the so-called "fracture disease". This is accomplished by early, active, pain-free mobilization of the muscles and joints adjacent to the fracture, without interfering with bone union.

These four **biomechanical** *principles are vital to a method of internal fixation to produce optimal fracture healing.*

In *multiple fractures* one must aim to mobilize all joints early. Example:

Fig. 1

a	Patient with a comminuted fracture of the left femur (a′), supracondylar fracture of the right femur (a″), and a compound fracture of the left tibia (a‴).
b	Function four weeks after operative treatment. Normal function of hip, knee and foot. The legs are symmetrical and partial weight bearing is possible.
c	Four months after internal fixation using condylar plates.

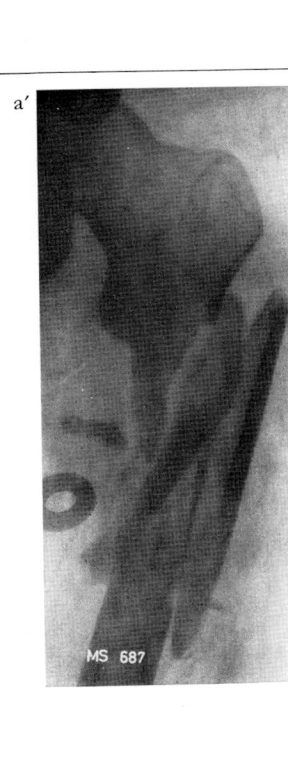

a′

MS 687

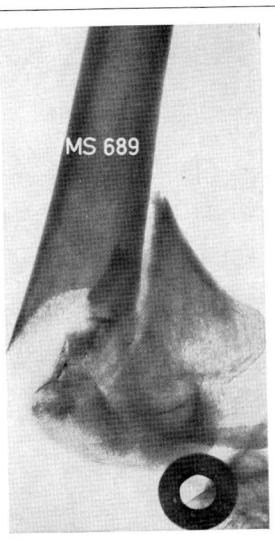

a″

MS 689

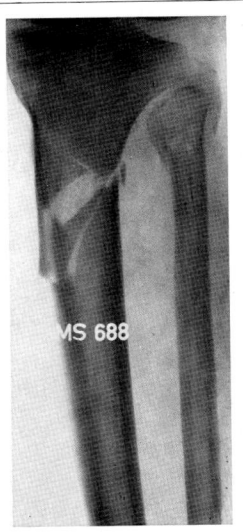

a‴

MS 688

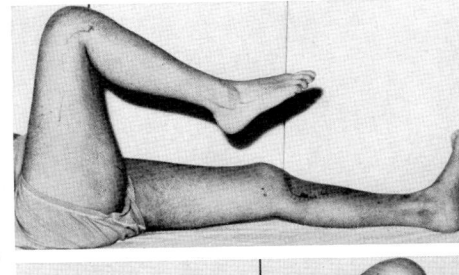

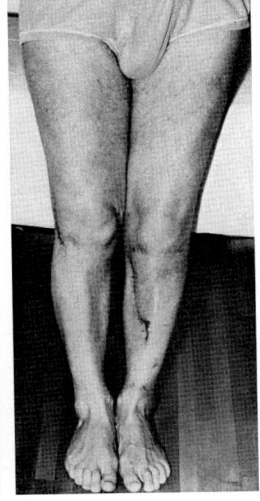

b

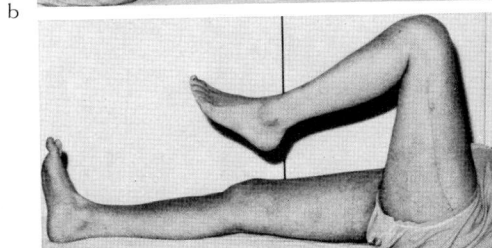

c

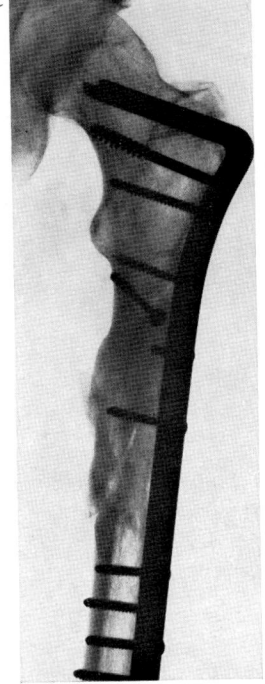

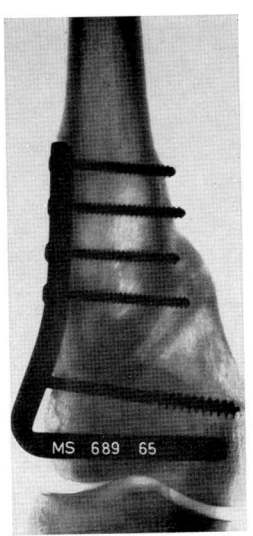

MS 689 65

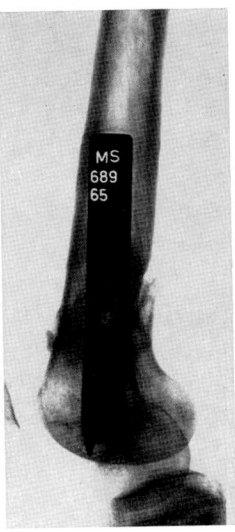

MS 689 65

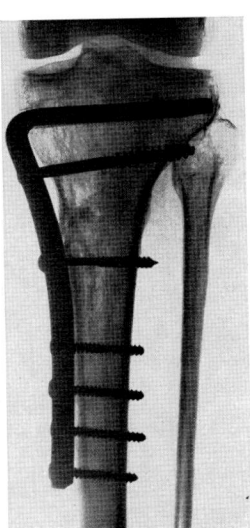

In intra-articular fractures, reconstruction of the joint surfaces and secure fixation of the many fragments which are often present, is of the utmost importance if early movement is to be instituted. A knowledge of the anatomy and joint mechanics, a three dimensional appreciation of the problem and technical ability, are all basic requirements if a perfect result is to be obtained.

In fractures involving the joint, the damage to soft tissue must be considered when early movement is contemplated. In the early period of healing it is wise to support the limb in a removable splint, either plaster, plastic or sponge rubber. This helps in soft tissue healing (Fig. 86). But also in the splint active mobilization may often be possible within the first few days.

In *comminuted intra-articular fractures* rigid internal fixation is usually possible, but to obtain a full range of movement it may be necessary to sacrifice part of a joint surface.

Fig. 2

a	Severe comminution of the upper ends of both forearm bones, first after injury and then nine months later. The comminuted radial head was resected. For technical details see Fig. 122.
b	Result nine months after surgery.
c, d	The return of movement at the end of the first month: Full extension, bilateral flexion to 30°, pronation 90°, supination 105°. This represents a full return to normal function.

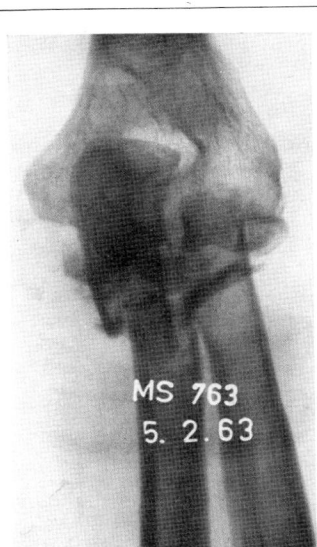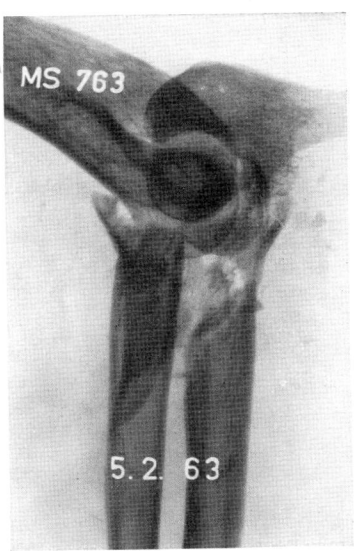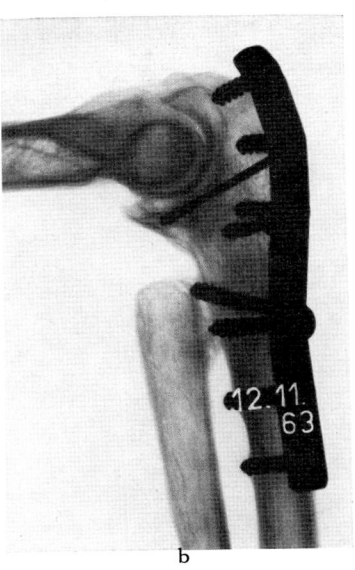

a

b

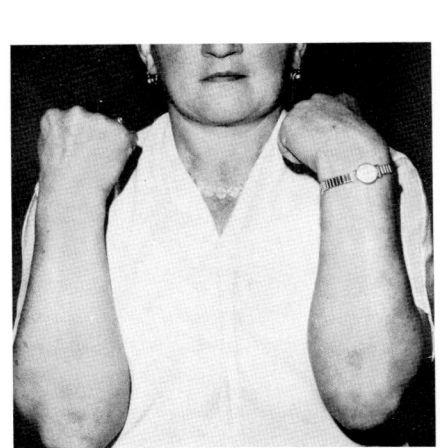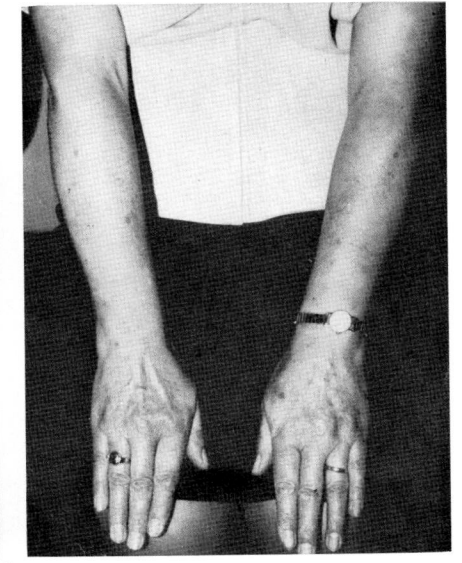

c

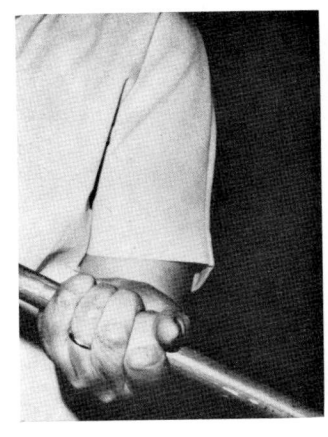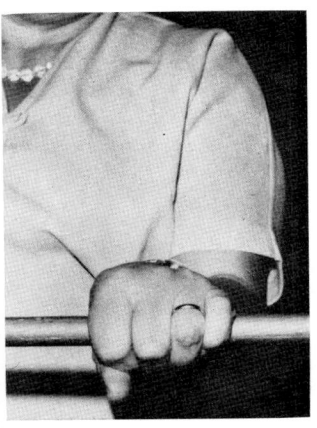

d

B. Basic Principles

The First Basic Principle

Reaction of Bone to Metal Implants

Stable internal fixation necessarily involves a lasting fixation of the implant in the bone. WAGNER was able to show that the AO screws obtain a lasting hold in animal and human bones for periods of several months. The following aspects of the screws and their use are critical:

1. Austenitic steels have no toxic effect on directly adjacent bone tissue.

2. The choice of the thread profile is critical. The AO screw reduces damaging shear forces on the loaded bone component and obtains its hold almost entirely by pressure. The bone from such pressure areas shows signs of functional adaptation on histomorphologic study.

3. Pre-threading of the screw-hole with a tap assures a good fit of the screw-thread without damaging the bone. Self-tapping screws, on the other hand, give rise to multiple micro-fractures and subsequent connective tissue formation in the region of necrotic bone. The fibrous tissue offers the screw a poor hold.

Fig. 3   Condition of a commercially obtainable, self-tapping bone screw, in a hole which was not pre-tapped. After 90 days the splintered bone has been replaced by connective tissue.

Fig. 4   *Condition of an AO cortex screw.*

a   The bone tissue is closely applied to the saw-tooth profile of the thread. The blood-forming marrow is separated from the metal only by a fine bony lamella. Neither bone resorption nor marrow fibrosis are present. The screw was two months *in situ.*

b   Living osteocytes are present even in the bone which is directly adjacent to the metal. Their fine cell processes extend to the screw surface. No osteolysis is present. Screw was nine months *in situ.*

Fig. 5   *Functional adaptation of bone to the lag screw.*

a   A cancellous screw in the head of the tibia of a young dog is subjected to the growth pressure of the epiphysial plate. Adaptation to the sustained pressure takes the form of a load sclerosis of the bone around the screw thread.

b   Cross-section of the trough area of an embedded screw, showing direction of tension of the screw (←, from right to left). Enlargement of the trabeculae on the right side, which is exposed to the pressure from the screw.

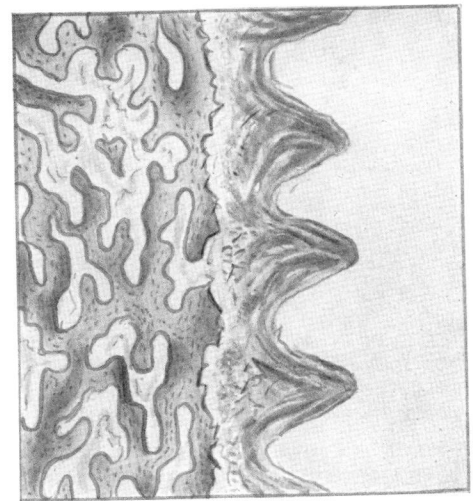

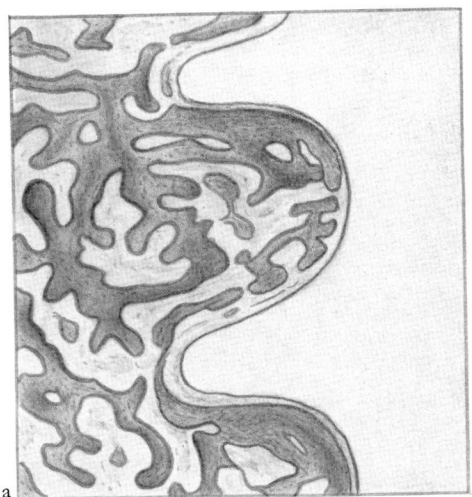

a

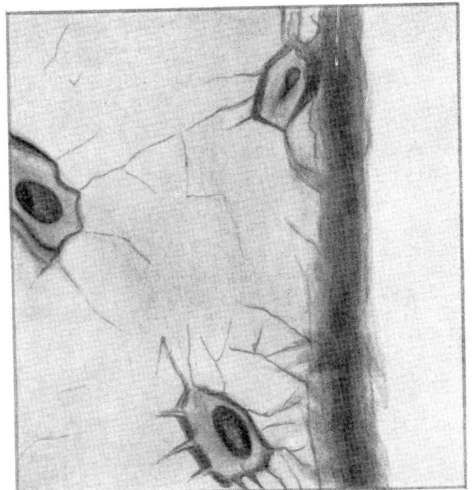

b

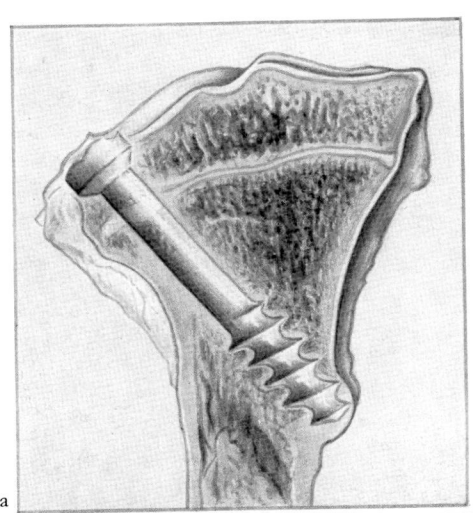

a

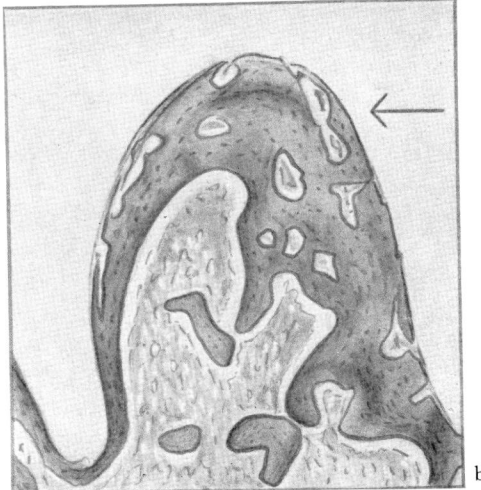

b

The Second Basic Principle

Clinical and Empirical Findings in Internal Fixation with Compression

When two vascular bone fragments are rigidly fixed under compression so that no shearing or torsional forces can act, no resorption of the fragments takes place, but direct bony union occurs without any radiologically visible periosteal or endosteal callus.

This so-called *primary bone union* is a sign of perfect internal fixation of vascular viable bone fragments.

According to BOEHLER, the bone fragments not only die but are resorbed. Thus the bone must shorten so that the fracture surfaces may be opposed to allow union. It is on these grounds that he developed his principle of the "necessary shortening" which has been the main point of his recent work. Such resorption after internal fixation with compression is only seen under two circumstances, firstly when the fragments are devitalized over a long segment; secondly when movement occurs, especially torsion or shear, even if these are only of microscopical dimensions.

In contradistinction we observe the so-called *cloudy, irritation callus* which may develop during bone healing. This is a warning sign and indicates some movement occurring at the fracture line.

The healing of a tibial fracture fixed with compression showing no visible periosteal or endosteal callus nor any widening of the fracture gap.

Fig. 6   Screw fixation of a fracture of the tibia with a butterfly fragment, (a) shown before and (b) thirteen months after surgery.

Fig. 7   Screw fixation of a tibial fracture with the addition of a neutralization plate. Before operation and seventeen weeks and thirteen months afterwards. This illustrates the socalled *primary bone union*.

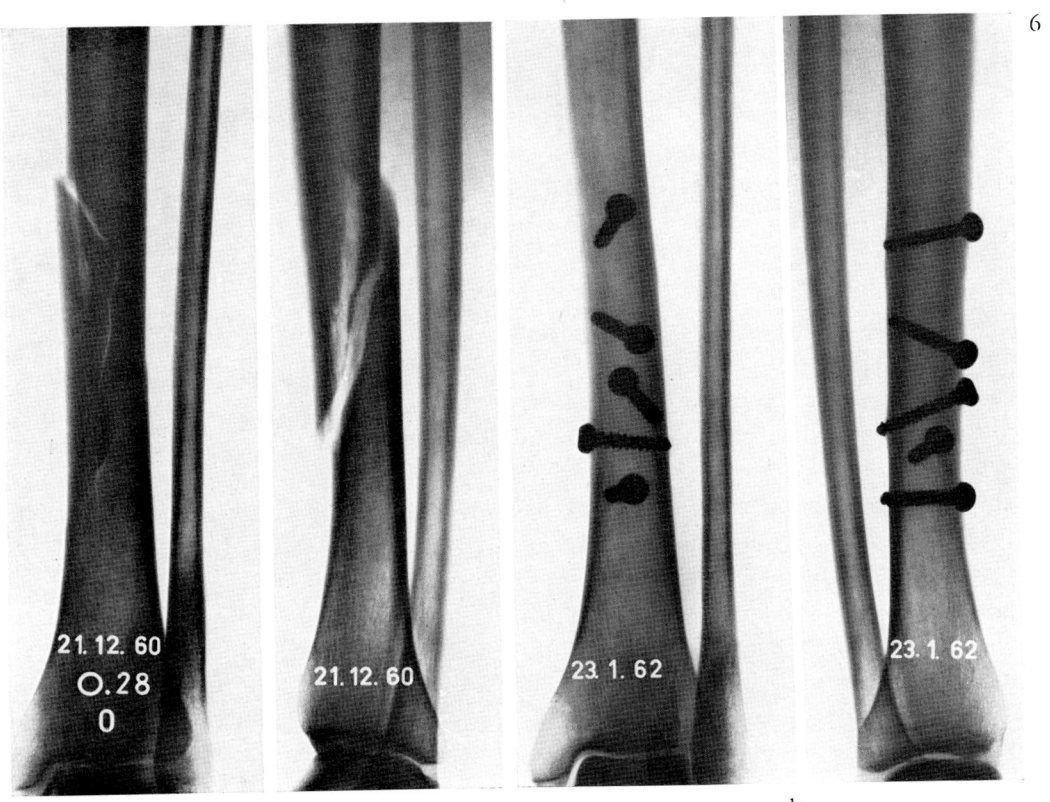

6

a   b

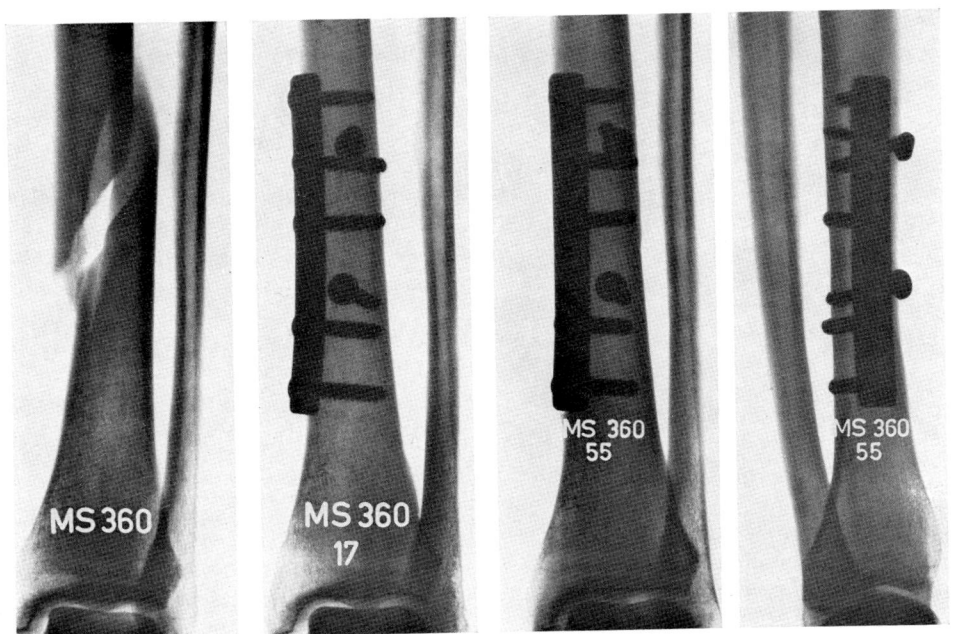

7

9

The Third Basic Principle

The Histology of Bone Union Occurring under Compression

In 1935, KROMPECHER showed in his experiments on the skulls of embryo rats, that in an area free from mechanical forces, primary vascular bone formation could occur without any cartilagenous or desmoid precursors. He postulated that this primary bone union was also possible after fractures, if these were completely immobilized. In 1949, DANIS claimed on radiological evidence that rigidly fixed fractures of the forearm bones were capable of producing primary bone union (soudure autogène).

In 1964, SCHENK showed, first in a dog and subsequently in humans, that fractures healed by primary bone union, as long as certain biomechanical conditions existed. The necessary factors were real rigidity and an intact blood supply. As long as the bone was not devitalized over a large area and the fragments were rigidly fixed, *resorption and bone formation did not occur one after the other, but happened simultaneously.*

In the experimental model done by SCHENK which involved a transverse osteotomy of a dog's radius, rigid stability was obtained using compression plates. In a clinical series this was achieved with lag screws and neutralization plates. Thus experimental and clinical evidence showed that bone was able to withstand high static loads without surface resorption at the fracture line. The blood supply must be very carefully considered. Clinically rapid post-operative revascularization of bone can be achieved in two ways. Firstly, it is important not to strip bony fragments, so that they maintain their normal blood supply. Secondly, a good vascular soft tissue covering must be maintained, so as to allow easier anastomoses of these vessels to those of the bone.

Fig. 8   *The healing of an osteotomy of a dog's radius under compression.* (Drawn from photographs by SCHENK).

a   Because of the physiological bow of the radius, after osteotomy and fixation a very small gap exists in the cortex next to the plate, and a much wider gap in the opposite cortex. The osteotomy surfaces show a very irregular zone of necrosis.

b   After eight days the small gap (*b'*) has not changed, while the wider gap in the opposite cortex (*b''*) now contains a number of vessels that have grown in, both from the periosteum and from the medullary canal. Osteoblasts have migrated from the vessel walls and have begun to lay down osteoid on the necrotic edges of the fragments, thus joining them together.

c   In the third stage of healing (8–10 weeks) revascularization of the necrotic fragment is occurring in two ways. In the cortex next to the plate where there was a minimal gap, the vessels are growing in from the widened Haversian canals. In the opposite cortex where there was a wider gap, the vessels are coming from the Haversian canals as well as from the outside. Under compression the close apposition of cortical fragments next to the plate does not allow any vessels to grow in from either the endosteum or the periosteum, while in the opposite cortex the vessels are growing in from both these sites. Both gaps, however, heal by primary vascular bone formation.

d   Magnification of a capillary bud arising from the Haversian canal, shows that bone resorption is immediately followed by bone formation. At the head of the column of penetrating cells are multinucleated osteoclasts (*a*) which are resorbing necrotic bone (*e*) and are making room for the capillaries (*b*) and their accompanying osteoblasts (*c*) to grow in. The osteoblasts lay down osteoid (*d*) and soon change into concentrically arranged osteocytes.

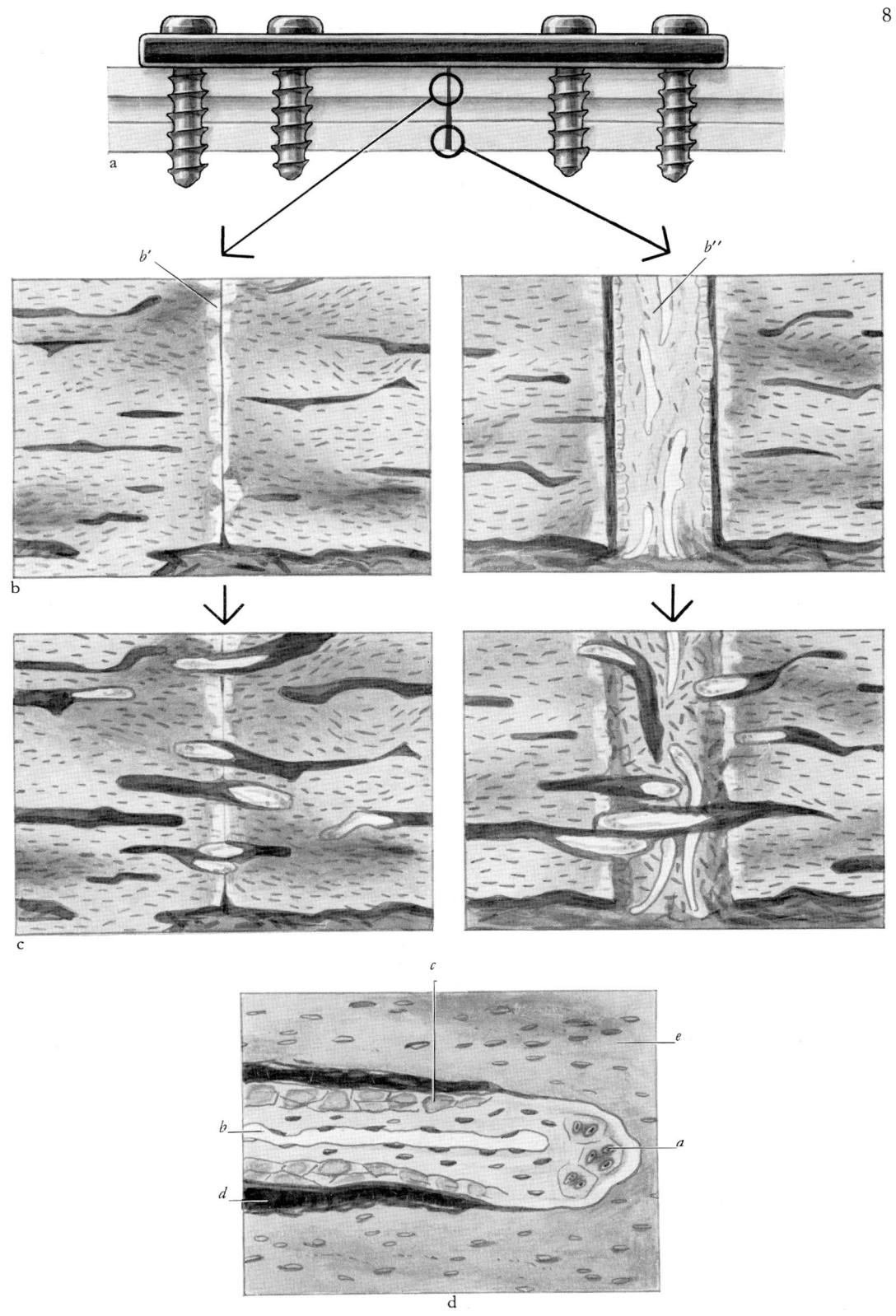

8

The Fourth Basic Principle

The Biomechanical Experiments for Measuring the Magnitude and Duration of Compression between Fragments

PERREN performed osteotomies of both the tibia and the metatarsals of sheeps. These were fixed with plates provided with strain gauges so that the existing compression could be recorded daily. He showed that an initial compression of over 100 kilograms diminished by 50% over a period of two months. This fall in compression is not related to resorption but to remodelling in the Haversian system.

As it is clear that under favorable biological and mechanical conditions the pressure between fragments diminishes very slowly, it is evidently safe to use the mechanical advantages of compression without incurring any biological disadvantages. Compression greatly increases the rigidity of the internal fixation.

Fig. 9   *Biomechanical experiments of* PERREN.

a   A plate fitted with strain gauges measuring up to 300 kg ($\pm$1.5 kg).

b   Such a plate can be put under tension with a tension device (Fig. 31). The tension in the plate is directly proportional to the compression at the fracture site.

c   This type of plate is applied to the osteotomized tibia of a sheep. The leads from these gauges run subcutaneously to a point on the animal's back.

d   A standard curve derived from dozens of measurements show a gradual fall in pressure over a period of four months.

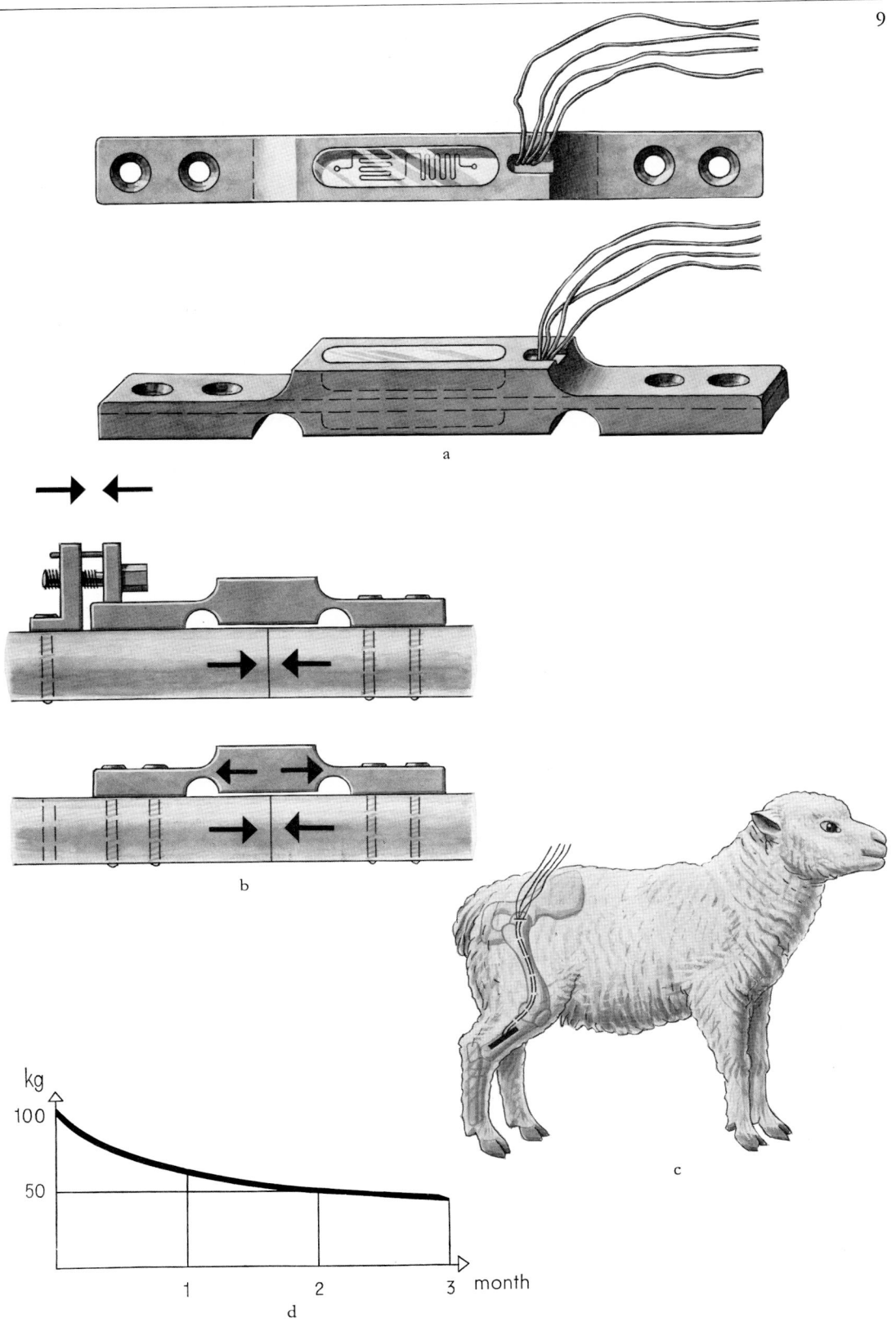

a

b

c

d

The Fifth Basic Principle

The Development of Standard Bone Instrument Sets which Have Made it Possible to Overcome most of the Problems of Internal Fixation of Fresh Fractures, Pseudarthroses, Osteotomies and Arthrodeses.

The surgeons of the AO responsible for the development of these implants and instruments, developed them as did DANIS, with the objective of applying *compression to bone fragments*. After their development these instruments have been put to extensive tests over the years. The ideas of other instruments have been borrowed, such as the compression apparatus of CHARNLEY and the medullary nail of KÜNTSCHER and HERZOG. These have been modified. The respective procedures have been made more simple, certain and versatile. Additional instruments such as bone holding forceps, spreaders, HOHMANN retractors and a series of compressed air machines have all helped to make internal fixation easier.

These instruments (known as the Synthes instruments) were first developed in 1958, and in the following years they were improved and supplemented by both orthopaedic and general surgeons, who, in their daily work practise internal fixation. Without the personal contributions and ideas of Mr. R. MATHYS, Mr. F. STRAUMANN and Mr. S. STEINEMANN, none of these ideas could have been implemented.

Copies: The AO instrumentation has been copied all over the world by most of the main manufacturers of surgical instruments. Although these copies observe only a few of the AO principles they nevertheless help to disseminate the AO method. The AO has tested both the quality and the design of the Synthes instruments but cannot accept responsibility for any of the copies. We strongly advise against using mixtures of implants of different origin.

Fig. 10   *The synthes instruments.*

1. *Sets for internal fixation using compression:*
   a Basic instrument set for screws and plates,
   b Instrument set for angled plates,
   c Screw set,
   d Standard plate set,
   e Small fragment set,
   f Angled blade plates.

2. *Sets for medullary nailing:*
   a Instrument set for medullary reaming, for insertion and extraction of medullary nails,
   b Reaming rod, guide rod, flexible reamer shafts, medullary tube, femoral and tibial nails.

3. *Additional instruments:*
   Bone holding forceps, hammer, chisels, Hohmann retractors.

4. *Compressed air machines:*
   a The universal drill and the small air drill,
   b The compressed air drill for medullary reaming,
   c The oscillating bone saw.

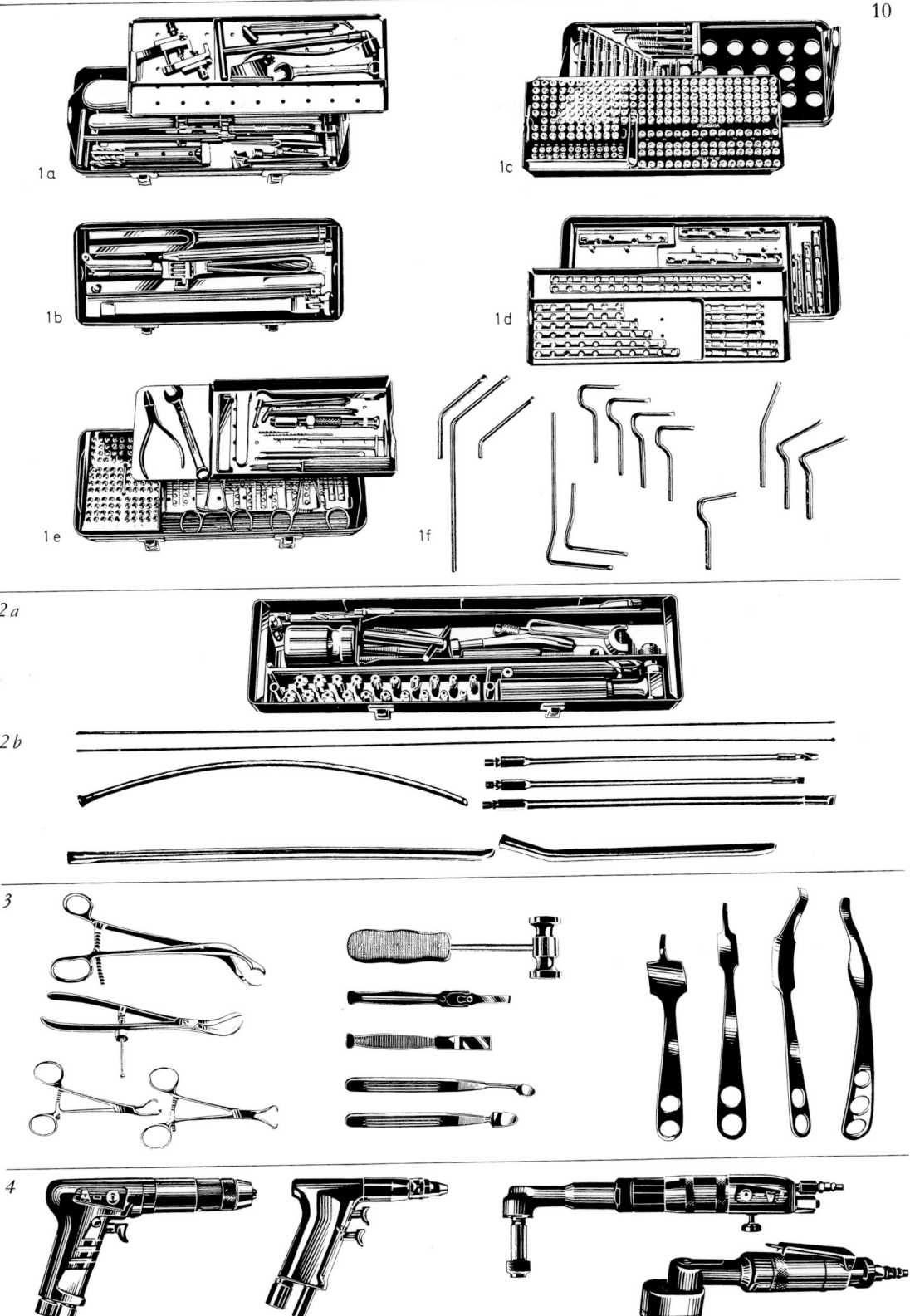

The Sixth Basic Principle

The AO Documentation Center

The backbone of the AO method is the careful documentation of over 14,000 operative cases that have been carefully followed up. Thousands of code cards were filled up and fed into computers. Over two hundred thousand X-rays, both before and after operation, as well as those taken at four and twelve months after surgery, were micro-filmed, printed and fixed on to punch cards. It is only by this detailed documentation that members of the AO were able to assess the potential and the results of the method, and to eliminate certain mistakes. This kind of follow-up system requires great patience and excellent organization, besides needing large financial backing. All of this is very worth-while however, because we are now able to prove or disprove any hypotheses. The study of failures was particularly valuable. Our rule has been that a single failure which has certainly resulted from the method itself and not from its misuse, requires re-evaluation and redesign of the technique. Over the years many procedures have been gradually improved, enlarged or standardized. The results of treatment, and discoveries by AO members are discussed every year during the AO course on operative fracture treatment that is held at Davos.

Systematic analysis of our failures has shown that these have mostly been due to a disregard of biomechanical principles. This means that most failures are preventable. *When a special surgical procedure has been in use for long enough to predict success or failure, it will then follow that success can always be achieved as long as sufficient care is taken.* This is why we feel that our procedures can be considered as safe and certain. It does not mean, however, that they are without difficulty nor that anyone is capable of carrying them out.

Anyone using the AO method should conduct follow-up examinations at four months and at one year on all their cases. It is only by such a review that the value of the method in the hands of any particular surgeon can be established.

Fig. 11   *AO Documentation.*

     a   A full series of enlarged prints of 35 mm negatives taken of all x-rays of one case.

     b   Punch cards showing all the necessary information on one side with the microfilms of the X-rays on the back.

     c   Code cards—those of the first period in hospitalization, those at four months follow-up and those of the final review.

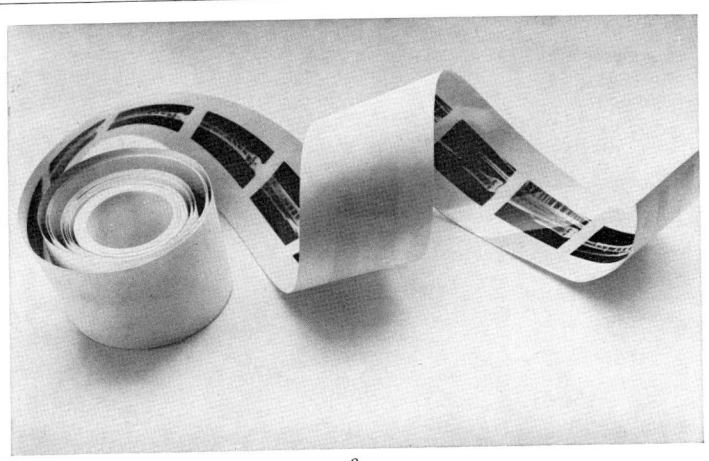

a

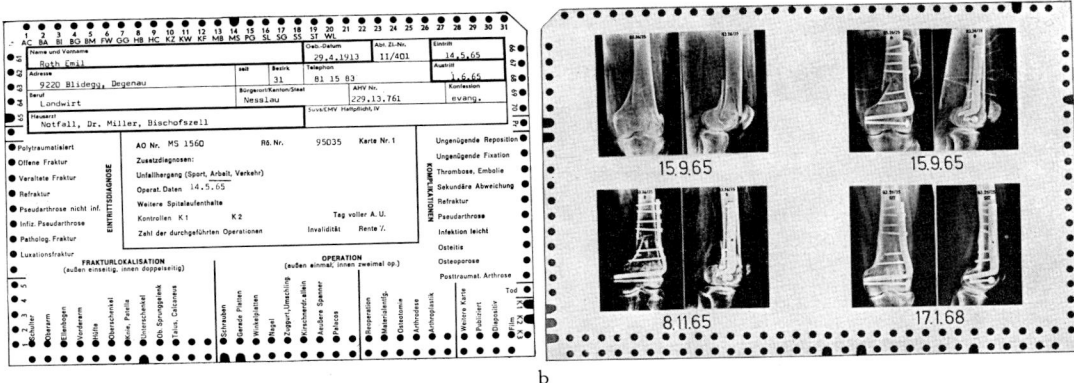

b

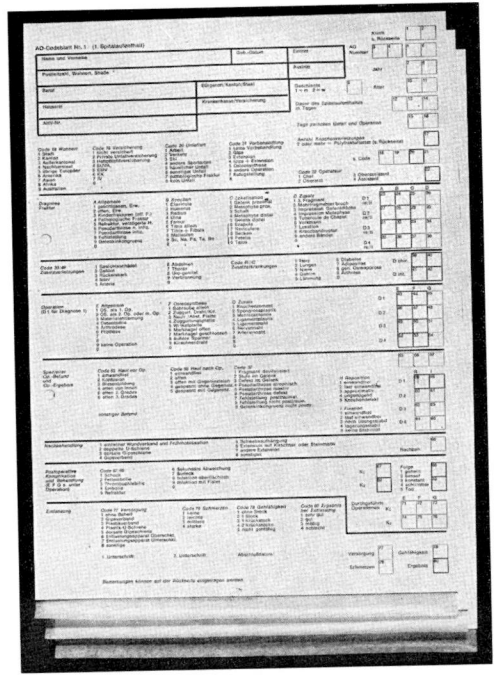

c

To page 19:

B. Medullary Nailing

Medullary nailing is reserved almost exclusively for fractures of the lower limb, especially for the middle third of the femur and the tibia.

> The so called *"compression plates"* are either *"tension band plates"* when they act as tension bands on the tensile side of the bone or *"neutralization plates"* when they are used to neutralize the forces acting on a stabilized fracture.

Remark: The word "compression plate" is a misnomer because the plate is actually under tension, however it has come into common use and will likely persist. It refers to a plate used in such a way that the fracture fragments are put under compression.

II. The Internal Fixation —
Method of the AO

Rigid internal fixation can be accomplished by either:

A. *Compression* (axial, interfragmental by itself or in combination with neutralization or buttress plates) or

B. *Medullary nailing.*

Though there are specific indications for each method, there are some types of fracture and some post-traumatic conditions which may be treated by either method with equally good results.

> Our experience with compression has led us to conclude that compression does not have any mystical osteogenic properties; it does, however, provide the most rigid form of internal fixation.

A. Compression

1. *Interfragmental compression* acts on the whole fracture surface and is achieved by means of lag screws. *Cancellous screws* are employed in the epiphyses and metaphyses and *cortex screws* in diaphyses. Interfragmental compression is used alone in most fractures involving cancellous bone as well as in those oblique fractures in cortical bone where the length of the fracture line is at least twice the diameter of the shaft at that level.

2. *Axial compression* is achieved by means of the *tension band principle* (tension band cerclage wiring in avulsion fractures, straight plates in shaft fractures, and special plates for fractures involving the ends of bones) or with *double compression* which is applied by means of either two plates or two to four Steinmann pins and a Charnley type of compression apparatus.
   When the tension band principle is applied, it is vital that it is used on the side of the bone that is under a distraction force. Double compression, on the other hand, is useful only in the metaphysis or epiphysis or in shaft pseudarthroses.

3. The combination of *interfragmental and axial compression.* Compression between cortical fragments is used in combination with a neutralization plate in the treatment of tibial shaft fractures for instance, or in cancellous bone in combination with a buttress plate.
   Continuation see page 18.

1. Interfragmental Compression

Cancellous Screws

To compress fragments of epiphyseal or metaphyseal bone the thread of the cancellous lag screw must not cross the fracture line. After drilling a hole the thread is cut with a cancellous tap. In pure cancellous bone as in the malleoli, the malleolar screw may be inserted without predrilling or tapping.

> *The principle of the cancellous screw:* the thread of the screw must never cross the fracture line.

N.B.: Screw fixation of cancellous bone is only effective if the fracture surfaces are in close apposition. If a gap is present this must first be filled with an autogenous cancellous bone graft (see Fig. 87/88).

Fig. 12	*AO cancellous screws.*
a	The standard cancellous screw is threaded for 32 mm of its length. The diameter of thread is 6.5 mm. The head of the screw has a hexagonal recess.
b	The cancellous screw with a short thread, being only 16 mm in length. In all other details it is the same as a.
c	A special small cancellous screw with a thread diameter of 4 mm and a Philips head.
d	A malleolar screw with thread and head identical to that of the cortex screw. The thread extends, however, only over the distal half of the screw and its tip is triangular so that predrilling and tapping is not necessary.
e	Washer for use on the neck of a screw if there is danger of the screw head sinking into the bone.
Fig. 13	*Some typical indications for the use of cancellous screws.*
a	Fracture of a femoral condyle. Use two long threaded cancellous screws—one with a washer.
b	Fracture of the posterior lip of the lower end of the tibia (Volkmann's triangle). Use a cancellous screw with a short thread. Introduce it from the front backwards, so that it lies parallel to the ankle joint and just above it.
c	Long oblique fracture of the lateral malleolus. This may be stabilized with two small cancellous screws.
d	Fracture of the medial malleolus. Fix this fracture with one malleolar screw in combination with a second screw or a Kirschner wire to prevent rotation.
e	Fracture of the lateral malleolus. A short spiral fracture can be fixed with one malleolar screw which is introduced so that it lies obliquely in both planes and so that the tip penetrates the proximal cortex.
f	A Y-fracture of the lower end of the humerus. The first step is fixation of the humeral condyles with a malleolar screw.

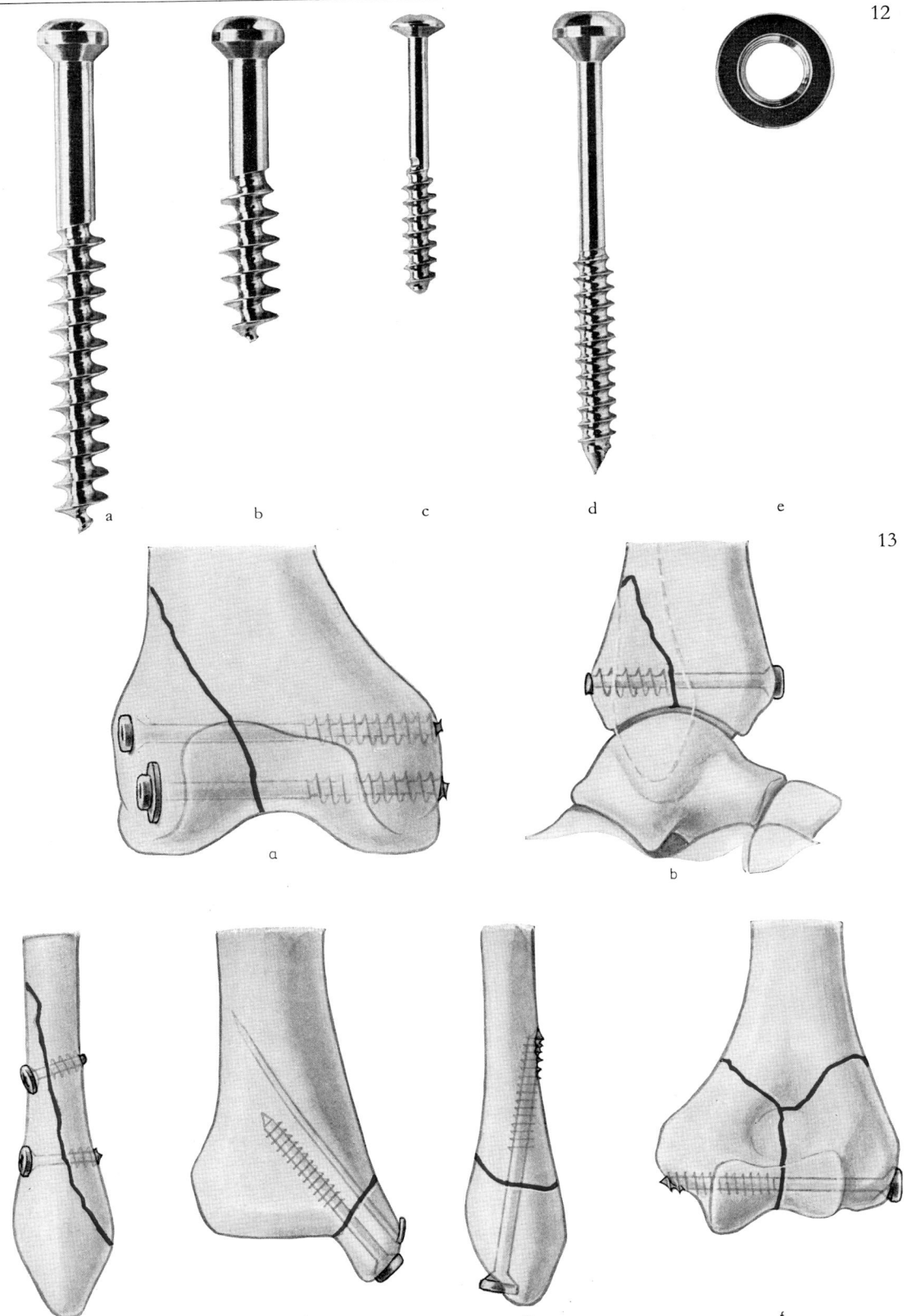

a   b   c   d   e

a

b

c   d   e   f

The cortex screw will act as a lag screw only when it can obtain a grip in the far cortex and not in that nearest to the screw head. This requires a larger hole to be cut in the cortex nearest to the screw head, and a smaller one the far cortex, which should also be tapped. The large hole is referred to as the "gliding hole" and the far one as the "thread hole".

Fig. 14	*The AO cortex screws and their taps.*
a	A standard cortex screw has a thread of 4.5 mm diameter. The screw head has a hexagonal recess and a core of 3 mm diameter. (The figure shows it at twice its normal size.)
b	A small cortex screw with a thread diameter of 3.5 mm and a Philips head.•
c	A special small cortex screw to be used for small bones in hand and foot surgery. This has a thread of 2.7 mm diameter and a Philips head.
d, e, f	Taps for a, b and c (one-third of their normal size).
Fig. 15	*The specifications of the standard AO cortex screw.*
	The screw head has a shallow cylindrical flank (*a*) which allows a better contact with the hole in the plate. The hexagonal recess in the head (*b*) affords a better grip for the screwdriver (*c*). Philips screwdriver (*d*) with its screw holding sleeve (*e*).
Fig. 16	*Details of a standard AO cortex screw compared with those of an ordinary commercially available self-tapping bone screw.*
1	The thread of the AO screw (*a*) is at right angles to the axis and represents the pressure bearing surface. The thread is of equal diameter throughout so that even the last turn of the thread (*b*) can get a full grip on the bone. The tip (*c*) is round without any flutes. This makes it necessary to cut the thread for the screw with a tap. The drill hole (*d*) is only 0.2 mm greater than the core of the screw. This is possible because this is a non-self-tapping screw and the thread is precut for it with the tap.
2	In comparison, many commercially available screws are self-tapping (*e*) and for this reason the drill hole (*f*) must be made relatively wide so that only the tips of the narrow round threads (*g*) get any purchase on the bone.

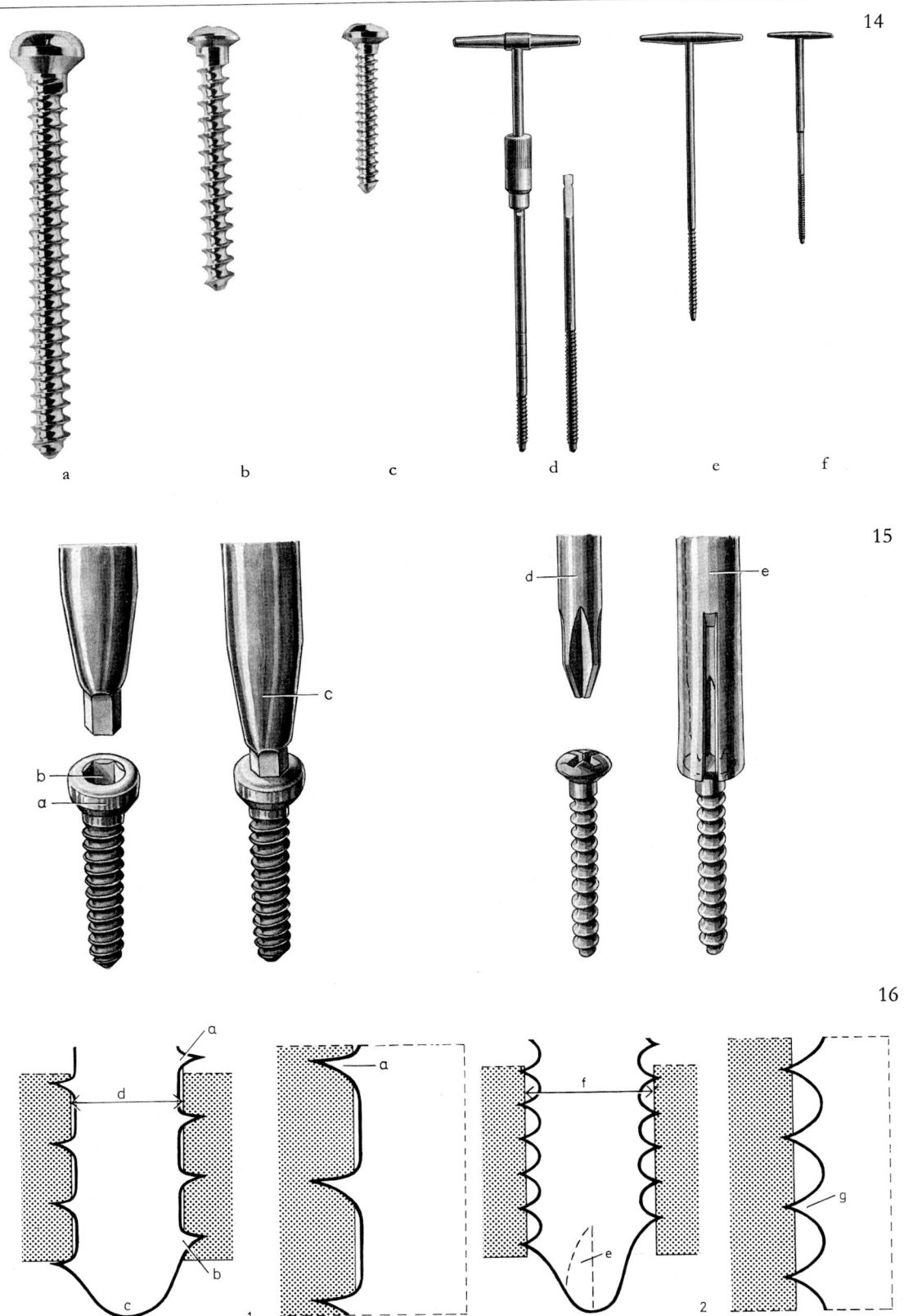

14

15

16

1

2

23

Standard method of internal fixation with compression of cortical fragments using a cortex screw.

Fig. 17   *The principle.*

a   The hole in the cortex nearest to the screw head (*gliding hole*) is cut so that the threads can pass freely through it without getting a grip, and so that the screw only gets a hold on the far cortex (*thread hole*). As the screw is tightened, the fragments are compressed. This is how *compression between fragments* is obtained.

b   If, on the other hand, a drill hole goes through both cortices and the thread is tapped in both, then the fragments can never be compressed relative to each other. The screw will break long before the slightest approximation of the fragments.

Fig. 18   *Screw fixation after the fragments have been reduced.*

a   Drill the near cortex with a 4.5 mm drill, using the 4.5 mm tap sleeve which acts as a drill guide.

b   Insert the special drill sleeve which has an outer diameter of 4.5 mm and an inner diameter of 3.2 mm into the hole that has just been drilled, and push it until it meets the opposite cortex. This drill sleeve will now allow an accurate hole to be drilled in the far cortex, even if the hole is placed obliquely.

c   Now drill the far cortex with a 3.2 mm drill, fitted with a stop.

d   Measure the required screw length with the depth gauge.

e   Tap out the thread in the far cortex with the short 4.5 mm cortex tap.

f   Using the special countersink tool, cut a proper countersink in the near cortex for the screw head.

g   With the screwdriver screw in the AO cortex screw but do not tighten it. The screws are finally tightened when they have all been inserted.

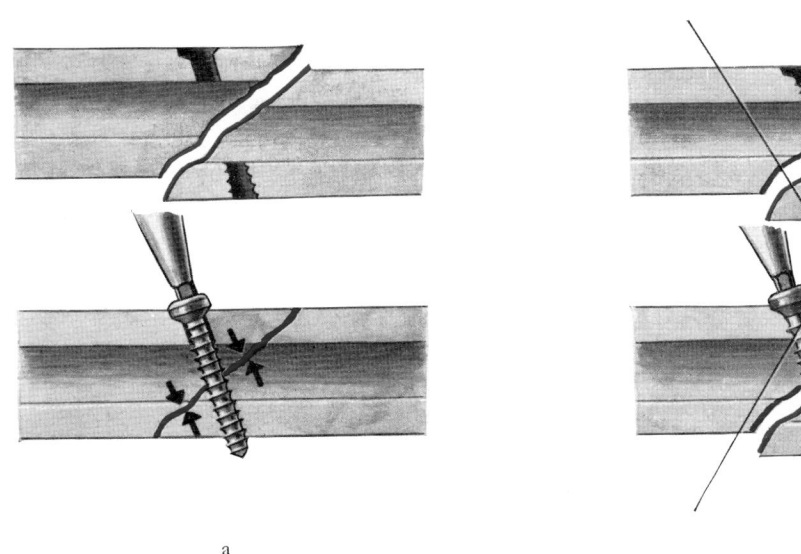

a   b

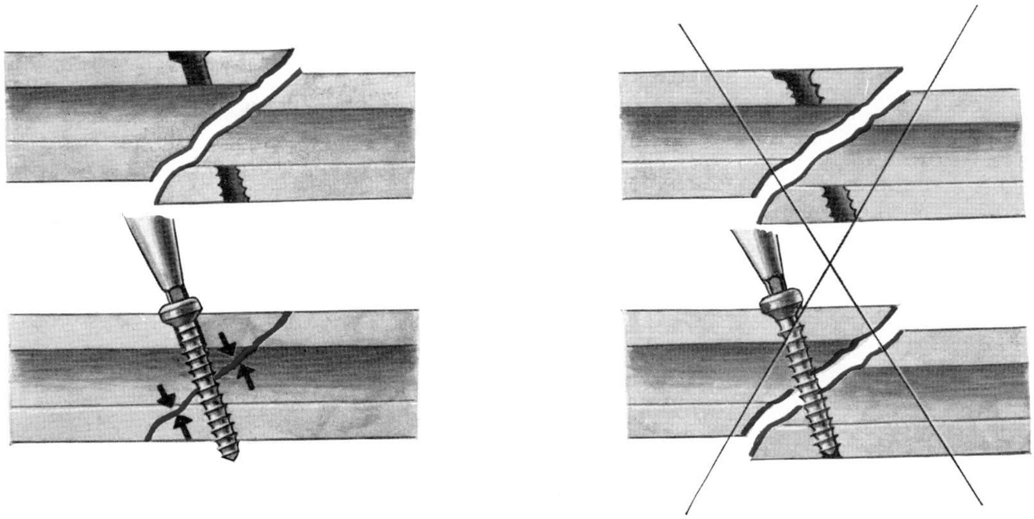

17

18

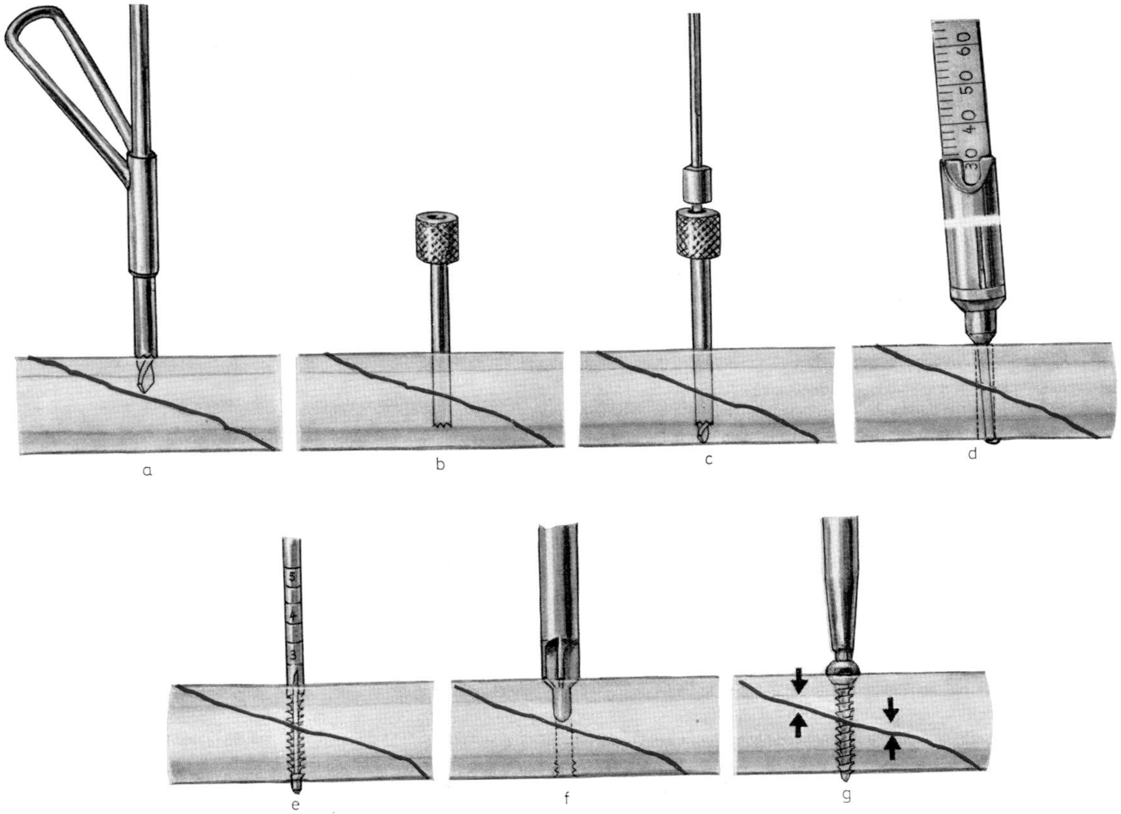

a   b   c   d

e   f   g

Fig. 19   *The drilling of the near cortex (gliding hole) from the outside inwards with a 4.5 mm drill prior to reduction.*

a   Use the 4.5 mm drill with its sleeve and drill the near cortex before reduction, aiming for the middle of the medullary canal ("*gliding hole*").

b   The fracture is now reduced and held with bone holding forceps. The drill sleeve with an outer diameter of 4.5 mm is now inserted into the hole and the opposite cortex is drilled with the 3.2 mm drill. The thread is now tapped in this far hole ("*thread hole*") and the screw inserted as described in Fig. 18 (d–g).

Fig. 20   With the special AO reduction clamp it is possible to grasp both borders of the tibia without devitalizing either the posterior or the lateral surfaces. This method results in the least damage to the blood supply of the bone.

Fig. 21   First drill two of the three required drill holes. After reduction of the fragments and temporary fixation with one or two reduction clamps, drill the thread holes in the opposite cortices as shown in Fig. 19. In the middle, the two main fragments are held together by one lag screw. The remaining two lag screws are inserted so that their direction lies halfway between perpendiculars to the axis of the limb and to the fracture plane (see also Fig. 25).

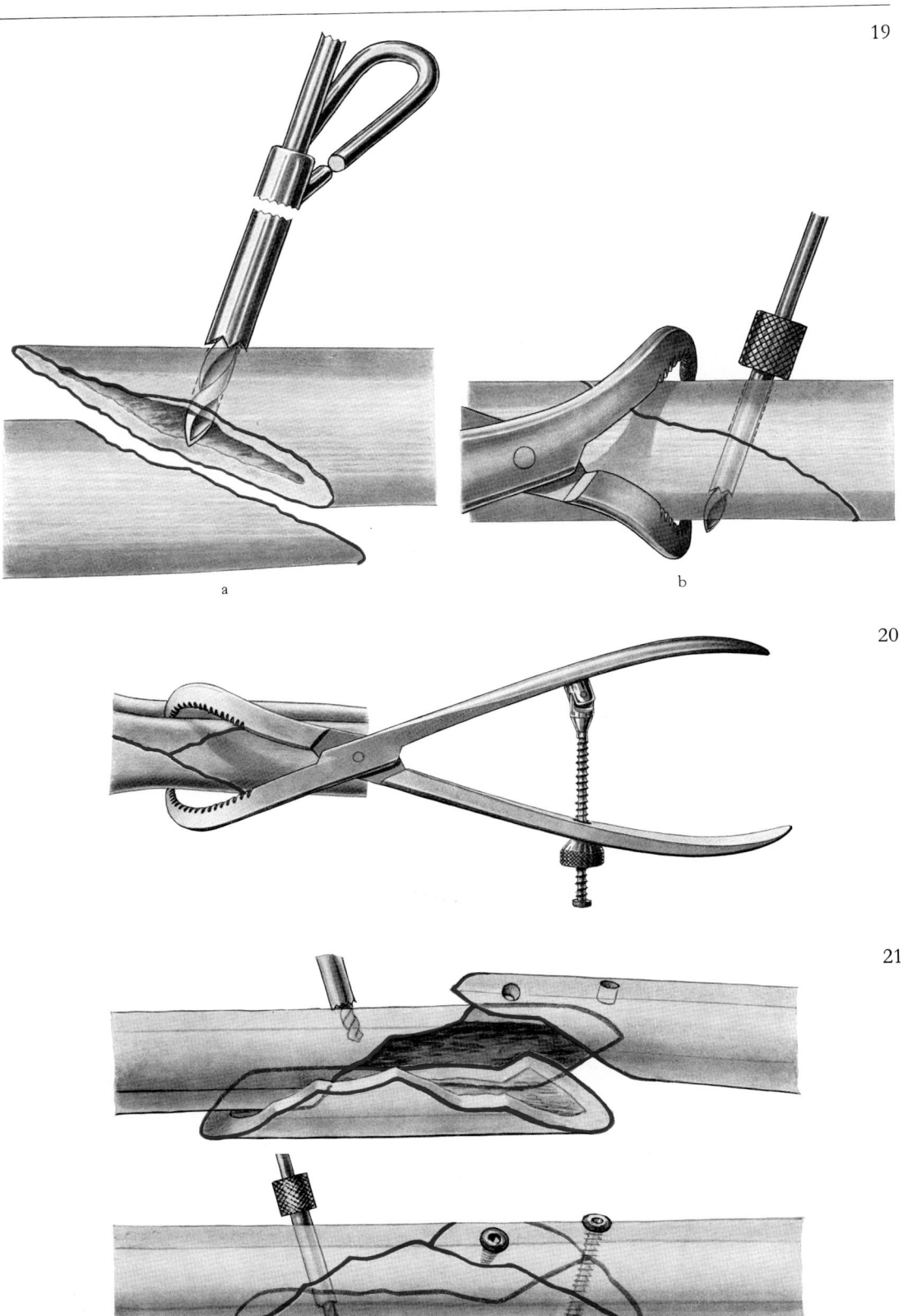

a

b

Another type of screw fixation technique.

Fig. 22   *Drilling of the thread hole in the far cortex with a 3.2 mm drill prior to reduction.*

With a 3.2 mm drill a suitable thread hole is made in the center of the cortex of the posterior fragment (a). Now take the special aiming device (b) which has a 3.1 mm tip (c) and a 4.5 mm drill sleeve, pass it round the bone and let it slip into the hole that has just been drilled. This will correctly aim the 4.5 mm drill in the near cortex to make the two holes coaxial. Reduce the fracture. Drill the gliding hole with the 4.5 mm drill. Finish the screw fixation as in Fig. 18 d–f.

This procedure conditions an undesirable stripping of the posterior plane of the bone, but is often the only possibility to place the thread hole in one fragment end optimally.

Fig. 23   After reducing a shaft fracture in the tibia, temporary cerclage wire fixation is helpful (see page 182). The AO discourages this because it leads to devitalization of the posterolateral aspect of the tibia.

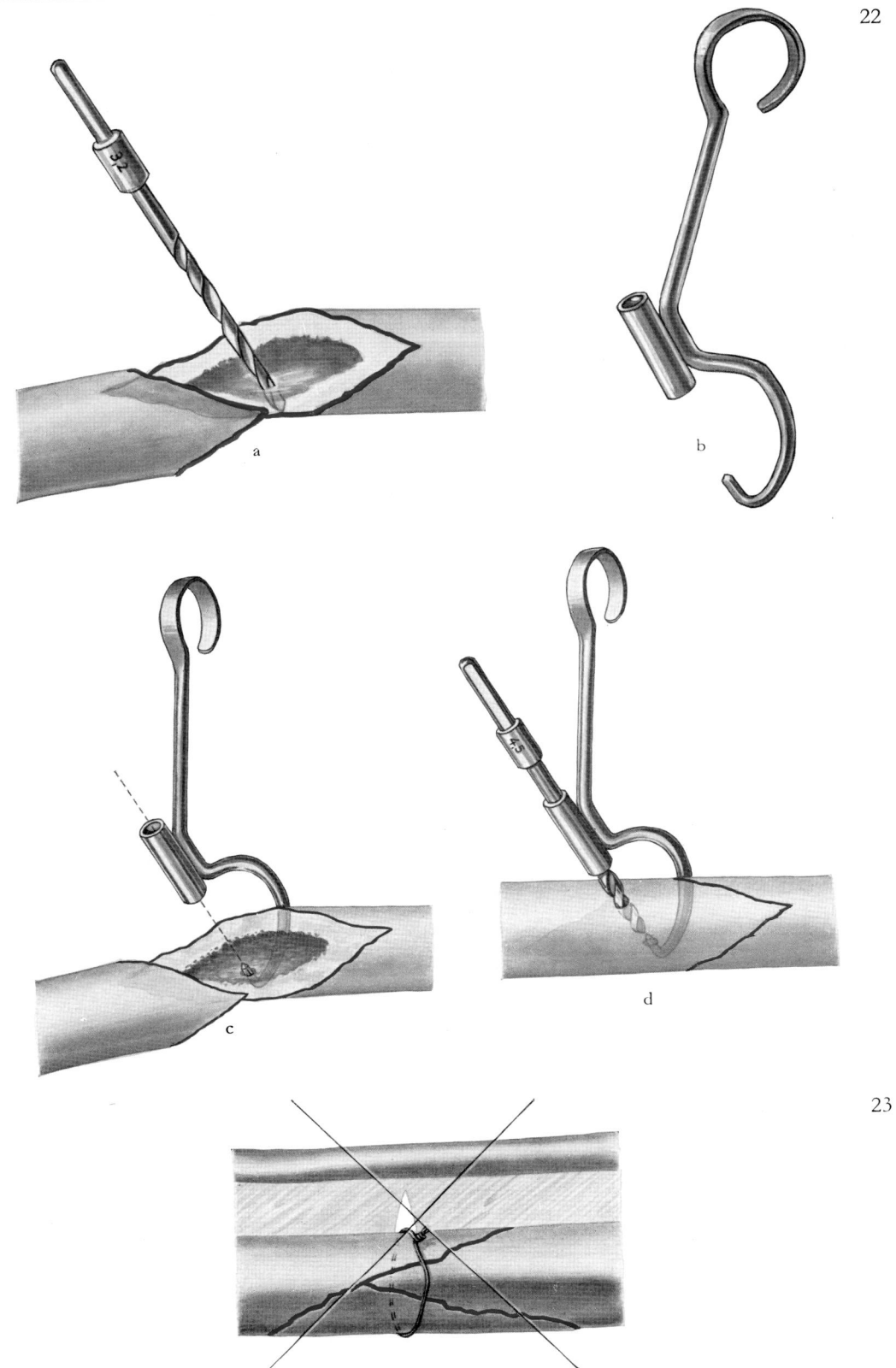

a

b

c

d

If screws only are used for fixation, the direction of each screw is of the utmost importance

Fig. 24   *The direction of the screws.*

a   In a spiral or long oblique fracture at least one screw should be inserted at right angles to the shaft of the bone. The other screws should be inserted in such a way that some will come to lie anteriorly, and others posteriorly to the middle screw in order to exert interfragmental compression at right angles to the fracture plane and overcome all shearing or torsional stresses.

b   A cross-section shows why screws placed in different directions get the best compression between fragments.

c   If a single screw is used for fixation and is placed at right angles to the plane of the fracture, then, under axial compression, the fragments glide easily upon each other and displacement may occur.

d   If, on other hand, the screw is placed at right angles to the long axis of the shaft, displacement can only occur if the head of the screw penetrates the cortex, which is not very likely, or when the threads strip out of the bone.

Fig. 25   Simple spiral fracture with a butterfly fragment: One screw (a) fixes the two main fragments. The other screws (b) are inserted so that they bisect the angles between a perpendicular to the long axis of the shaft and a perpendicular to the fracture plane. The screws should not be tightened until the very end.

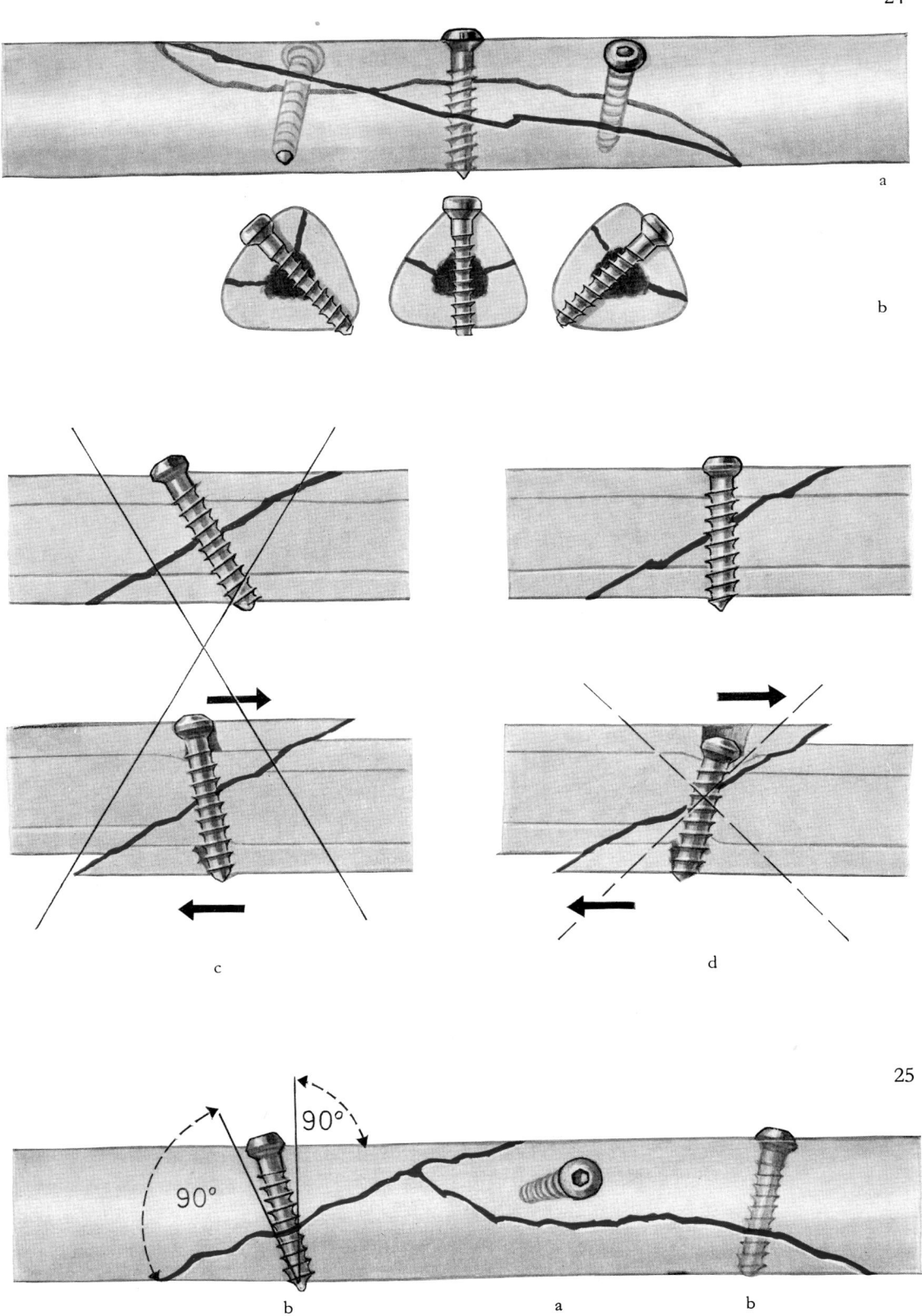

a

b

c

d

90°

90°

b   a   b

2. Axial Compression

The Tension Band Principle

The term "tension band" has been borrowed from engineers and was first defined by PAUWELS as a system to be used in the treatment of pseudoarthroses, fractures of the patella, and intertrochanteric osteotomies. With a tension band, the acting tensile forces are counteracted and are converted into compressive forces. To employ this principle we use, as did PAUWELS, 1.2 mm wire, straight plates, T-plates and angled plates, which are placed under tension with our tension device. Similarly, the standard and small semi-tubular plates are employed as tension bands and so are Schanz screws when held with two external compression clamps.

Fig. 26	PAUWELS' *diagram to show the difference between load and stress as well as the tension band principle.*
a	If a column is loaded so that the weight lies in its center, then within the column there are only compressive stresses (D = 10).
b	If the weight is applied eccentrically, then in addition to compressive stresses (D = 10 present in a) we introduce a bending moment. This results in additional compressive stresses (D = 100) and equal and opposite tensile stresses (Z = 100).
c, d	These additional bending stresses, the result of eccentric loading, can be neutralized by means of a *tension band*, which in the diagram is respresented by a chain (c). This neutralization of the bending stresses acts as if an additional compression were exerted by a second weight (d), placed at an equal distance from the center of the axis of the column, but on the opposite side. Although the load is increased (D = 200 kg) the total stress is reduced to a fifth (20 kg/cm²) because the bending stresses are completely neutralized.
Fig. 27	*The use of the tension band in internal fixation. Three examples taken from* PAUWELS.
a	*Fracture of the patella:* If a cerclage wire is placed posteriorly to the center of the patella, then the fragments must open up anteriorly. This is a phenomenon which can often be observed in simple circumferential wiring. If, however, the wire is placed anteriorly, as shown (a') then tensile stress is converted into a compressive stress.
b	*Intertrochanteric varus osteotomy:* A varus osteotomy can be adequately fixed by means of two Kirschner wires and a tension band wire. The Kirschner wires prevent rotation and the tension band wire prevents any further varus displacement.
c	*Longstanding pseudarthroses of the femur:* The simple insertion of a tension band wire just in front of the linea aspera, will result in consolidation without resection of any tissue between the fragments, but as the tension band wire cannot overcome all rotational stresses it is necessary to supplement this form of fixation with a hip spica for two months.

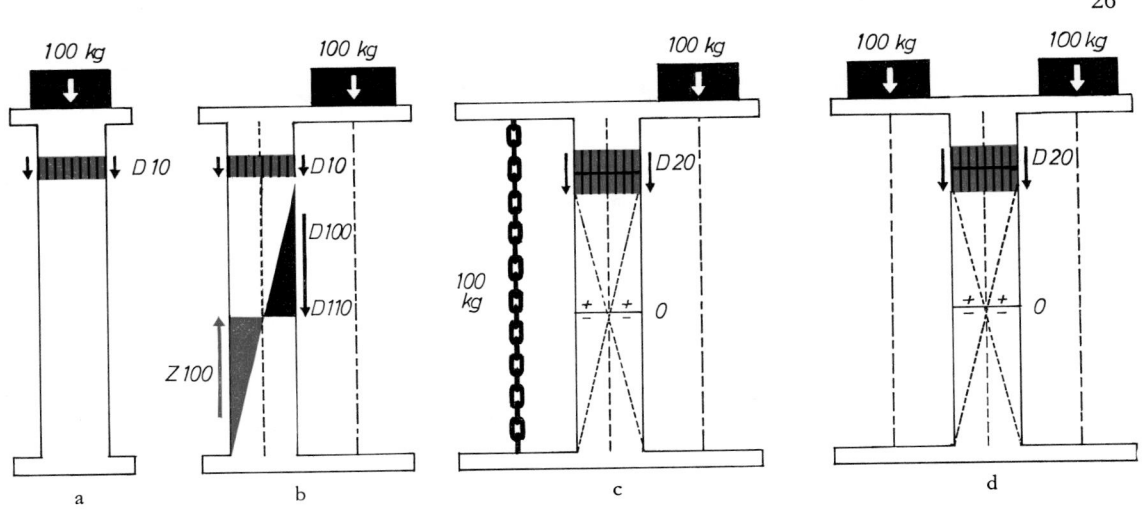

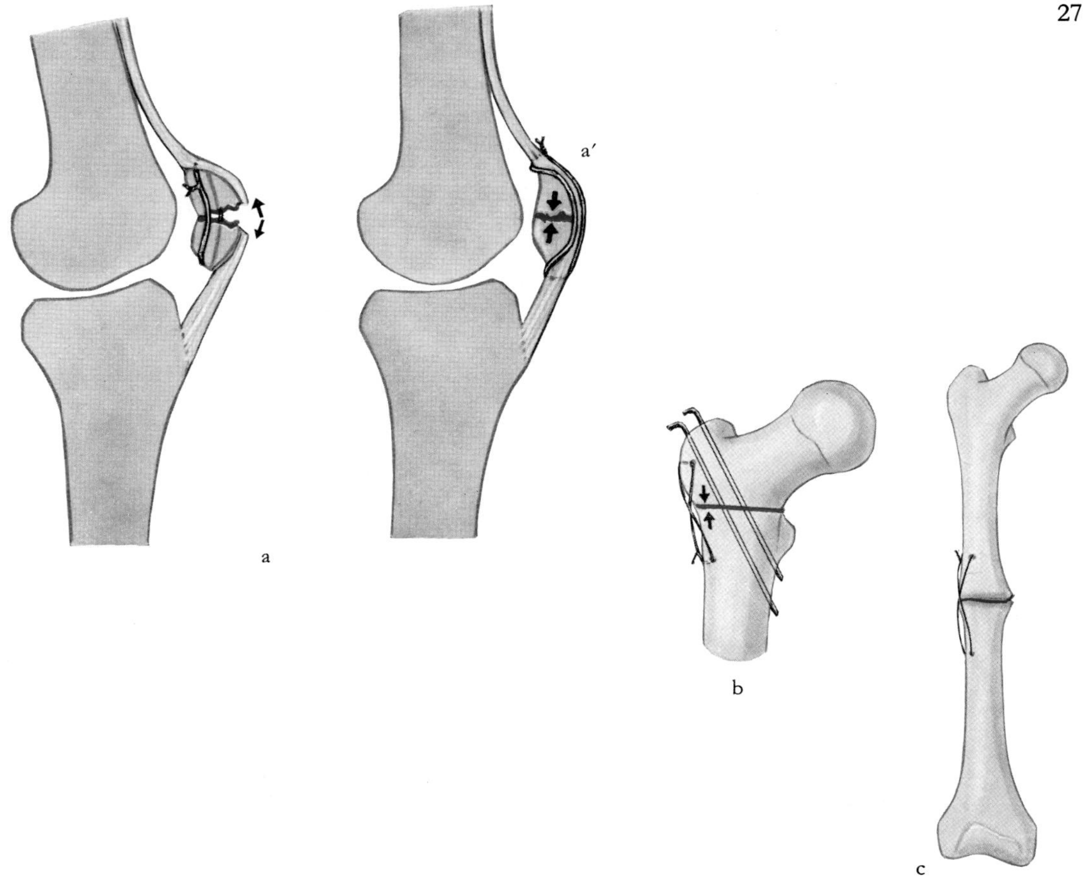

Tension bands which are made of 1.2 mm soft wire, are chiefly indicated in the treatment of avulsion fractures at the insertion of muscles, tendons or ligaments. If, in addition, one has to deal with a rotational component or when accurate reduction of the fragments is vital, two parallel Kirschner wires should be introduced before the insertion of the tension band. The tension band is then passed round the wire ends.

The best illustration of the tension band principle is a transverse fracture of the patella. As the wire is applied anteriorly and placed under tension, it results in an over-correction of the fracture. As soon as the knee is bent, however, counter-pressure of the femoral condyle results not only in the closure of the fracture but also in compression of the fragments. A tension band will result in axial compression of the *whole fracture* only then when the bone surface opposite to the tension band provides a counter resistance.

Fig. 28	*Tension band internal fixation of the patella.*
a	Use a 1.2 mm wire. Pass this wire round the insertion of the ligamentum patellae and the quadriceps. Tighten the wire until the fracture is slightly over-corrected. Supplement this fixation with a second wire, passed more superficially.
b	On flexing the knee or contracting the quadriceps, the pressure of the condyles against the patella compresses the bony fragments together.
c	The view from the anterior aspect. The wires shown in the illustration were placed under tension with the AO wire tightener and the wire ends were then bent with pliers. This type of wire fixation is much better than just twisting the ends, for it is not only simpler but the wire does not break.
Fig. 29	If conventional cerclage wiring of the patella is carried out with the wire running circumferentially round the middle of the patella (seen from in front), then on flexing the knee the fragments invariably come apart on the anterior surface. We therefore advise against using this procedure.
Fig. 30	*Tension band internal fixation combined with Kirschner wires.*
a	In fractures of the olecranon, especially transverse ones, the Kirschner wires must be introduced parallel to each other and in line with the acting forces. If reduction is anatomical and the fragments are impacted, the Kirschner wires are not necessary.
b	In fractures of the greater trochanter, particularly if comminuted, a tension band wire is inserted above the insertion of the gluteus medius and minimus, opposing their distraction forces. The Kirschner wires add further stability to this fixation.
c	This may be used in avulsion of either the medial or the lateral malleolus, if these cannot be screwed back into place (see Fig. 201). The tension wire is placed deep to the collateral ligament. The disadvantage of this otherwise excellent method, is the wide exposure needed, especially when removing the metal. Therefore, even with small avulsion fragments we prefer to fix them with one or two small cancellous screws.

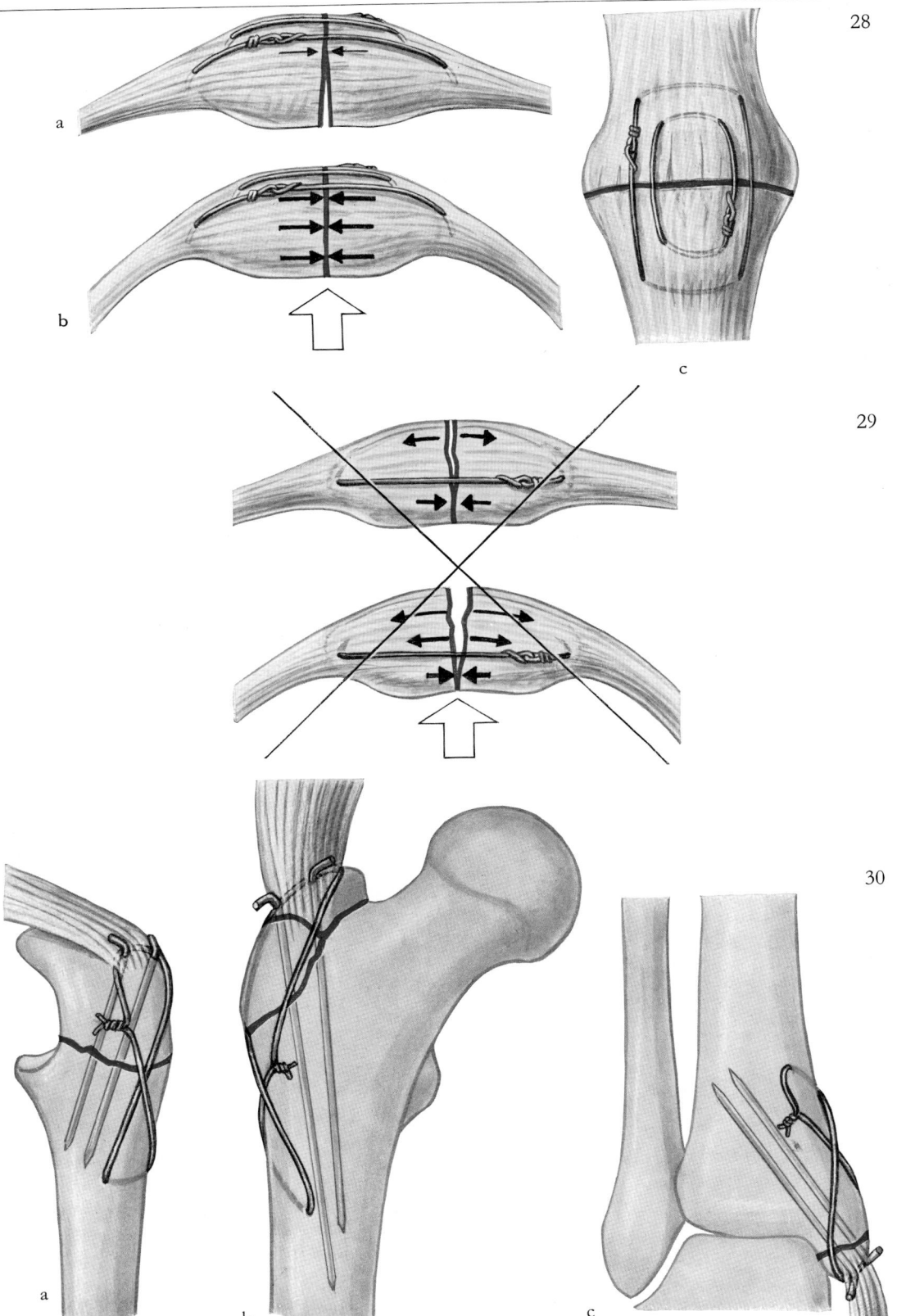

These plates are intended to convert tensile forces into axial compressive forces, just as in tension band wiring of the patella. The plate is placed under tension with the help of the tension device. This plate can be relatively weak, as it is not intended to withstand any bending or shearing stresses. In the tibia the tension band principle is only used in the treatment of those non-unions which are not suitable for medullary nailing, and never in the treatment of fresh fractures. In non-union, the plate is applied on the convex side, which is most often on the lateral surface of the tibia and less often at the back (Fig. 34c).

A wide and strong tension band plate is indicated when great torsional forces have to be counteracted, as in fractures of the middle or lower third of the femur, or when fragments are osteoporotic as in non-unions of the humerus. The use of the wide plate leads to a much more rigid fixation without danger of splintering the bone.

All straight AO plates have two holes at each end, threaded so that they will accept cancellous screws.

Fig. 31	*The long tension device* for use with straight and angled AO plates. Its two metal pins are so designed that they do not get in the way of the screwdriver when tightening up the fixation screws.
Fig. 32	*The technique for applying a straight tension band plate* (for non-union of a long bone shaft, or for fractures of the ulna).
a	Drill a 3.2 mm hole 1 cm from the fracture line. Tap out the thread, reduce the fracture, apply the plate and fix it gently with the first screw. Maintain the reduction by holding the plate and bone together with a rubber-covered bone holding clamp. Use the drill sleeve now to drill a hole 18 mm from the end of the plate using a 3.2 mm drill bit, to fix the tension device to the bone and again tap out the thread with the tap.
b	Insert the hook of the tension device into the horizontal slot made in the end hole of the plate and screw the tension device to the bone. If then bone is of good quality it is sufficient to fix it to the near cortex only, but if not, then the crew should be inserted through both cortices. Now tighten up the nut with the socket wrench with universal joint until reduction is complete.
c	Now insert the remaining screws into the first fragment. It is important to use the drill guide to make sure that the 3.2 mm drill bit is inserted exactly in the center of each plate hole. When the holes are being tapped it is often helpful to use the 4.5 mm tap sleeve to protect the soft tissues from being caught on the tap itself.
d	Now further compression can be applied by using the open-end wrench. With the universal jointed socket wrench one can obtain only 40–45 kg of compression between the fragments but with the open-end wrench this can be increased to 150 kg.
e	Once the fragments are fully compressed and therefore rigidly fixed, the reduction is checked again. If it is perfect the remaining screws are inserted as described above.
f	Finally the tension device is removed by first loosening the compression and then removing the cortex screw. The last screw must now be inserted into the last hole of the plate, and this may be a short screw in order to smooth out the gradation between the normal elastic bone and the rigid segment deep to the plate. In the tibia at least five cortices and seven in the femur must be grasped by the screws on each side of the fracture line, assuming that the cortex is normal and not porotic. This method of plate fixation only applies to tension band plates and not to neutralization plates which are discussed later (page 53).

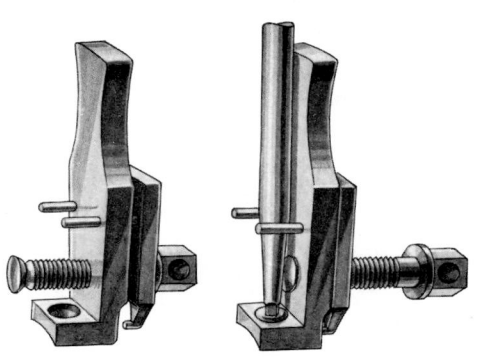

31

32

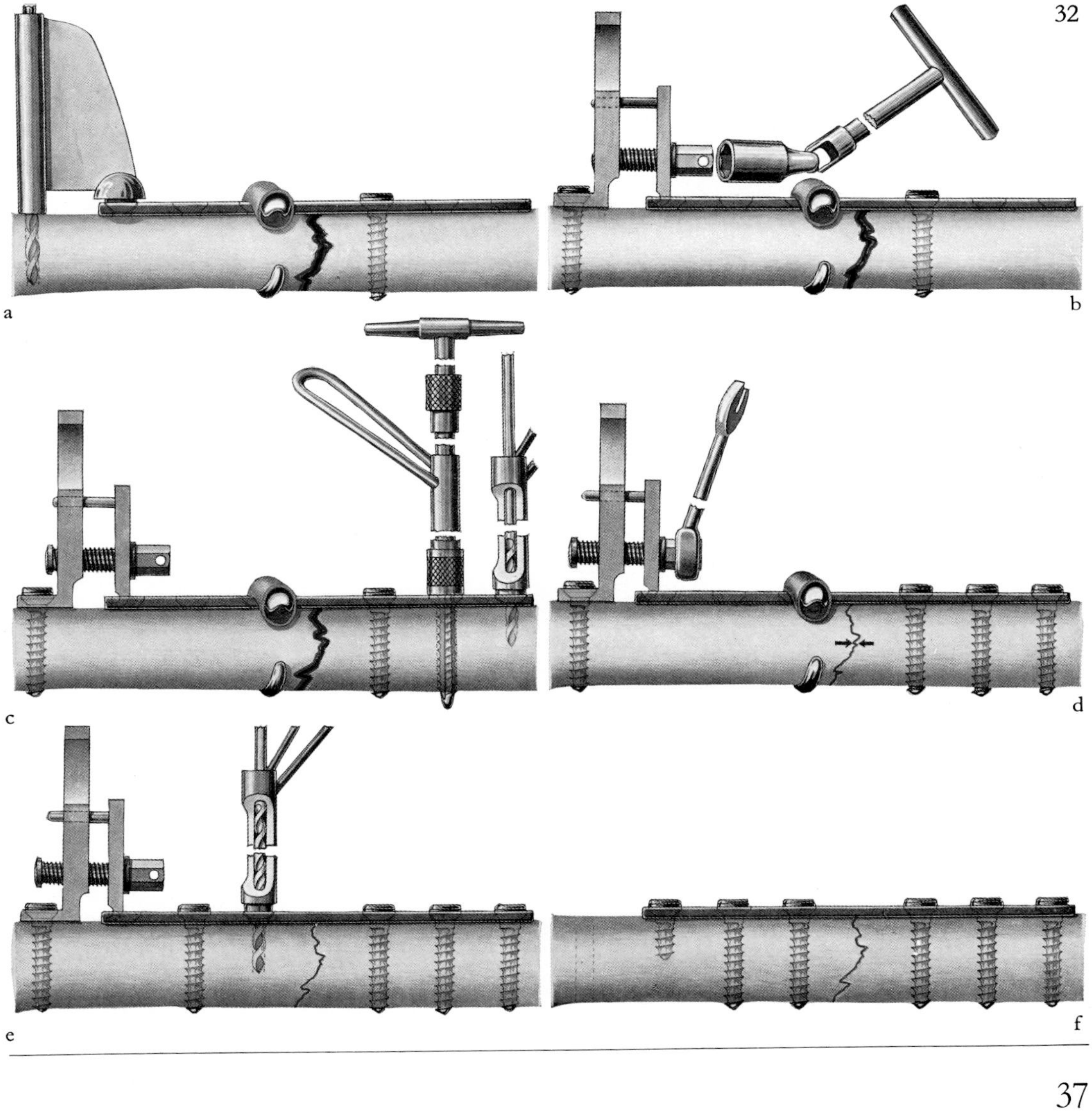

a

b

c

d

e

f

If a plate is placed on a side where compression forces are acting then it cannot act as a tension band to immobilize the fracture, but it fatigues and soon breaks because of the tremendous bending forces it is continually subjected to. Its ability to provide rigid fixation is directly proportional to its distance from the fulcrum of the bending moment. In the femur a plate applied laterally only acts as a tension band as long as the medial cortex is intact and acts as a counter-strut (Fig. 93).

A comminuted shaft fracture cannot be stabilized with a tension band plate. Such a plate becomes subject to bending stresses and the metal fatigues and breaks (see page 104).

> The principle of a tension band plate: It must be inserted only on the tensile side of the bone.

Fig. 33   *The principle of the tension band plate.*

Long bones are subject to eccentric loading. One must know which side of the bone is under tension so as to decide where to apply the plate. The femur (a) for example, can be compared to a bent column (b). The plate which is applied to the outer or convex side can then counteract all tension forces (c) and provide rigid internal fixation. If it were applied on the inner or concave surface, it would give no fixation at all (d) and such a plate would come under excessive bending stresses and would soon show a fatigue fracture.

Fig. 34   *In non-union of the tibia, the tension plate must always be placed on the convex side, which is the one under tension.*

a   Very often in non-union of the tibia there is a varus deformity, and for this reason the plate should be put on the lateral side (a'). Such a plate applied under high tension, not only corrects the deformity but also compresses the fragments on the lateral side, which was the side originally under tension. An osteotomy of the fibula is seldom necessary, because correction of the varus deformity lengthens the tibia (see Fig. 250).

b   In the rare valgus deformity a plate must be applied on the medial side.

c   When there is much backward bowing a plate must be applied on the posterior surface of the tibia. (For the approach see Fig. 174/4.)

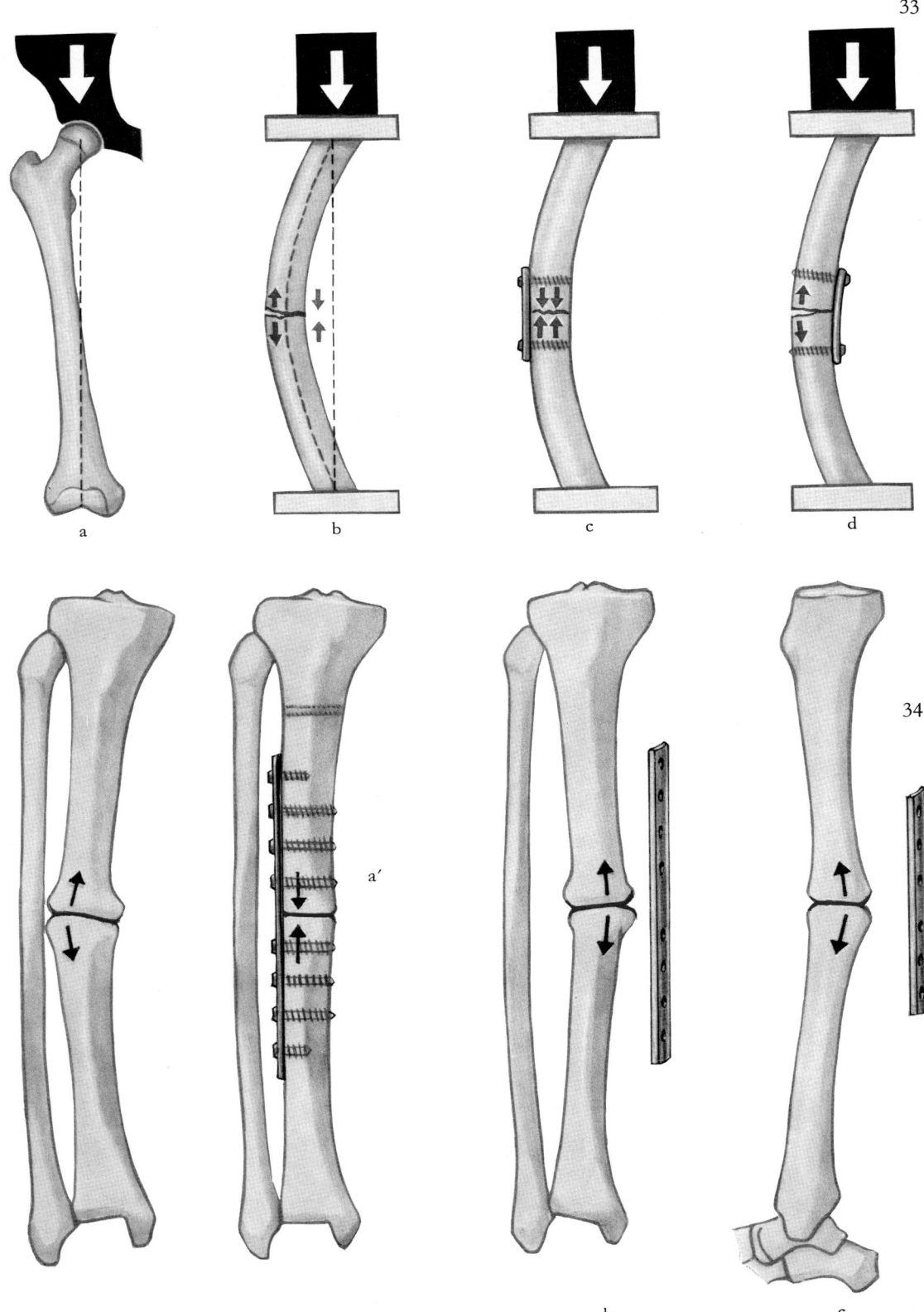

a

b

c

d

a′

a

b

c

In the upper limb the side under tension is determined by the arrangement of the muscles. Therefore transverse fractures of the humerus and of both forearm bones may be adequately fixed by tension band plates, and do not need plaster fixation.

In the femur the side under tension is opposite to the femoral neck and is $1-1^1/_2$ cm anterior to the linea aspera. It is here that all tension plates must be applied.

In the tibia the side under tension is only obvious in non-union (Fig. 34). In a fresh fracture one cannot determine which side is under tension or compression and for this reason a different principle altogether must be employed (see page 53).

Fig. 35	If the elbow is not stiff, then to fix a fracture of the lower humerus, the plate must be applied posteriorly.
Fig. 36	If the elbow is stiff, then a plate is applied to the anterior surface.
Fig. 37	In the forearm the posterior surface is the one under tension, which is why dorsal bowing and a gap on the dorsal surface occurs. The plates should therefore be applied on the posterior surface.

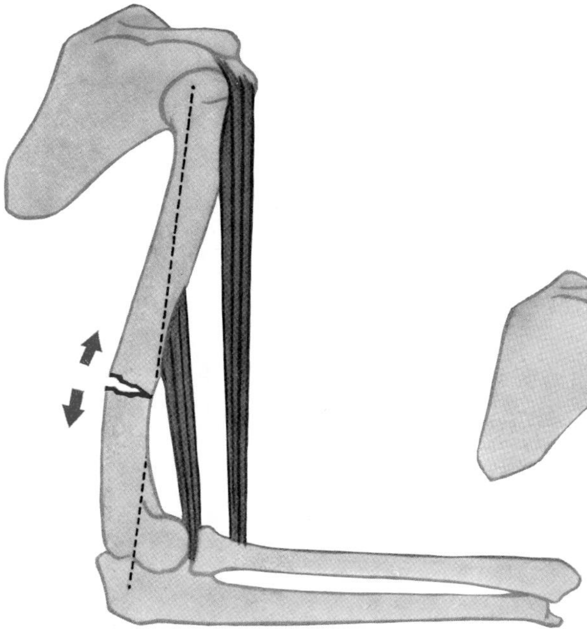

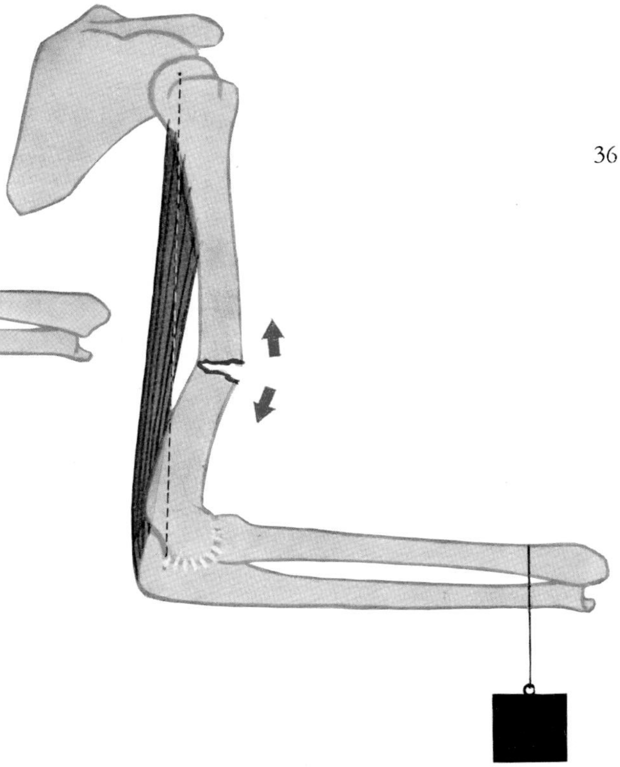

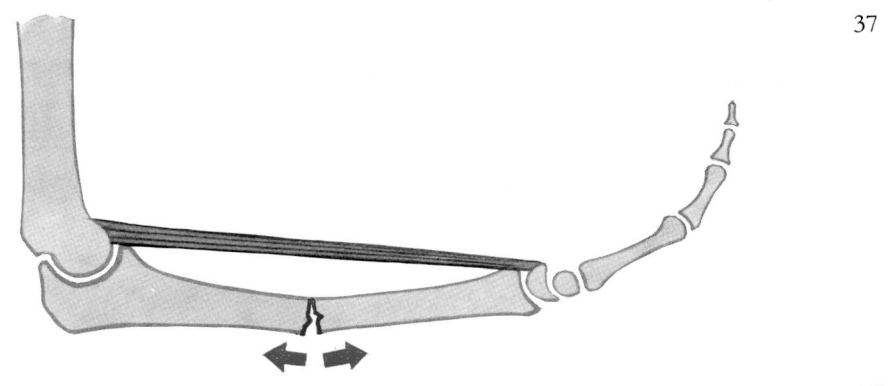

A tension band plate has to counteract only tensile forces and therefore does not need to have any resistance to bending. In some round bones, such as the radius, there is not enough room to apply the tension device owing to danger of injury to the interosseous nerve in fractures of the upper third. For this reason we have developed the semi-tubular plate with oval holes. This plate, which is made from medullary nail material, having a thickness of about 1 mm, may be screwed firmly to the bone and the edges press themselves into the cortex and give further resistance to rotation. Provided reduction is perfect, the oval holes enable the plate to be placed under tension. This is done by inserting the screws at one end of the oval i.e. eccentrically. As the conical head of the screw engages the plate, it places the plate under tension. These plates are fixed to the bone with standard AO cortex screws which have conical heads.

The small semi-tubular plates are useful when applied to subcutaneous bone where a bulky plate would be undesirable. It is best fixed to the bone with a small cortical screw (3.5 mm in diameter) as, for example, in a fracture of the lower fibula.

Fig. 38   *Internal fixation using compression with a semi-tubular plate.*

a   Drill the first hole 1 cm from the fracture, tap the thread, apply the plate and insert the first cortex screw, tightening it so that its head just touches the plate. Now reduce the fracture accurately. While an assistant pulls on the plate with a hook so that the edge of the oval hole is firmly pressed against the screw, the second hole is drilled eccentrically as far from the fracture as possible. Use a 3.2 mm drill guide to avoid damaging the plate with the drill. As seen from the side and face on.

b   Tap out the thread, insert and tighten the second screw. Now tighten the first screw. Because the first one is also placed eccentrically, tightening will press the conical head of the screw down thus pushing the first fragment up against the second. In this way the fragments are compressed.

c   The remaining screws are inserted in the center of each oval hole. If further compression is desired, the remaining screws are also inserted slightly eccentrically, away from the fracture line, so that with the tightening of each screw compression will increase.

38

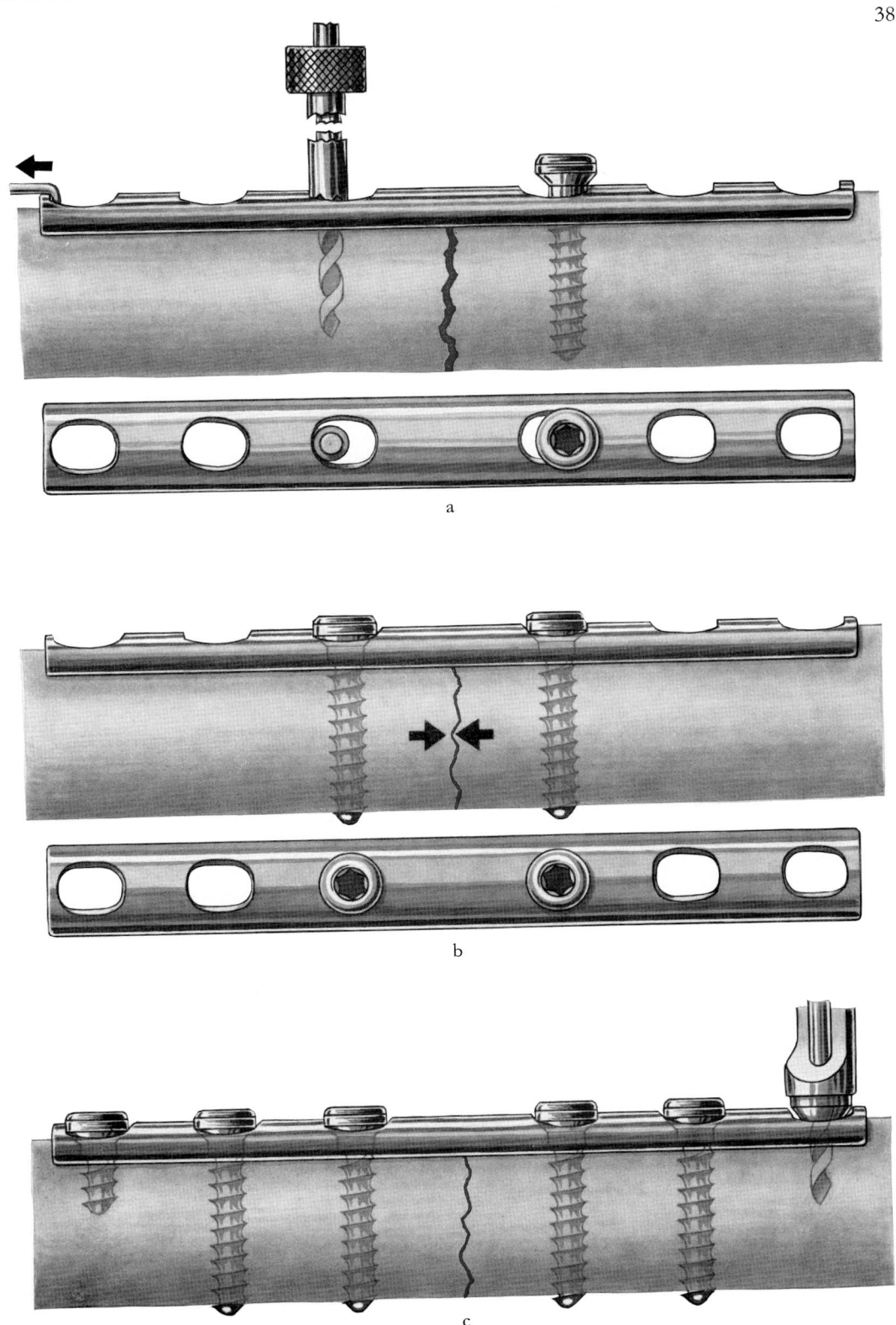

a

b

c

43

The chief indication for the standard semi-tubular plate is in fractures of the radius or the upper end of the ulna, and especially in comminuted fractures of the olecranon.

The small semi-tubular plate is especially useful in comminuted fractures of the lateral malleolus. This maintains full length of the bone in difficult fractures. It has also been used in the treatment of metacarpal and metatarsal fractures.

Both the small and standard semi-tubular plates may be used in double-plate fixation (see Fig. 44).

Fig. 39	*Examples of the use of the standard semi-tubular plates as tension band plates.*
a	All fractures of the radial shaft can be successfully treated with a semi-tubular plate (5–7 holes).
b	Comminuted fractures of the olecranon are best stabilized under compression with the standard semi-tubular plate.
Fig. 40	*Examples of internal fixation with the small semi-tubular plate.*
a	The small semi-tubular plate is most useful in comminuted fractures of the lateral malleolus.
b	The small semi-tubular plate is used in treatment of fractures of the fifth metatarsal.

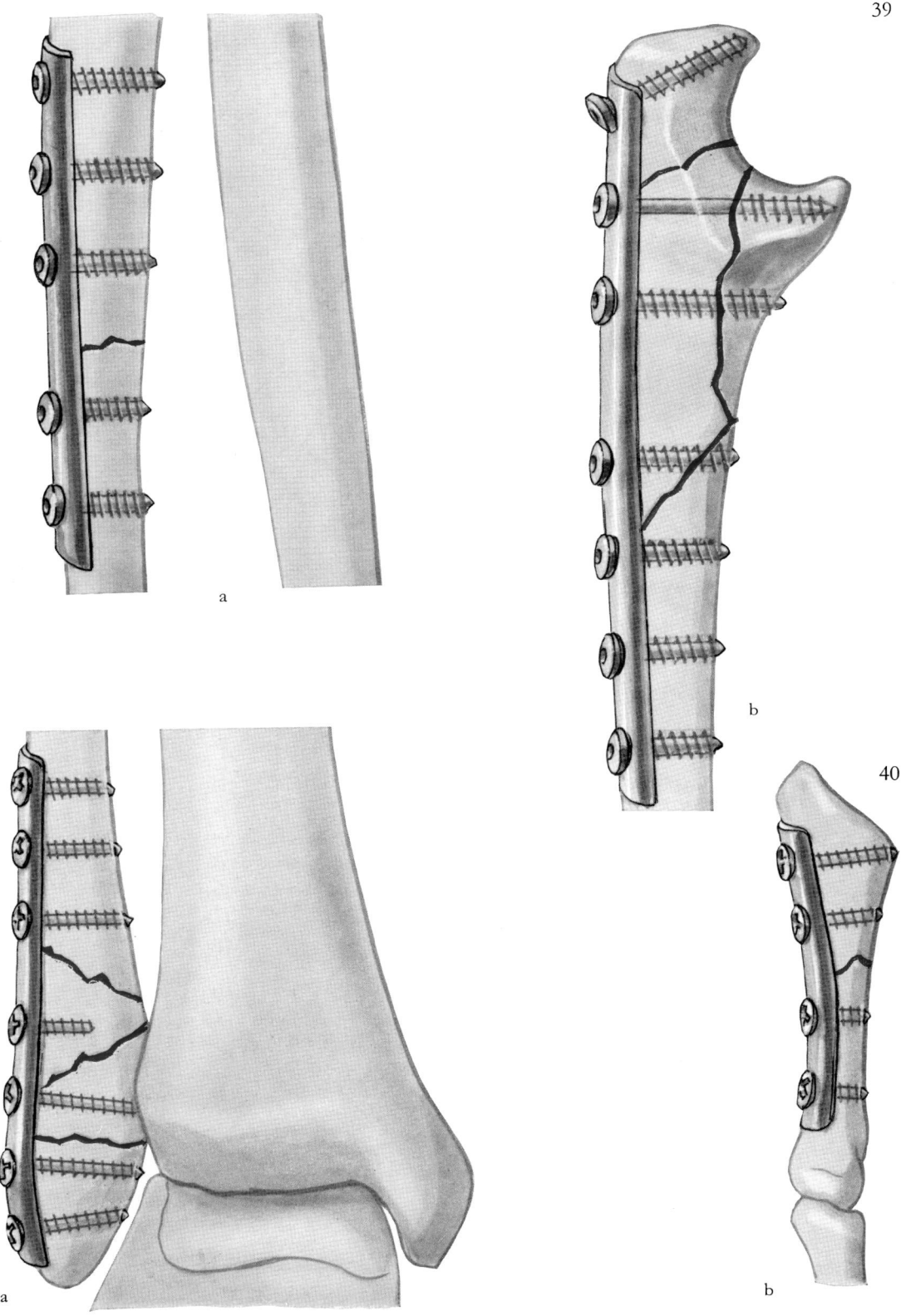

Other Forms of Tension Band Internal Fixation

The T-plate which is used for fractures through the anatomical or surgical neck of the humerus spans with its proximal end the groove for the long head of the biceps. One screw is inserted into the lesser tuberosity and the other into the greater tuberosity. The oval hole gives temporary fixation of the fragments before compression is applied. The main indications for the T-plate are in treating irreducible fracture dislocations of the upper humerus, badly displaced fractures through the anatomical or surgical neck and subcapital pseudarthroses.

A hip arthrodesis combined with an osteotomy of the pelvis can be so rigidly fixed with the cobra-head plate that post-operative hip spica fixation is unnecessary and the patient can be up and about within a few days.

With the *external compression clamps* (Charnley) it is possible to apply the tension band principle and axial compression as well—as for example in an intertrochanteric osteotomy in a child. Thus, if the Schanz screws are correctly positioned, displacement of the fragments becomes impossible.

Fig. 41   *Internal fixation of a fracture of the humerus with the T-plate.*

a   Reduce the fracture and if necessary stabilize the different fragments with Kirschner wires. Now apply the T-plate so that it spans the sulcus between the tuberosities. Drill the pilot holes for the two cancellous screws with a 3.2 mm drill. Tap the hole with the cancellous tap. In a pure subcapital fracture use the fully threaded cancellous screw. If the head itself is fragmented, then a cancellous screw that is only partly threaded is indicated. Now, using the 3.2 mm bit, drill a hole in the cortex through the oval hole of the plate as far from the fracture as possible.

b   Tap the thread and insert the first cortex screw but do not tighten it.

c, d   Apply the tension device and tighten it until the first cortex screw has moved and the oval hole is as far proximal as possible. Now tighten the first cortex screw in the oval hole and insert a more proximal cortex screw. Remove the tension device and insert the last screw.

Fig. 42   *The cobra-head plate* (a) used in hip arthrodeses is placed under tension after the upper part of the plate has been fixed to the pelvis (b). For this technique see page 282.

Fig. 43   *The external compression clamps* are slid over the Schanz screws one after the other. As soon as the compression clamp closest to the body is tightened and the one further away from the body is loosened, the osteotomy interfaces become compressed. This technique is only used in children under the age of five for fixation of intertrochanteric osteotomies.

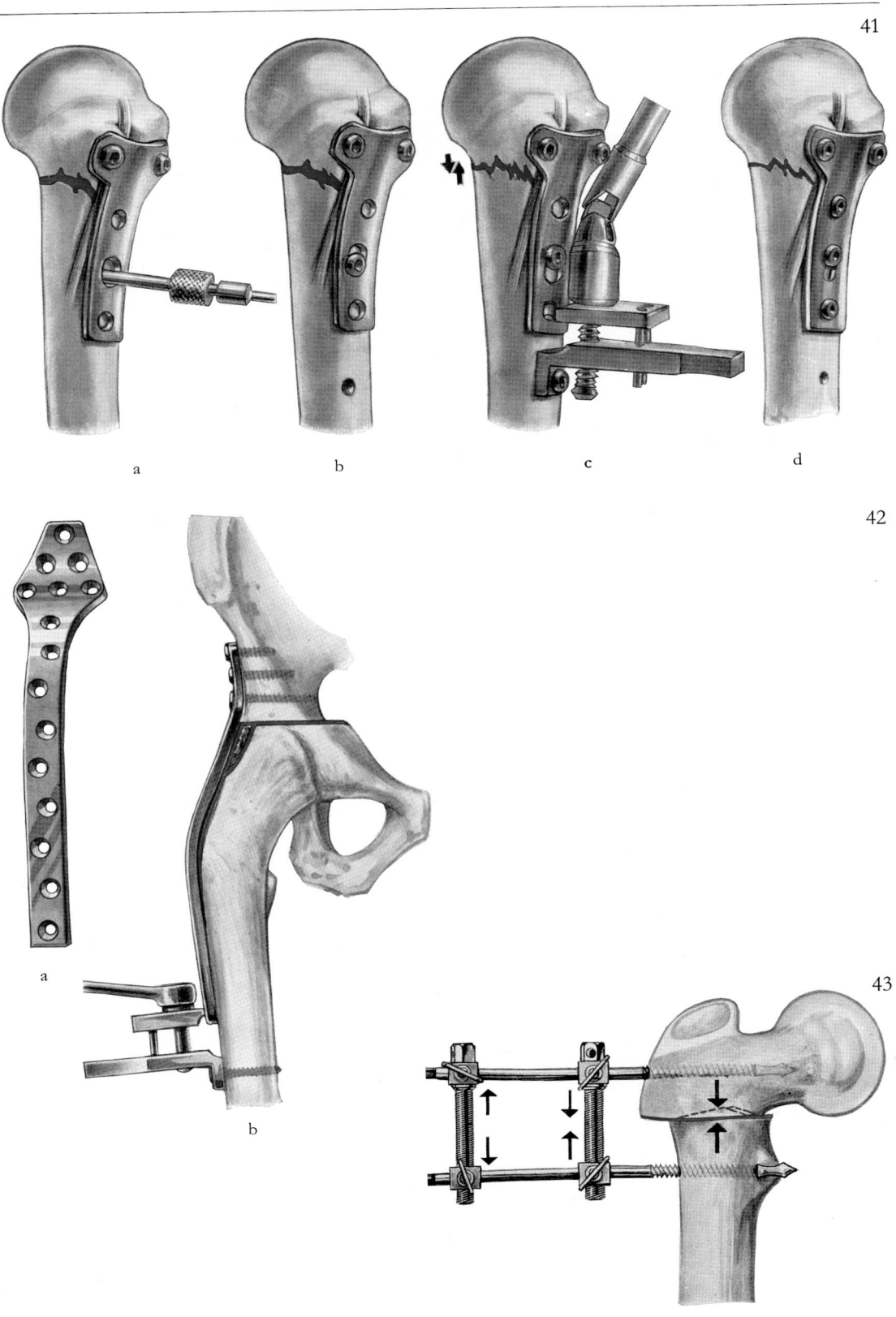

a   b   c   d

a

b

Double compression can be applied with two plates or two to four external compression clamps. Double-plates must never be used in fresh shaft fractures because they neutralize any tensile or compressive stresses so much that no stress is exerted on the underlying cortex. Because bone is constructed in accordance with the principle of minimal material for maximum strength, once the underlying cortex is relieved of all stress it becomes thinner and thinner and turns into cancellous bone. This phenomenon explains why femoral shaft fractures fixed with double plates may refracture soon after removal of the plate.

Double plates are therefore only to be used in the metaphyses, as in fractures of the tibial plateaus or for non-union of the femur where such massive callus has been produced that there is no danger of inducing osteoporosis.

Certain fractures, such as those of the lower ends of the humerus or tibia, are best stabilized with compression using the small or standard semi-tubular plates.

An exception to the rule governing the use of double plates in the treatment of fresh fractures is discussed on page 186 under the heading of Short Comminuted Fractures of the Shaft of the Tibia.

Double external compression clamps are used in arthrodeses of the knee and ankle (Fig. 45), in supramalleolar osteotomies of the tibia or in the treatment of infected non-union of the tibia accompanied by bone loss (Fig. 46).

Bilateral compression using two plates.

Fig. 44

a   For osteotomy of the upper tibia to correct valgus or varus deformity we most often use a T-plate and a straight plate, or two straight plates. For the technique see Fig. 294. The example we have chosen is a varus rotation osteotomy of the upper tibia.

b   In treatment of non-union of the femur between the middle and distal thirds in the presence of abundant callus, where medullary nailing is contraindicated. In such a case there is no danger from secondary osteoporosis because there is so much callus. The double plate fixation under compression results in a much more rapid ossification of the pseudarthrosis. The lateral plate is wide, the anterior narrow and shorter.

c   In transverse fractures through the lower end of the tibia one can use two semi-tubular plates with short screws.

d   In Y-fractures of the lower end of the humerus we have found it most useful after reduction and fixation of the articular components, to employ two small semi-tubular plates for fixing the supracondylar component. We stabilize the intercondylar fracture with a malleolar screw, inserting it if possible from the radial side.

a

b

c

d

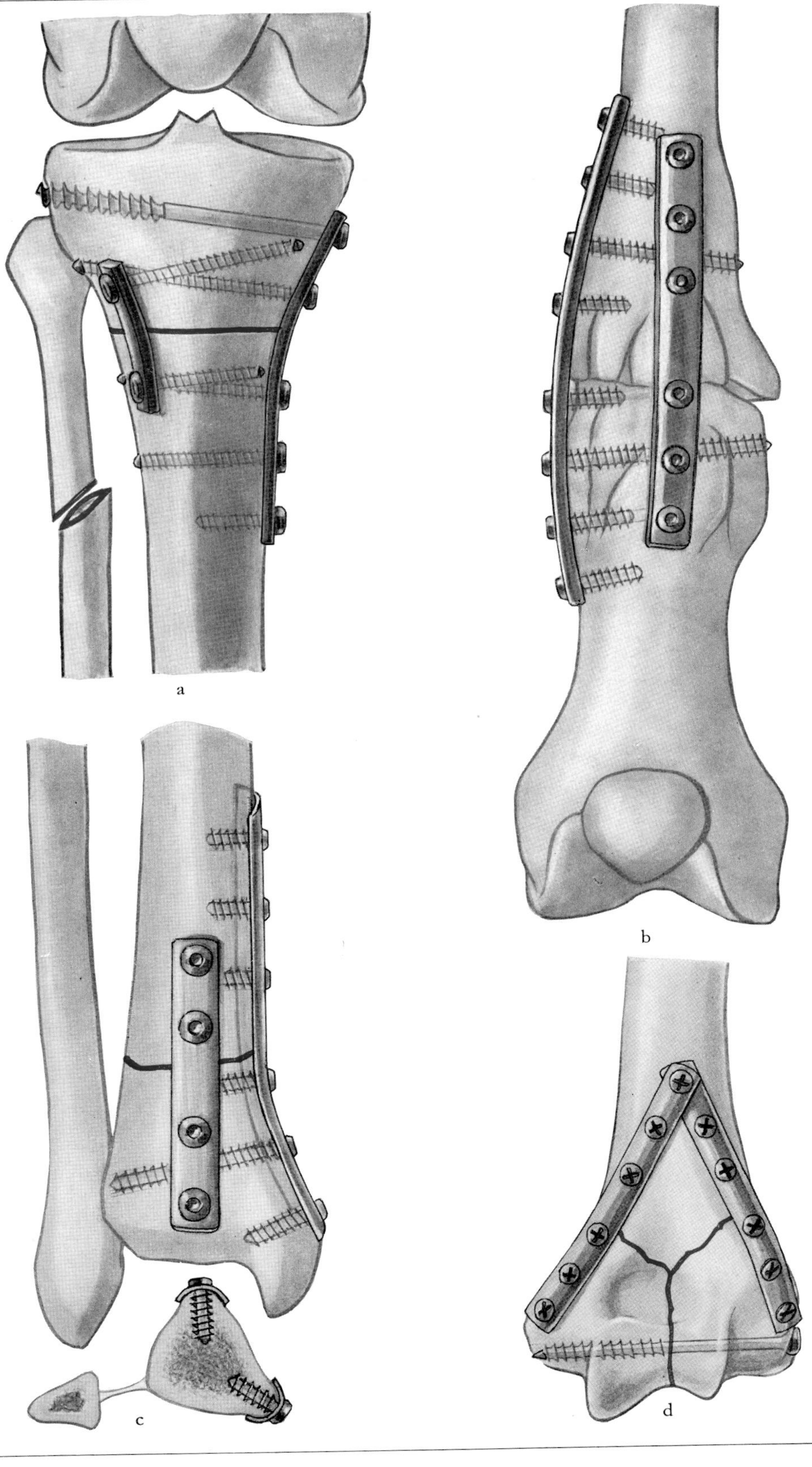

Fig. 45

    a   Double external clamp fixation using four Steinmann pins and four external compression clamps in arthrodeses of the knee.

    b   Fixation of arthrodeses of the ankle.

Fig. 46

    a   Simple method of fixation of osteotomy through the upper tibia using external compression clamps (see Fig. 293).

    b   Osteotomy through the metaphysis of lower tibia.

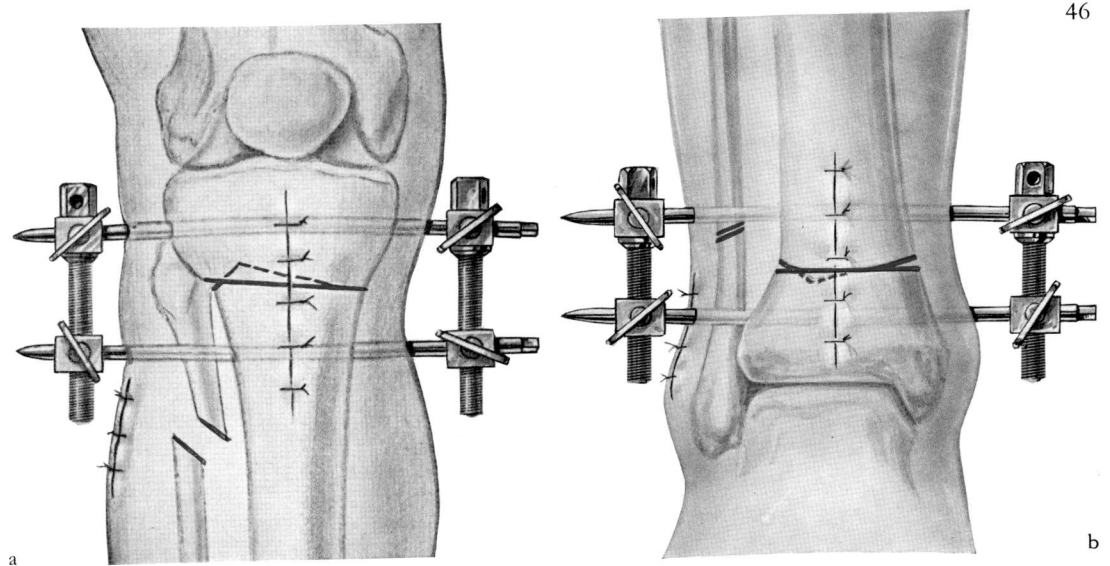

a

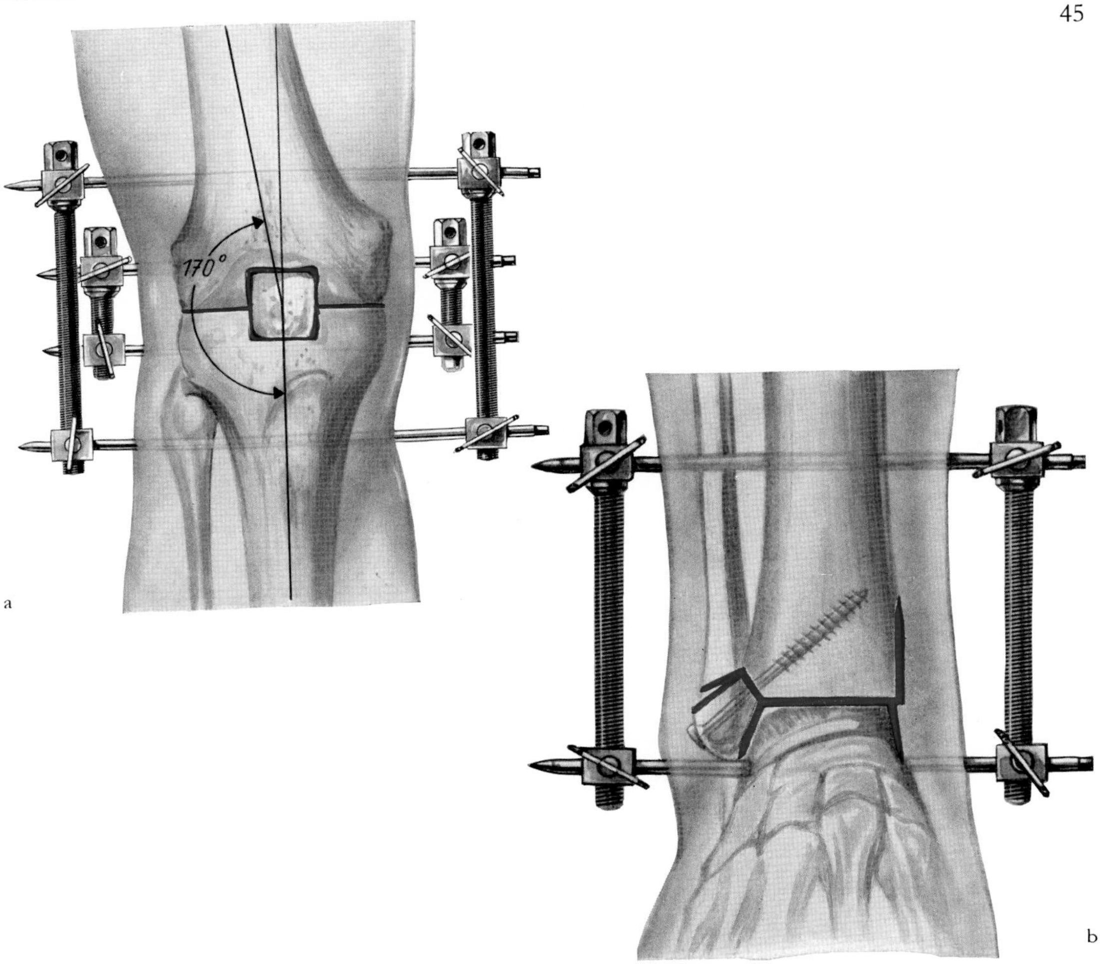

b

a

b

3. Interfragmental and Axial Compression Combined with Either the Neutralization or Buttress Plate.

a) The Neutralization Plate

In suitable fractures (in cancellous bone, long spiral and oblique fractures through the cortex), bending or torsional forces acting on the fractures surfaces can be completely neutralized by lag screws applying compression between fragments. In those cases in which the direction of bending forces is known, it is possible to neutralize bending stresses with axial compression on the tension side (tension wiring or tension band plates). Where bending moments may change in response to loading changes, as in the tibia, neutralization by mere tension band plates would be inadequate. The same holds true for the more comminuted fractures. Though internal fixation may seem to be rigid, microscopical movements are occurring between the fragments. They will result in bone resorption, delayed union and eventually fatigue fracture of the plate.

To counteract these harmful forces we add a *neutralization plate* to the standard *interfragmental compression* using lag screws. This plate is fixed to the two main fragments and bridges the comminuted area. *This neutralization plate transmits all torsional and bending forces from the proximal to the distal fragments and thus prevents these forces from acting on the fracture surfaces.*

The neutralization plate is chiefly used in treating tibial fractures. The plate we employ in fractures of the shaft is the narrow plate which, for practical purposes, is almost always applied to the medial side of the tibia (page 84).

N.B.: A neutralization plate applied to a bone without axial compression or compression between fragments, results in inevitable movement at the fracture site.

> A neutralization plate is always placed under tension. In this way it also exerts axial compression.

> Never use a broad plate as a neutralization plate on the tibia.

Fig. 47   *Method No. 1: The insertion of a lag screw through the plate.*

a   After reduction of the fracture hold it reduced with the reduction clamp and drill a 4.5 mm hole in the near cortex at 90° to the long axis of the bone. Insert the 4.5 mm drill sleeve and drill the second cortex with a 3.2 mm drill. Remove the drill sleeve and use the tap to cut the thread in the far cortex.

b   Now fix the plate to the bone with this lag screw which at the same time results in compression between the fragments. The second screw must be short so that it does not damage the tip of the second cortical fragment.

Fig. 48   *Method No. 2: Reduction and screw fixation of a small butterfly fragment before applying a neutralization plate.*

               After fixing a small butterfly fragment by means of two lag screws, the neutralization plate is applied so that it bridges the butterfly and is fixed at each end to one of the main fragments with two or three screws in its end holes. No screw should be inserted into the fracture line. Occasionally it is possible to fix the butterfly fragment to the plate either with a short screw or with a lag screw, but one should avoid clustering screws together.

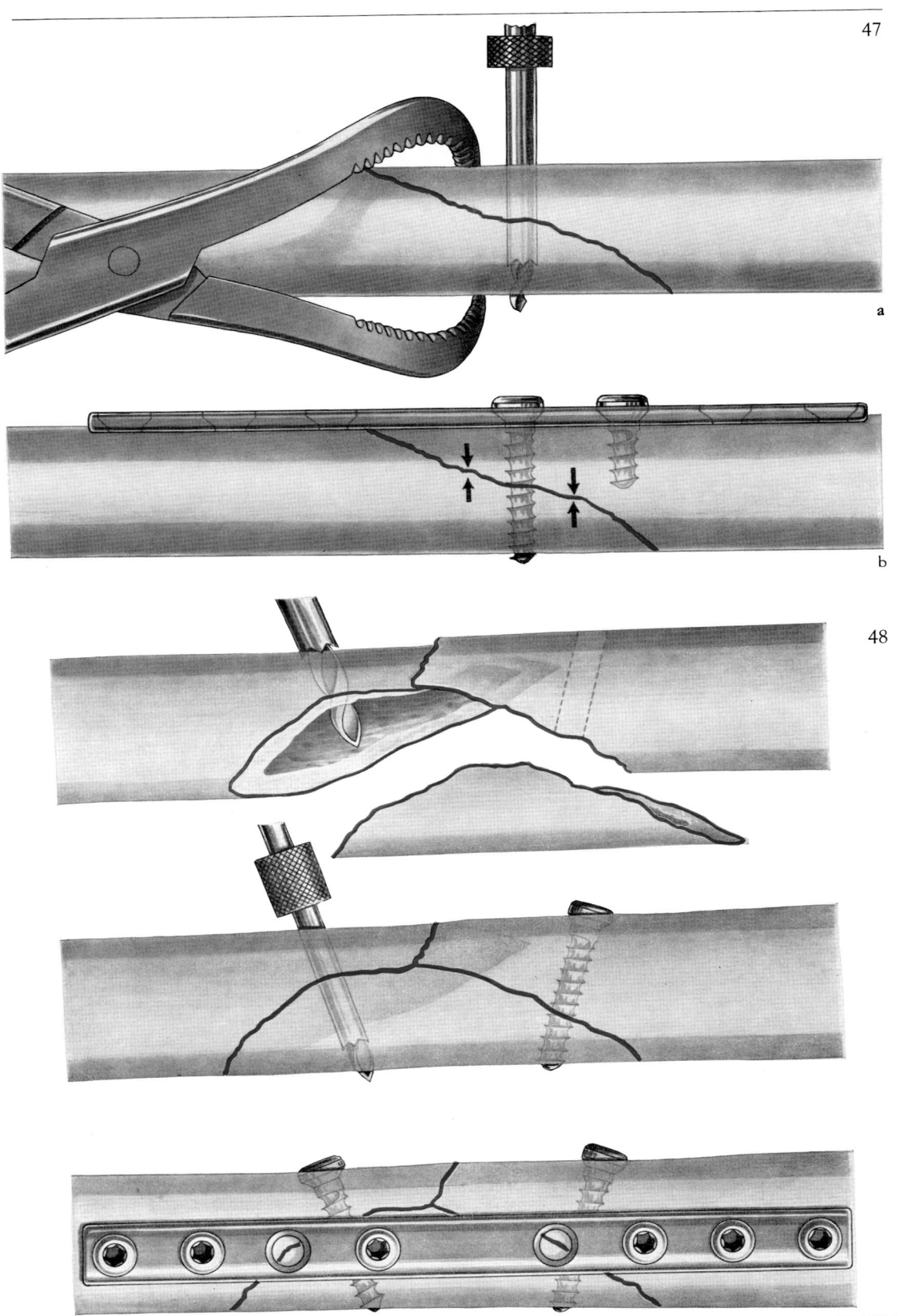

47

a

b

48

55

The main object in a very comminuted fracture is to convert multiple fragments into a fracture with two main fragments. Each fragment is fixed separately with one or more lag screws (see Fig. 21).

The orientation of the fracture planes must be carefully considered as it is useless simply to aim a drill into the open medullary canal. One must be sure that the intended screw will get a sure hold on the far cortex through its center. To achieve this *each fragment must be considered separately while carrying out the open reduction*. Thus, each fragment should be first screwed down lightly and only at the end should all the screws be tightened up, when all fragments have been reduced and fixed in their appropriate position. The neutralization plate is now applied so that it spans the area of comminution and joins the two main fragments together.

> In a comminuted fracture the fragments are reduced and fixed with lag screws before the neutralization plate is applied.

Fig. 49   *Technique.*

a   Drill the gliding hole in the main fragment before reduction.

b   Pass one jaw of the reduction clamp round one cortex, reduce the fragment and hold it with the other jaw. Insert the 3.2 mm drill guide into the gliding hole and drill the second cortex with the 3.2 mm bit. Countersink the hole, measure the required length of screw with the depth gauge, tap the thread and insert the screw but do not tighten it.

c   The second fragment is then fixed in the same manner, and a gliding hole drilled in the other main fragment.

d   The neutralization plate spans the comminuted area. The two middle screws are short.

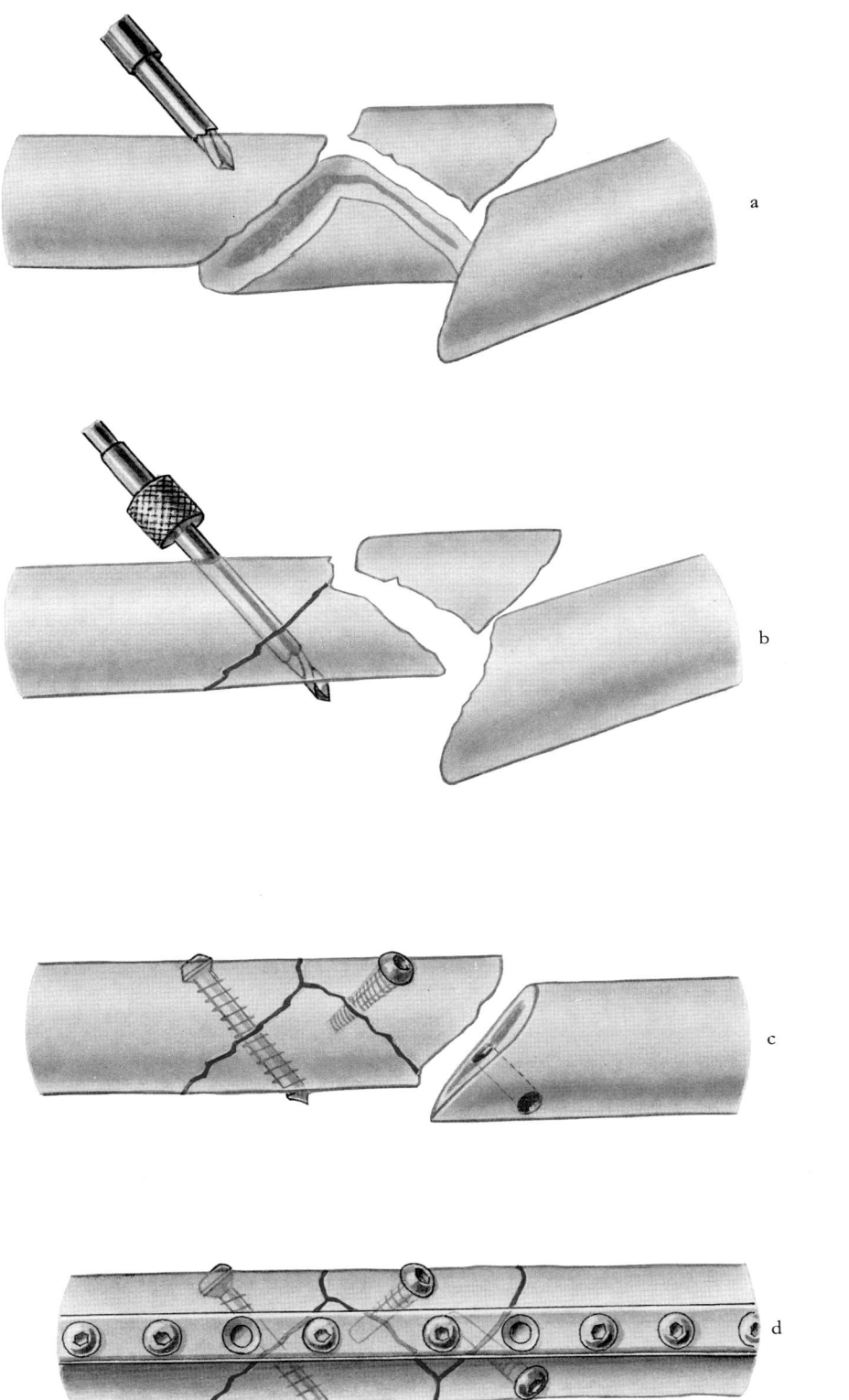

Contouring the Narrow Plate when Carrying out Internal Fixation of the Fracture of the Lower Tibia

When dealing with the lower third of the tibia it is absolutely essential to twist the plate in order to adapt it to the contour of the medial border of the tibia, as this part does not run parallel to the upper part.

Fig. 50

a	Twisting of the plate with two bending irons.
b	Fixing the plate after bending to the medial surface of the tibia.
b', b''	Cross section of the tibia made through the upper and lower end of the plate, showing why contouring of the plate is essential.

Fig. 51 *The AO bending instruments.*

a	*Bending press*, side view.
b	With this press the plate should be bent between the screw holes.
c	When the plate must be twisted, hold one end of the plate firmly in the press and then apply a bending iron, twisting it until the right shape is obtained. With some practice twisting may also be achieved by placing the plate obliquely in the jaws of the press.
d	Narrow plates can be quite easily bent and twisted with the *bending pliers*.

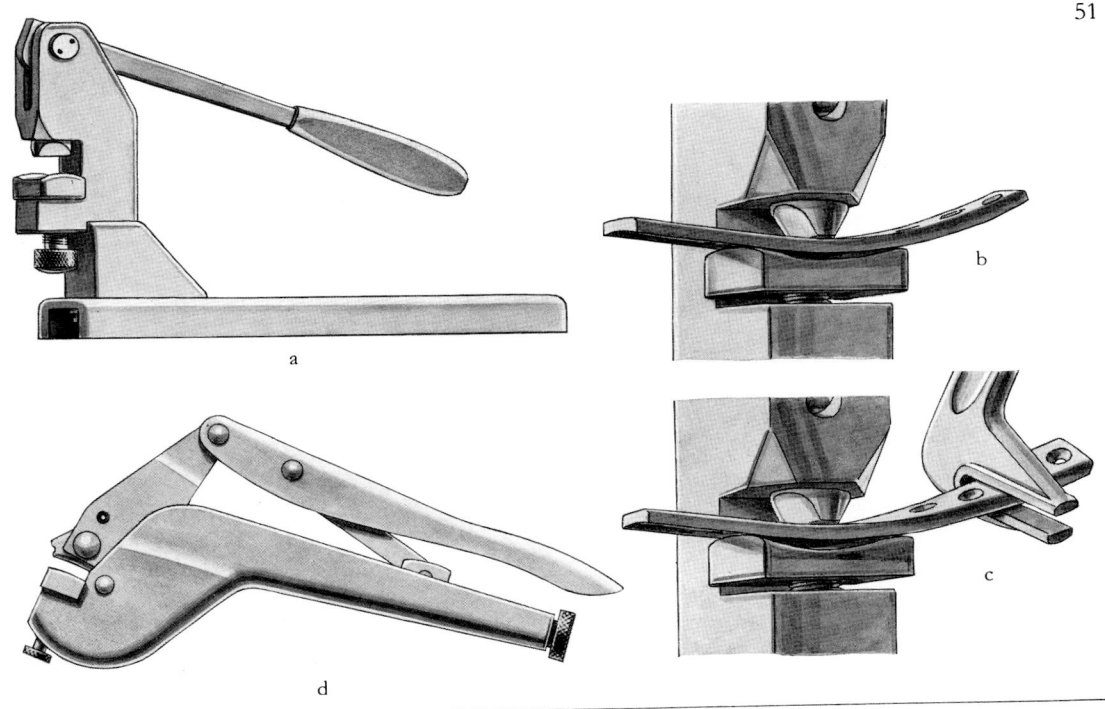

a   b

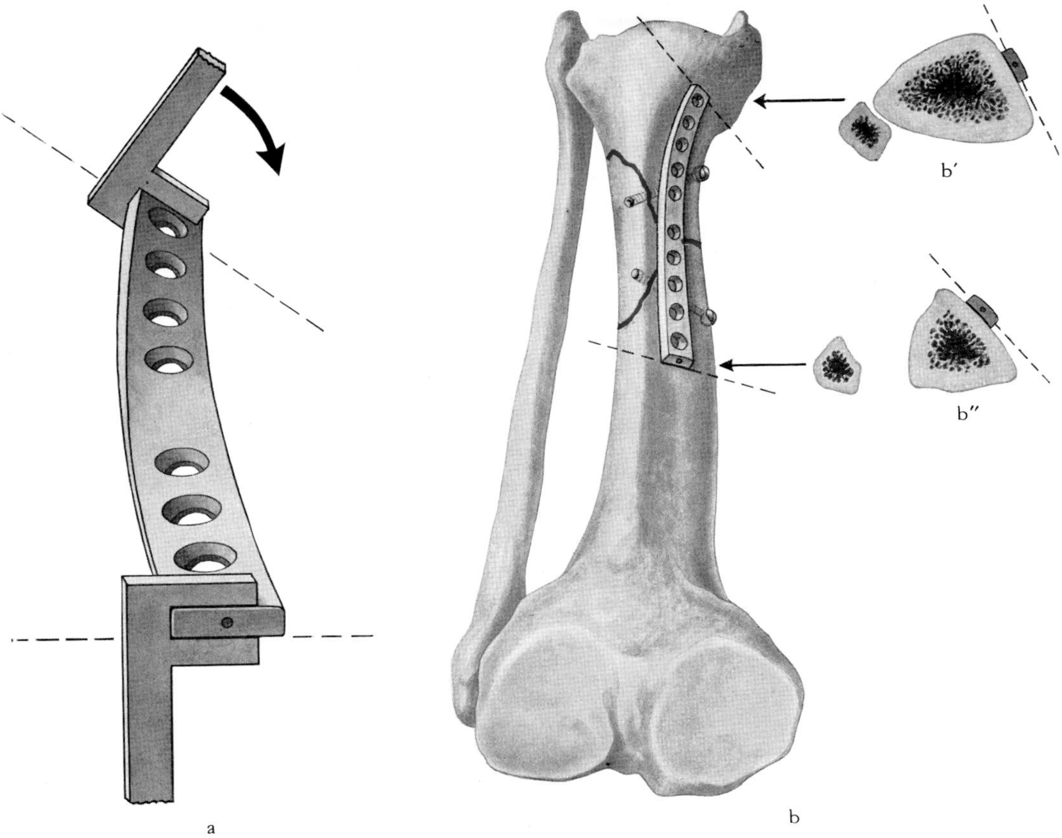

b′

b″

a

b

c

d

A neutralization plate can be placed under tension by special contouring and by fixing it in a special way to the bone, or by means of the tension device. This provides *axial compression* besides compression between fragments effected by lag screws. This not only increases the rigidity of the fixation but helps in reconstructing the internal architecture of the bone and its axial orientation.

A basic rule is that the plate should only be applied after the fracture has been anatomically reduced and held by means of lag screws applying compression between the fragments. The plate should be contoured, using the plate bending instruments, so that there is a distance of 1–2 mm between the middle of the plate and the bone. In the lower end of the tibia it is also necessary to twist the plate.

There are two alternatives:

a) In the metaphysis the plate is contoured in such a way that it is shorter than the bone beneath. This means, in fact, that the plate is somewhat straighter than the corresponding length of bone. When using this method the end screws are inserted first and the tension device is not needed.

b) For the shaft, the plate is bent to a slight bow so that it is somewhat longer than the corresponding section of the bone. Then the first screw is inserted next to the fracture line into the major fragment. Next, the tension device is fixed to the other main fragment and the plate is placed under tension, after which the remaining screws are inserted.

The result: Once the plate is under tension longitudinal axial compression in the bone results, in addition to the already applied compression between fragments obtained by means of the lag screws. The axial compression is exerted on both sides of the fracture, and this greatly increases the rigidity of the internal fixation. The tension in the plate, however, must not be too excessive, lest an axial deformity should result.

Fig. 52		*The two ways of applying a neutralization plate.*
	a	The plate is shorter than the bone. There is a gap of 1–2 mm between the middle of the plate and the bone. The plate is first fixed to the bone by driving in the end screws, without the need of the tension device. The plate must be bent less than the bend that is present in the bone.
	b	The plate is longer than the bone. This plate is first fixed to the bone with a screw close to the fracture line which is then tightened until the plate lies flush with the bone. The plate is now placed under tension by using the tension device on the opposite side of the fracture from the first screw.
Fig. 53		*The technique for applying a neutralization plate for a fracture of the lower end of the tibia.* First the different fragments must be compressed together by the use of lag screws. Axial compression is obtained by the special way in which the neutralization plate is bent and fixed to the bone. It must be so contoured, using the bending press or bending pliers, and bending irons, that at the center of the plate there is a gap of 1–2 mm between it and the bone. The plate is first fixed to the bone at either end. Insertion of the remaining screws draws the plate close up to the bone so that the plate is under considerable tension and the bone under corresponding compression. The tension in the plate, which is directly related to its distance from the bone, should not be too great, lest a varus deformity results. In our illustration, the distance between plate and bone (a) has been exaggerated for clarity. If this were the true position, the plate should be fixed first with the screws (c) and (d) leaving the end holes until the very last. The middle screw (b) is a lag screw and so the hole nearest to the plate (gliding hole) should be drilled with a 4.5 mm bit.

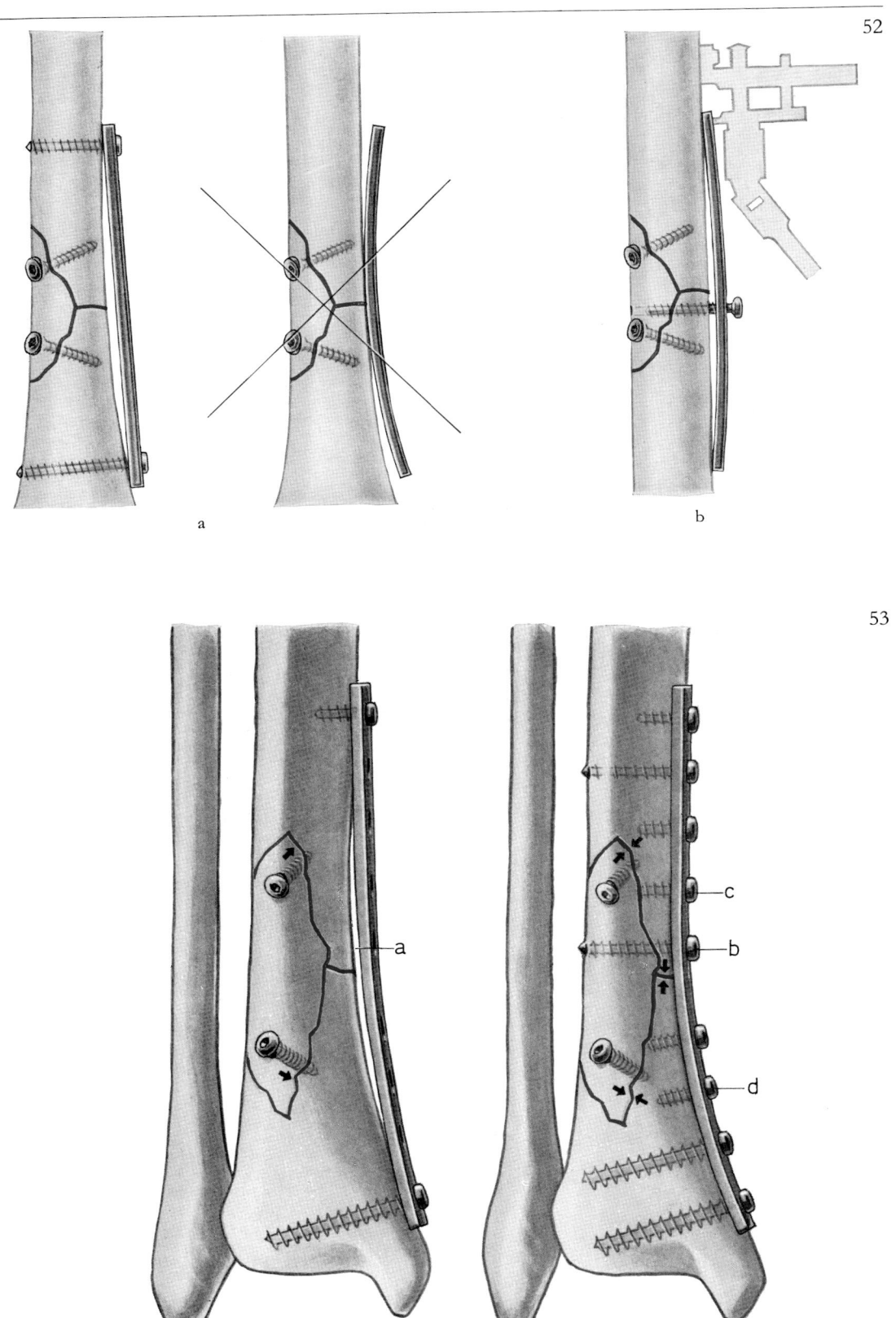

a

b

a

c

b

d

b) The Buttress Plate

The buttress plate is only used on cancellous bones to support the thin cortex that is present at the upper or lower end of the tibia, for instance. Its function is to prevent the occurrence of any slow progressive deformity.

Fig. 54   In a comminuted *fracture of the tibial plateau* after reduction and internal fixation with one or more cancellous lag screws, the cortex may be supported with a T-plate.

Fig. 55   Comminuted *fractures of the lower end of the tibia* involving the joint should be reduced, fixed with screws under compression, and any existing defect filled with autologous cancellous bone. It is then also necessary to *support the medial side* with a narrow buttress plate so as to prevent any varus deformity (see also Fig. 187).

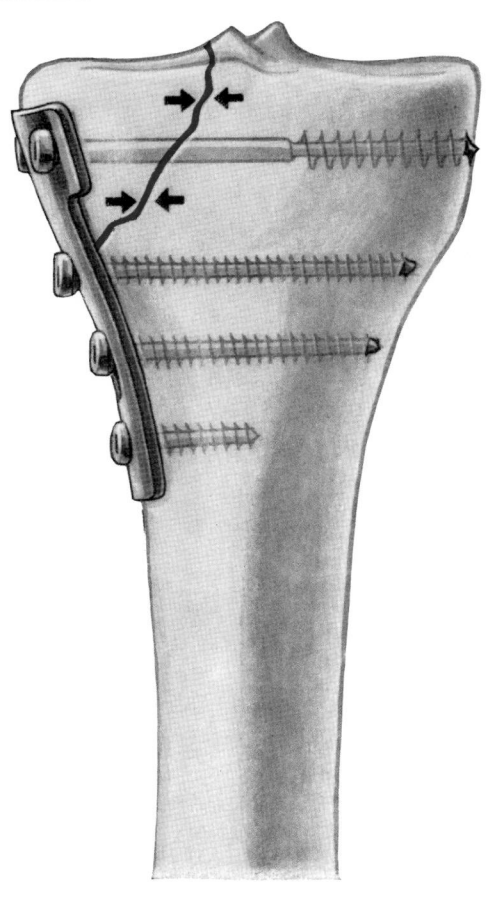

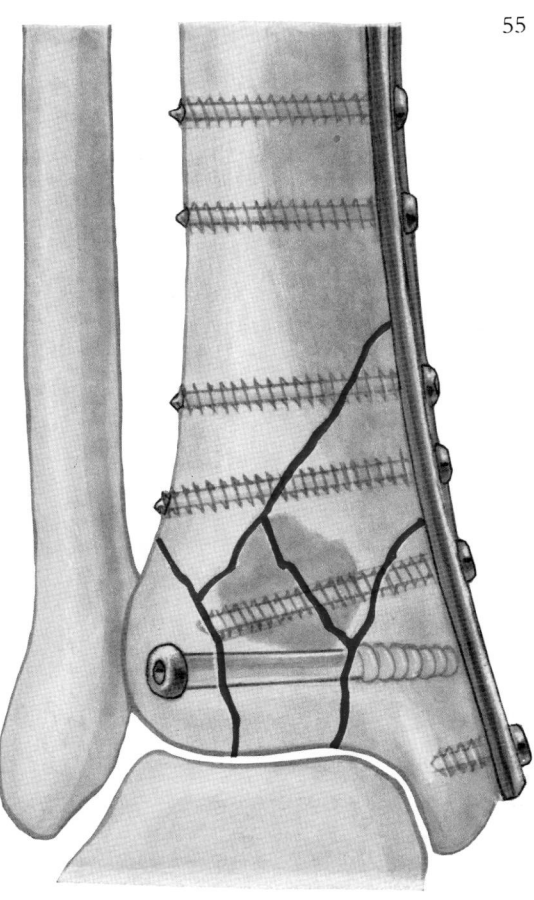

4. Angled Blade Plates as Means of Internal Fixation

Angled AO blade plates can be employed as *tension band plates*, *neutralization plates or buttress plates*. They have solved many postoperative problems in hip surgery by making it safe to start early movements and partial weight bearing. Their use eliminates the danger of fragments becoming displaced, as may happen for instance in intertrochanteric osteotomies. The use of angled plates raises a number of theoretical and technical questions which need to be discussed together. The whole of this chapter will therefore be devoted to a discussion of the use of these plates, although the basic principles of rigid internal fixation are still observed. These principles include axial compression with tension band plates, and the combination of interfragmental compression with neutralization or buttress plates.

The AO blade plates have a U-shaped profile and a fixed angle between the blade and the plate. This fixed angle gives greater strength and leads to less corrosion than may occur with two-piece nail plates. The fixed angle, however, makes them more difficult to use for inexperienced surgeons, because the blade must not only come to lie in the middle of the femoral neck (the so-called horizontal plane) but also must always be exactly right in the *coronal and sagittal planes*. It is therefore mandatory to *plan the position* of the plate accurately before operation, and to check its position afterwards. A preoperative drawing is recommended, even for the experienced surgeon. When all the different angles have been drawn in on the preoperative sketch, it is fairly simple to hammer in the special seating chisel in the right direction.

There are *four types of standard AO angled blade plates* and in addition a few special plates for use in difficult cases or under special circumstances. Before each operation the right plate, and especially in fractures, the right blade length must be selected.

The angled blade plates are used in the proximal and distal third of the femur.

The Principles of the AO Angled Blade Plates

The special feature of the AO angled blade plate is that the channel for the blade of the plate must be cut by the special seating chisel, which has an identical profile to that of the blade of the plate. A chisel guide with adjustable angle as well as three triangular positioning plates are used to set the seating chisel in the right direction.

Fig. 56 *The instruments used for inserting AO angled blade plates.*

a The special seating chisel for cutting the channel for the blade plate. During insertion it is held with the slotted hammer to prevent rotation. The hammer also serves as an extractor.

b The standard U-section of the blade of an angled blade plate.

c The chisel guide which helps in establishing the sagittal plane.

d Triangular positioning plates.

Fig. 57 *The use of the instruments and the determination of the three standard planes for inserting a 130° blade plate, for example.*

a *Femoral neck axis or the horizontal plane:* After exposing the intertrochanteric region and inserting three Hohmann retractors (Fig. 142), pass a Kirschner wire along the front of the femoral neck. This Kirschner wire marks the horizontal plane.

b *The frontal plane:* Using one of the triangular positioning plates with a 50° angle, the 130° between the axis of the shaft and the blade can be determined. A second wire is now inserted into the greater trochanter at 50° to the axis of the shaft and parallel to the first Kirschner wire, thus giving the horizontal plane.

c *The sagittal plane:* Prepare the hole for the seating chisel, first with the 4.5 mm drill and then with the 7 mm router and thin osteotome (Fig. 149). Then hammer in the special seating chisel with its guide. The shaft of the blade plate must come to lie flat on the femoral shaft. It is therefore vital that the flap of the chisel guide comes to lie parallel with the femoral shaft while the seating chisel is hammered in.

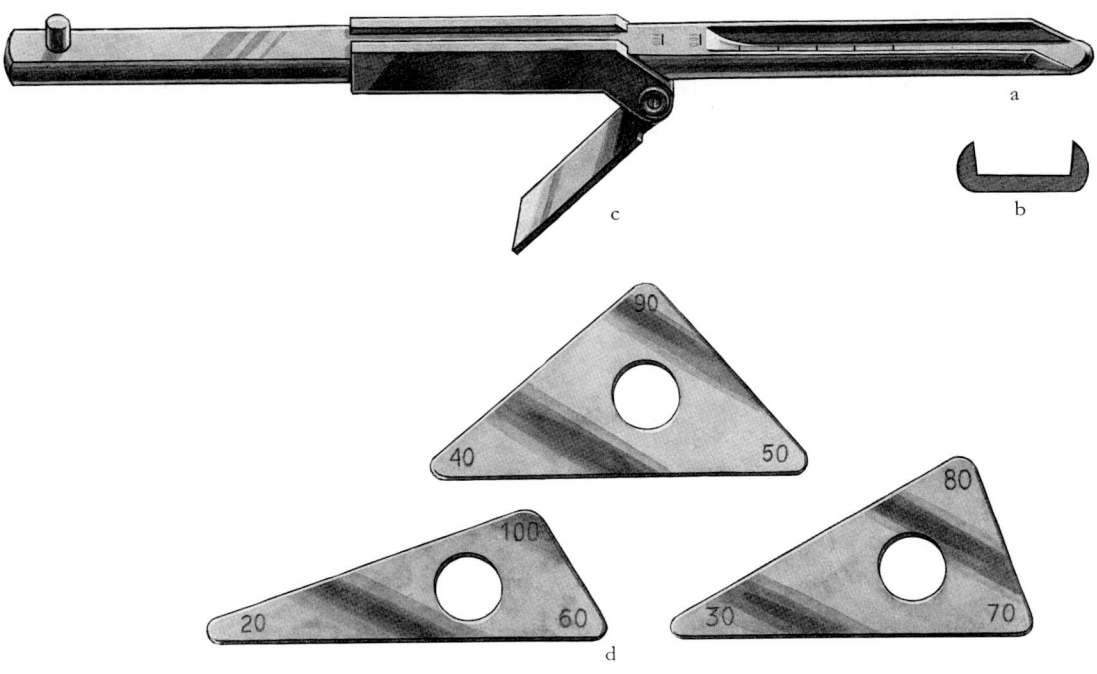

a

b

c

d

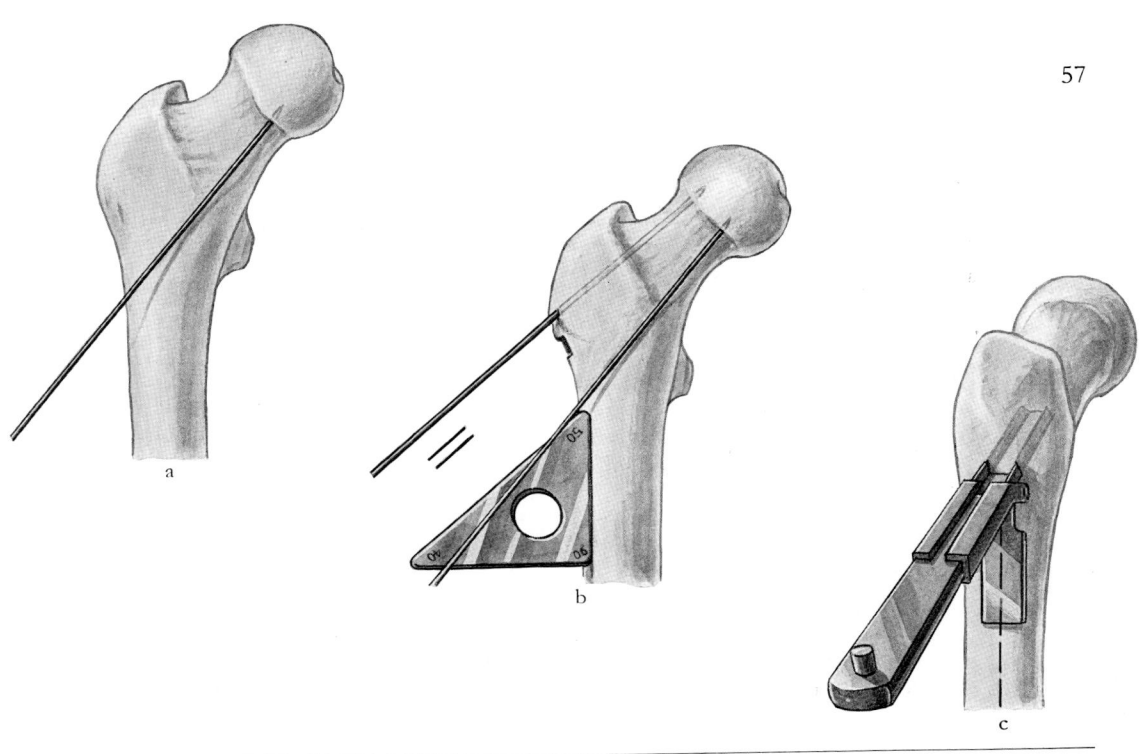

a

b

c

The 130° blade plate is used in fractures of the femoral neck and in some pertrochanteric fractures in which the greater trochanter is almost intact. The 130° blade plate with the extra long shaft can also be employed to fix subtrochanteric fractures.

Fig. 58   *The 130° blade plate.*

a   The standard 130° pertrochanteric plate is also useful for fixing femoral neck fractures.

b   The pertrochanteric plates with different shaft lengths.

c   The blade plate for femoral neck fractures.

d   The triangular positioning plate with 50° angle (complementary angle 180° —130° = 50°), used for marking the coronal plane for the 130° plate.

Examples of application:

e   An example of the pertrochanteric plate used as a buttress. Compression is achieved by means of two cancellous screws inserted parallel to the blade. It is important that the blade as well as the screws get a good grip on the head (Fig. 149).

f   Subcapital fractures should be over reduced into valgus and anteverted and *impacted* in this position. The plate then only acts as a simple buttress. The tip of the plate should come to lie below the point where tension and compression trabeculae cross over, which is the only really compact part of the femoral head and where the cancellous bone will give good support. Compression is supplied by the body weight and muscle pull.

58

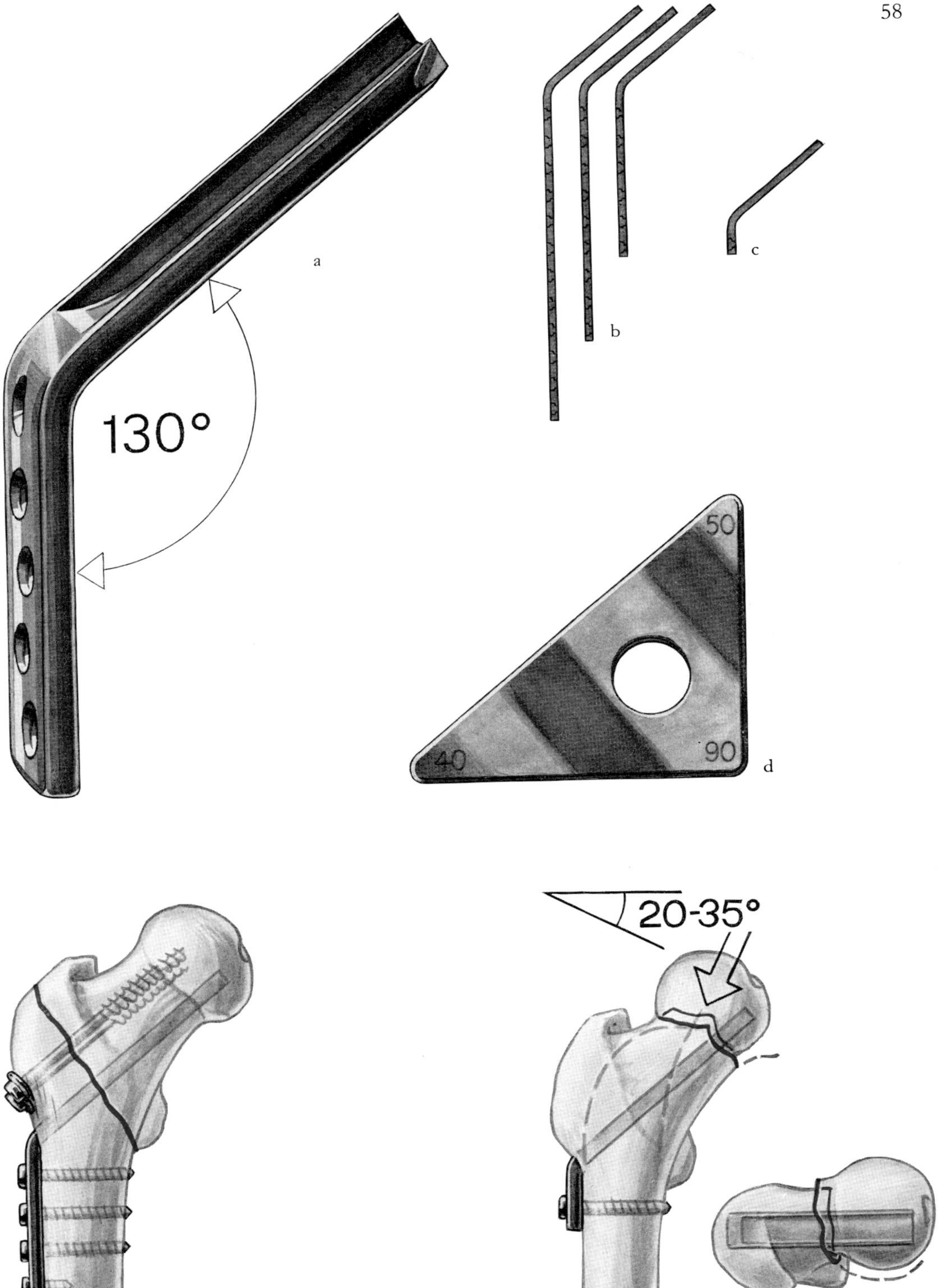

130°

a

b

c

50

40 90

d

20-35°

e

f

69

The 95° condylar plate is designed for use in supracondylar fractures of the femur. The blade of the plate is inserted parallel to the axis of the joint which is known to subtend an angle with the axis of the shaft of 81°. As the shaft is slightly conical the plate comes to lie along the cortex of the bone if the blade is inserted parallel to the knee joint, as long as there are no anatomical abnormalities. These plates can be used in supracondylar fractures of the femur, in valgus supracondylar osteotomy of the femur and in some pertrochanteric fractures. In these last, when the bone is much comminuted, the condylar plate is more useful than the 130° plate, but it must be placed under tension so as to withstand any bending stresses more firmly. They cannot, however, be used unless the calcar of the femur is intact.

Fig. 59		*The condylar plates.*
	a	The standard condylar plate with two holes for cancellous screws and three holes for cortex screws.
	b	The condylar plate of longer shaft lengths for comminuted fractures of either end of the femur, provided with five, seven, nine or twelve holes.
	c	The physiological axis of tibia and femur showing the angles they form with the knee joint itself.
	d	The special condylar plate guide which is shaped like a mould for the shaft portion of the condylar plate. (For its use see Fig. 164 and 291.)
Fig. 60		*The use of condylar plates.*
	a	In a supracondylar fracture the blade is inserted parallel to the articular surfaces of the condyles. The anatomical angle between the femoral shaft and the axis of the knee joint is 81°. The angle of the condylar plate is 95°. When the plate is placed under tension the angle increases to somewhere between 98° and 100°. The angle between the axis of the femoral shaft and the knee joint therefore measures about 99° as under physiological conditions.
	b	The use of the condylar plate in a pertrochanteric fracture in which the calcar is intact. Compression of the fracture is obtained by using cancellous (rarely malleolar) screws firmly biting on the intact calcar in addition to the compression obtained by placing the plate under tension.
	c	Condylar plates with a long shaft used in comminuted fractures of the upper end of the femur. For the technique of reduction of these comminuted fractures with the help of a long condylar plate, see Fig. 61.

70

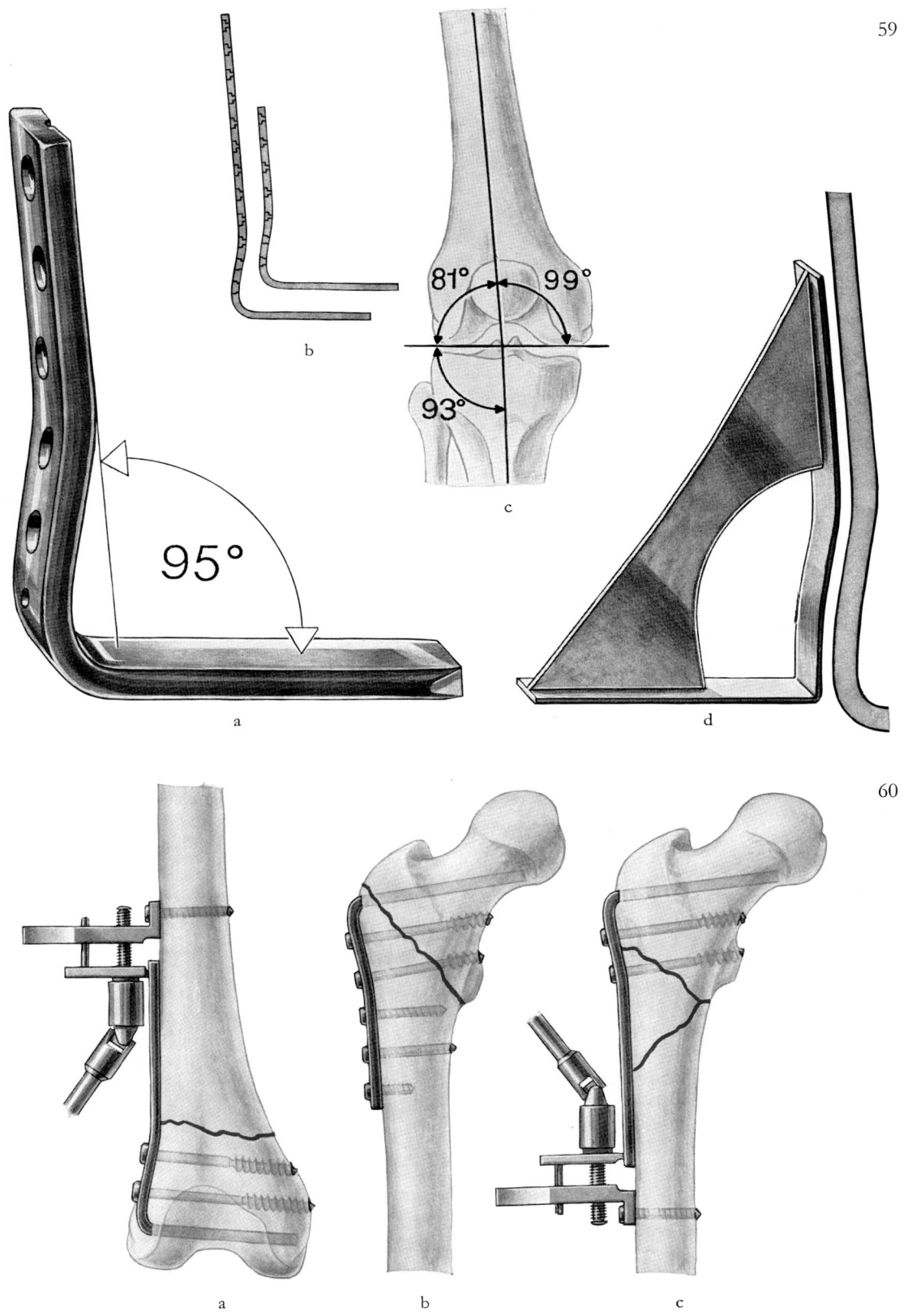

59

81°   99°

93°

95°

b

c

a

d

60

a   b   c

71

Special uses of the condylar blade plate.

Fig. 61   *Comminuted subtrochanteric fractures.*

The first step is to insert the condylar plate into the proximal fragment and secure it with two cancellous screws. The fracture can then be reduced and screwed to the plate. If loose fragments between the two main fragments are devitalized, autogenous cancellous bone graft should be inserted at the same time as the internal fixation (see Fig. 87/95b). (No weight bearing if the medial side of the bone is not stable!)

Fig. 62   *Supracondylar osteotomy.*

A supracondylar valgus osteotomy is best held with a condylar plate. Do the outer part of the osteotomy first and then insert the condylar plate and secure it to the distal fragment with one cancellous screw. Now complete the osteotomy, reduce the fragments and then place the osteotomy under compression.

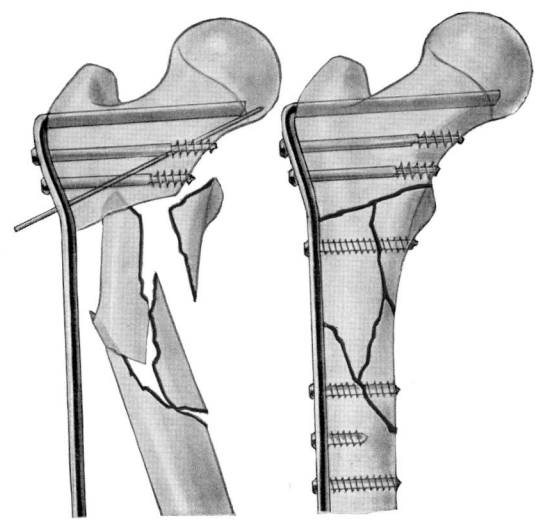

61

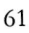

62

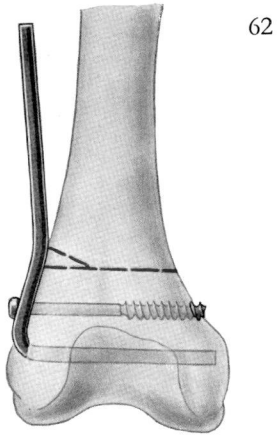

These 90° blade plates have a fixed angle of 87°. They are always used as tension bands. Under tension of about 100 kg the fixed angle opens up about 3°. Thus, when the required compression between fragment is achieved there is a 90° angle in the blade plate.

The blade of the standard plate has been shortened to 50 mm because the tension band effect is not enhanced by the use of a longer blade. On the contrary, we have found that bone resorption occurs deep to the blade as a result of recurrent changes in the axis between neck and shaft due to loading and unloading, and it has also been found that a longer blade is unnecessary.

Besides the standard 90° blade plate which projects 15 mm laterally, we have plates which produce a medial displacement of the shaft of 10, 15 or 20 mm. In teenagers, especially in a valgus osteotomy, it is best to employ a short 40 mm blade. The 100° blade plate is used when severe varus has to be corrected during the operation.

The 90° blade plates are particularly useful in such hip surgery as intertrochanteric osteotomy but they can also be used when undertaking a varus supracondylar osteotomy (Fig. 292).

For children there are smaller plates with chisels to match (Fig. 287).

Fig. 63		*The standard 90° blade plate for intertrochanteric osteotomy producing medial displacement of the shaft in the adult.*
	a	The plate has a double bend and a special slit for applying the tension device. At the bend there is a hole through which either a cortex or malleolar screw can be passed to get a purchase on the calcar. The depth of the bend is 15 mm and the plate length is 50 mm. The angle measures 87° so that after tension is applied, it will increase to the required 90°.
	b	Variants of the standard 90° blade plate are provided with the plate inset by either 10 or 20 mm in relation to the shaft, as well as 40 mm length of blade for valgus osteotomy in teenagers.
	c	A further variant with a 100° angle.
	d	The quadrangular positioning plate for use with varus osteotomy.
Fig. 64		*The use of the angled blade plate instruments before intertrochanteric osteotomy.*
	a	For a varus osteotomy of 20°, the appropriate positioning plate is selected. As in Fig. 57a the first Kirschner wire is passed along the front of the femoral neck then a second Kirschner wire is driven into the greater trochanter to indicate the frontal plane.
	b	For a valgus osteotomy, the perpendicular to the axis of the femoral shaft is found with the help of the quadrangular positioning plate for varus osteotomy, and then with the help of the triangular positioning plate one obtains the angle. In this case the valgus correction measures 20°.
	c	The flap of the chisel guide is set to 20° to the axis of the shaft, and to make sure that this angle does not alter while the chisel is inserted, the chisel should be held with the slotted hammer while it is being driven in.

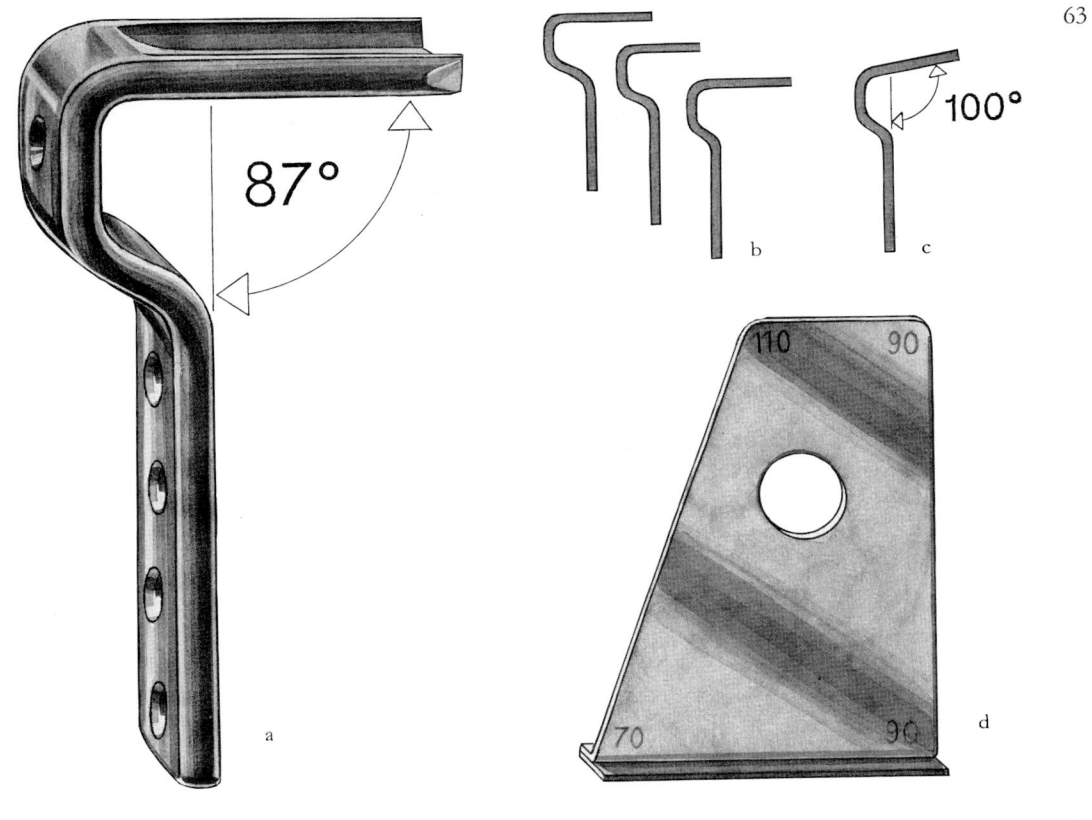

63

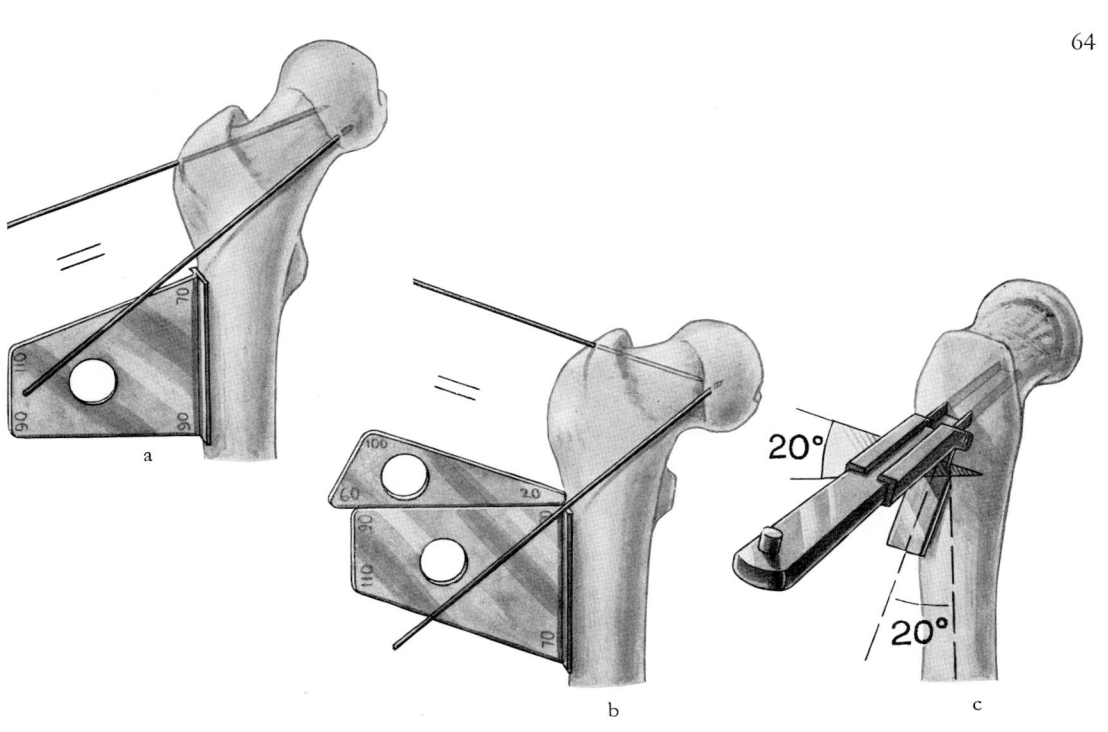

64

The right angled blade plate is always used as a tension band and is always placed under tension. In order to decrease the amount of shortening after the osteotomy, we use the oscillating saw (Fig. 285 3/4) and insert the bone wedge removed from the medial side into the lateral side. To reduce thermal injury to the bone ends resulting from the oscillating saw, the saw blade should be irrigated with cold saline or Ringer's solution during cutting.

Fig. 65   *Intertrochanteric varus osteotomy.*

a   In a varus osteotomy remove the medial wedge of 20°, reverse the wedge and place it on the lateral side between the main fragments.

b   Apply compression to the plate using the tension device (see also Fig. 285).

Fig. 66   *Intertrochanteric valgus and extension osteotomy.*

a   As before remove a wedge of 20°, but this time based laterally, the osteotomy being made parallel to the blade of the angled blade plate.

b   In an extension osteotomy with resection of a wedge of 20° based posteriorly this wedge should be reversed and inserted in the front.

Fig. 67   *Derotation osteotomy to correct excessive anteversion.*

a   After inserting the special seating chisel, drill in a Kirschner wire on each side of the planned osteotomy line. These two Kirschner wires should correspond to the required angle of correction. Insert the uppermost Kirschner wire at right angles to the chisel and determine the position of the second wire with the triangular positioning plate.

b   After the rotation has been carried out (as shown in this example with a correction of 20°) the two Kirschner wires come to lie parallel.
N.B.: In cases of severe osteoarthritis with stiffness, rotation must be checked in extension as well as in flexion after the blade has been placed under tension.

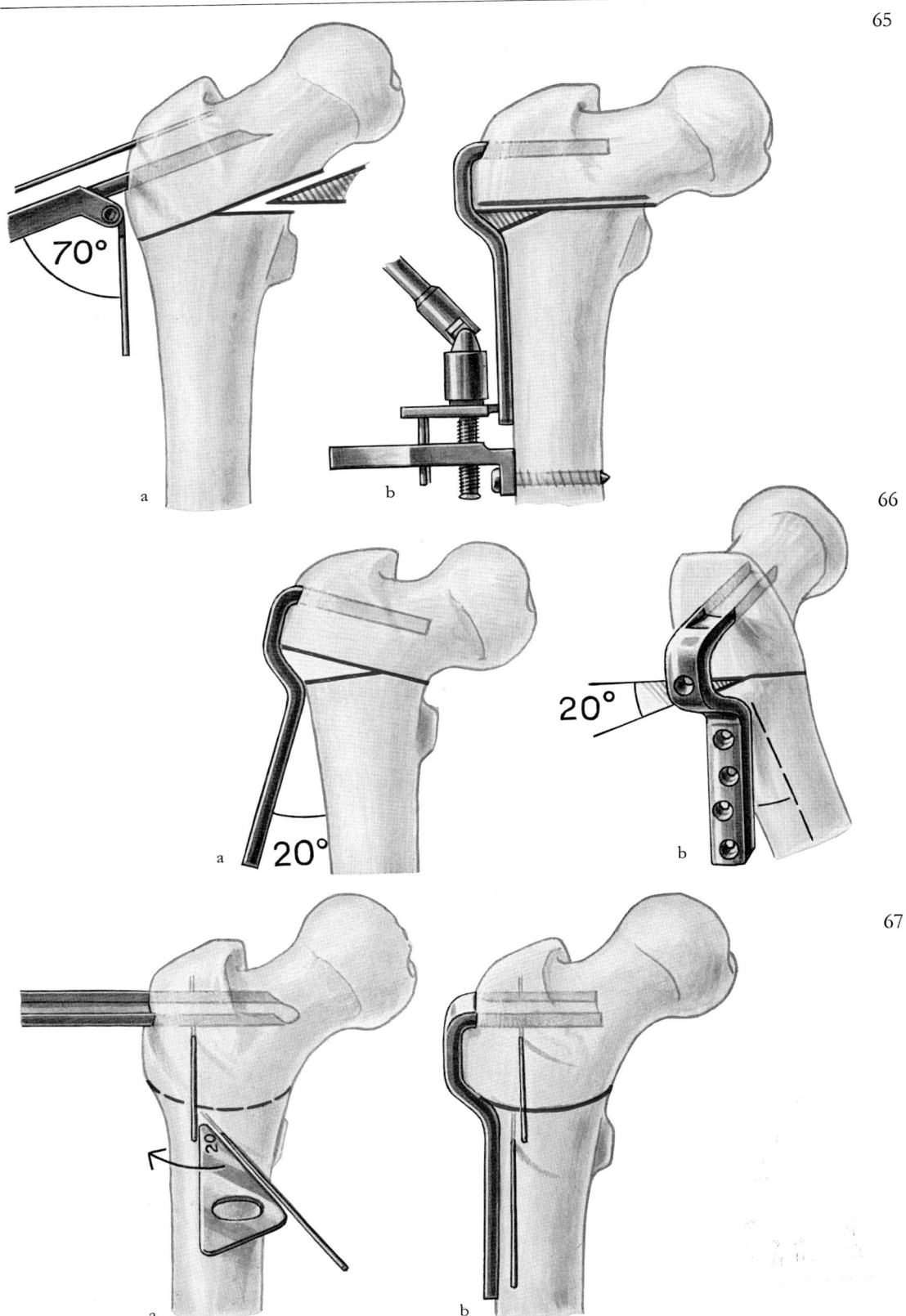

The Double Angled Plates for Repositioning Osteotomy

The 120° double angled standard plate is used for repositioning osteotomy for the treatment of pseudarthrosis in the femoral neck when the femoral head is viable. It may also be used for the treatment of femoral neck fractures with atrophic femoral heads in young patients.

The special 160° plate for valgus osteotomy which permits lateralization of the shaft is seldom needed.

With this plate, compression between fragments at the osteotomy is not achieved with the tension device, but by the maneuver of first placing the distal fragment in slightly greater abduction and then pulling it towards the plate with the screws. As the osteotomy surfaces are oblique they come under the required compression.

Fig. 68   *The special AO abduction blade plate.*

a   The standard 120° blade plate.

b   The special 110° model.

c   The special 160° model which brings the femoral shaft more laterally.

Fig. 69   *The technique of compression of the fragments after repositioning osteotomy.*

a   Insert the blade of the selected blade plate. Carry out the desired intertrochanteric osteotomy and remove the wedge of bone based laterally.

b   Reduce the osteotomy so that the femoral shaft only makes contact with the lower end of the plate and so that a gap of about 5 mm is left between the shaft and the plate. Now insert the lowermost small screw. When the proximal screw is inserted, the femoral shaft is pulled in towards the plate and the osteotomy is then impacted and compressed.

Fig. 70   *Valgus osteotomy with lateral displacement of the femoral shaft.*
The same maneuver is carried out in doing a valgus osteotomy to displace the femoral shaft laterally, using the 160° plate. (Also see Fig. 69b.)

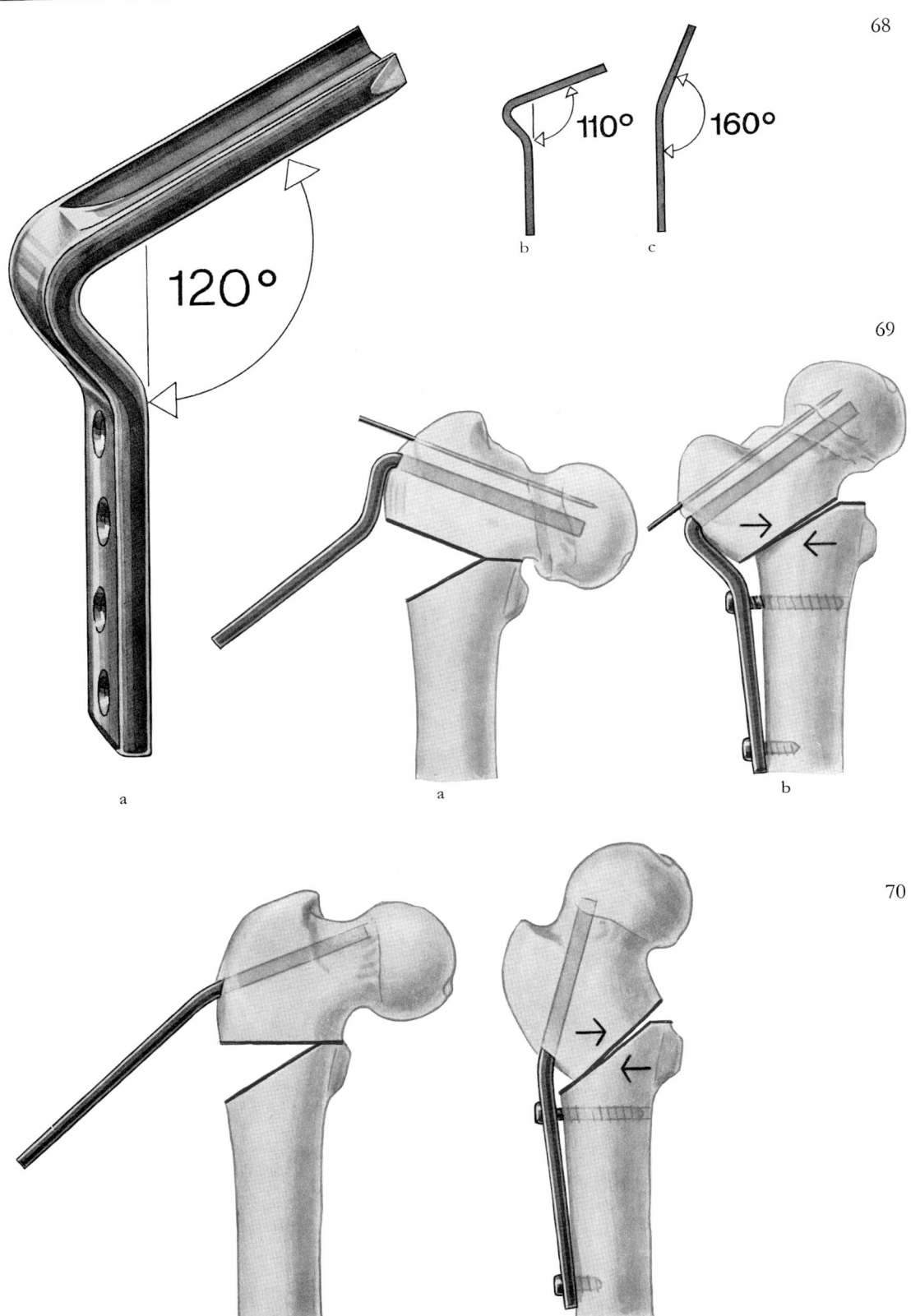

68

b   110°   c   160°

a

69

a   b

70

a

79

B. Intramedullary Methods of Internal Fixation

With intramedullary methods of fixation a medullary nail is relied upon to stabilize a fracture of the shaft of a long bone. Additional compression is not required but stability is secured by filling the medullary canal as completely as possible with the nail, with or without reaming.

1. The Intramedullary Nail

a) Indications for Intramedullary Nailing with Reaming of the Canal

The AO considers that intramedullary nailing with reaming of the canal is the method of choice in the treatment of all fractures of the middle third of the femur (see Fig. 160) as well as most transverse or oblique fractures of the middle third of the tibia (Fig. 74). The experienced surgeon can also use this method of internal fixation for certain fractures of the tibial metaphyses (Fig. 210). We believe that in cases of delayed union or non-union of femur or tibia, if alignment is good the methods developed by KÜNTSCHER and HERZOG result in the quickest and most spectacular results. We are opposed to intramedullary nailing of bones in the upper limb, as damage may occur to the shoulder or the wrist joint and it is often impossible to secure rotational stability in fresh fractures.

b) Indications for Medullary Nailing without Reaming of the Canal

Compound fractures, segmental fractures and some comminuted fractures of the tibia are nailed with narrower medullary nails without reaming.

c) Open or Closed Medullary Nailing

There are two basic methods. In the first the fracture is exposed, anatomical reduction obtained and the medullary canal then reamed and nailed. In the other method closed nailing is undertaken without exposing the fracture but reduction obtained under the image intensifier, followed by reaming and finally nailing.

Open medullary nailing has its advantages. It facilitates an exact anatomical reduction, precise control of rotation, the complete removal of any debris resulting from the reaming, and finally the evacuation of all haematoma. No special apparatus nor even a fracture table is required and radiation is kept to a minimum.

2. Medullary Wiring

This is only used to fix the fibula (Fig. 194d). In other bones the medullary canal is much too wide to give any stability by this method.

3. HACKETHAL's Method of Stacked Nails

This method is only useful for transverse fractures of the humerus. It gives better rotational stability than simple medullary nailing. Despite or possibly because of the existing slight elasticity of this type of nailing, we have found that rapid consolidation of the fracture occurs.

We have abandoned HACKETHAL's original method using the image intensifier and reduction apparatus, and prefer an open reduction through a posterior approach. If the fracture is below the spiral groove, the posterior incision which was made to introduce the nail is simply extended upwards. In fractures of the middle third and those above the spiral groove, the fracture is exposed from the lateral side.

As the techniques of medullary nailing and stacked nails are well known, we shall only enlarge on the modifications introduced by the AO. If further reading is required the works of KÜNTSCHER and HACKETHAL should be consulted.

To Make the Methods of Küntscher and Herzog more Dependable, the AO Has Modified these Methods of Medullary Nailing as Follows :

The medullary nail is lighter, more elastic and is made of thin tubes slit along the distal $^4/_5$ of their length. The proximal $^1/_5$ has been fitted with a thread on its inner surface to help in introduction and, more importantly, in extraction of the nails. The shafts of the reamers are flexible and the reamers themselves cut without jamming. We have also found that pneumatic motors, particularly those especially designed for medullary reaming, are better than electric ones (Fig. 10/4 b).

Fig. 71	*The features of the AO medullary nail.*
a	The nail for the tibia is made of a partially open tube with a curve at the proximal end (HERZOG curve).
b	The nail for the femur has a slight bow which corresponds to the physiological anterior curve of the femur.
c	The tip of the nail is shaped so that it will not bite into the cortex but will follow the guide rod.
d	On the inside of the upper end of the tubular part of the nail a thread has been cut which allows firm fixation of the conical bolt and prevents any damage to the nail at its impaction or, and this is more important, any difficulty in its extraction.
e	The AO nail, just like the Küntscher nail, has a clover-leaf profile.
f	For greater rotational stability in the tibia, a transverse screw can be passed through the upper slot of the nail.
g	At the lower end there are special side slots through which the HERZOG antirotational wires can be passed to prevent any secondary rotation, varus or valgus deformity.
Fig. 72	*Details of the AO insertion-extraction instruments and the guide rod.*
	The guide rod (a) with its curved end (b), ball end (c) for removal of any jammed reamers, the tibial nail (d), the femoral nail (e), the guide handle to prevent rotation of the nail during impaction (f), the guide rod for introducing the nail (g), the threaded conical bolt (h), the curved driving piece (i), the weight guide (k), the ram (l), plastic grip for fixing the weight guide (m), driving head (n) which can be fastened to the curved driving piece (i) when the weight guide (k) and the ram (l) are not employed.
Fig. 73	*The technique for the removal of a jammed medullary reamer.*
	The holder (a) is attached to the guide rod (b). Using the slotted hammer (c) impacted flexible reamers (d) or reamer heads (e) can easily be hammered out.

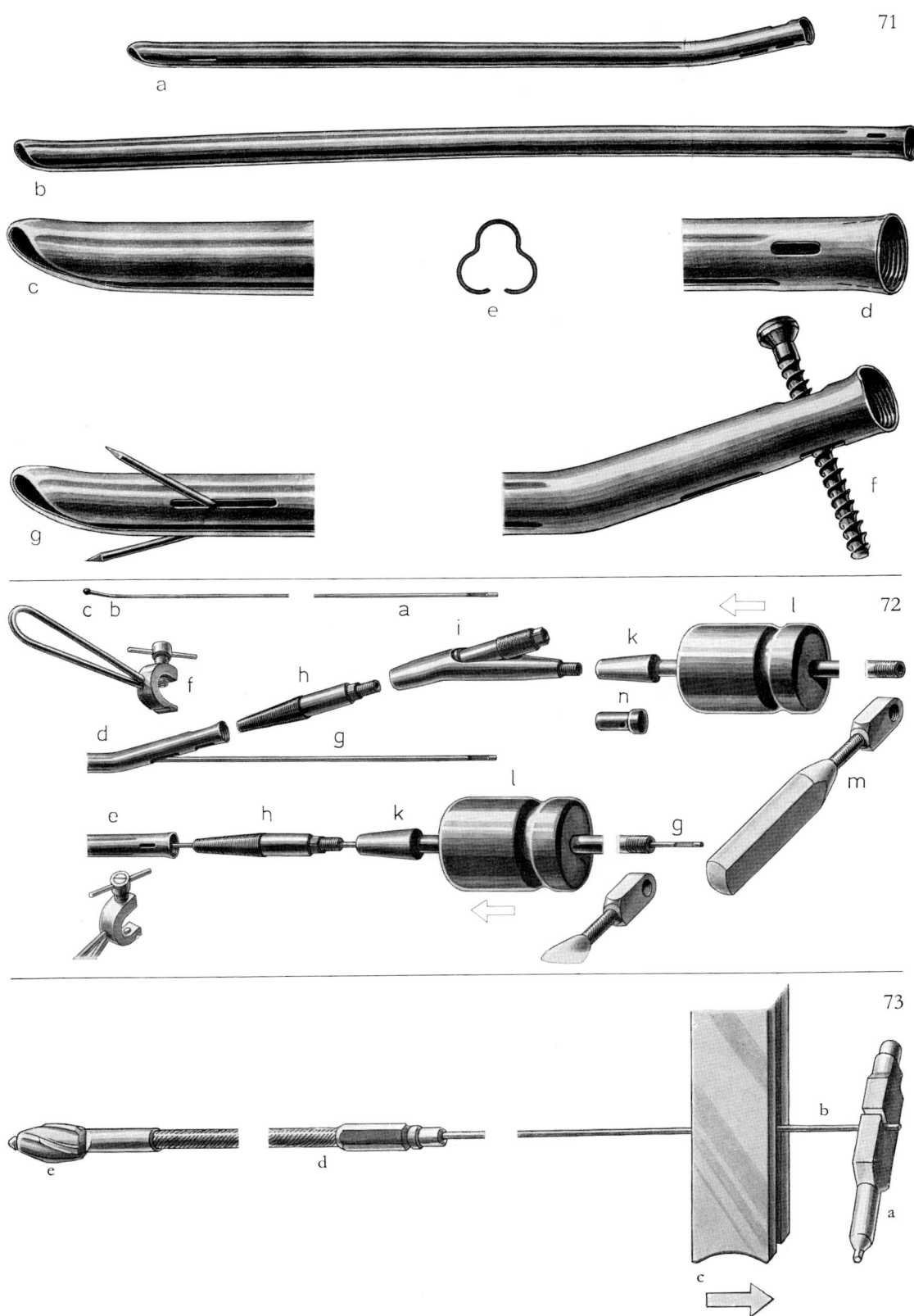

71

a

b

c

e

d

g

f

72

c b   a   i   k   l

f   h   n   m

d   g

e   h   k   l   g

m

73

b

e   d

a

c

83

Fig. 74   *The technique.*

a   Expose the fracture and reduce the fragments. The fragments are held in position with a semi-tubular plate and two Verbrugge bone clamps. If the image intensifier is not being used when nailing a tibia, the patient is placed supine on an ordinary table with the knee bent to an angle of 40–45°. The foot is supported. A transverse skin incision is made over the ligmanetum patellae and this is split longitudinally and held open with a self-retaining retractor (see Fig. 173c).

b   Perforate the cortex above the tibial tubercle with the awl, directing it first backwards and then downwards in order to enter the medullary canal.

c   Introduce the 3 mm guide rod. Note on this the length of the nail that was estimated before operation by measuring the normal side.

d   Reaming is begun with a 9 mm flexible reamer with its frontal cutting head. This head is used first to overcome any possible resistance in the medullary canal to the passage of subsequent reamers, as these only ream with their sides. Further reaming is carried out with flexible reamers, fitted with interchangeable heads. The heads are increased by 0.5 mm until the medullary canal is reamed to a diameter of 11.5 to 12.5 mm. The diameter should be 0.5 mm wider than the chosen nail. The skin and the patellar ligament are protected during reaming with a special metal tissue protector.

e   When reaming is complete, introduce the plastic medullary tube over the 3 mm guide rod. When the medullary tube is in position, remove the 3 mm guide rod and irrigate the medullary canal with saline or Ringer's solution until the fluid is returned clear.

f   Introduce the 4 mm rigid guide rod.

g   Remove the medullary tube and insert the appropriate 11 or 12 mm medullary nail. Prevent rotation of the nail during insertion with the special guide handle.

h   The nail should extend to within 1 cm of the ankle joint and its proximal end should lie flush with the cortex.

N.B.:   1. Bend the knee to an angle of 40–60° and support it on a padded roll. In this position, when the muscles are relaxed under anesthesia, simple longitudinal traction usually produces a good reduction. Additional manipulation is usually unnecessary. When the fracture is well reduced, it is easy to introduce the guide rod into the lower fragment. When resistance is felt to the passage of the guide rod, due to the cancellous bone of the lower end of the tibia, it is a sign that the guide rod has been passed for the required distance and an X-ray is usually unnecessary. Occasionally a small insision is required to check the reduction.

2. Occasionally wire cerclage is used in combination with intramedullary nailing. The cerclage wire must be removed within 6–8 weeks or avascular necrosis of underlying bone will result.

a

b

c

d

e

f

g

h

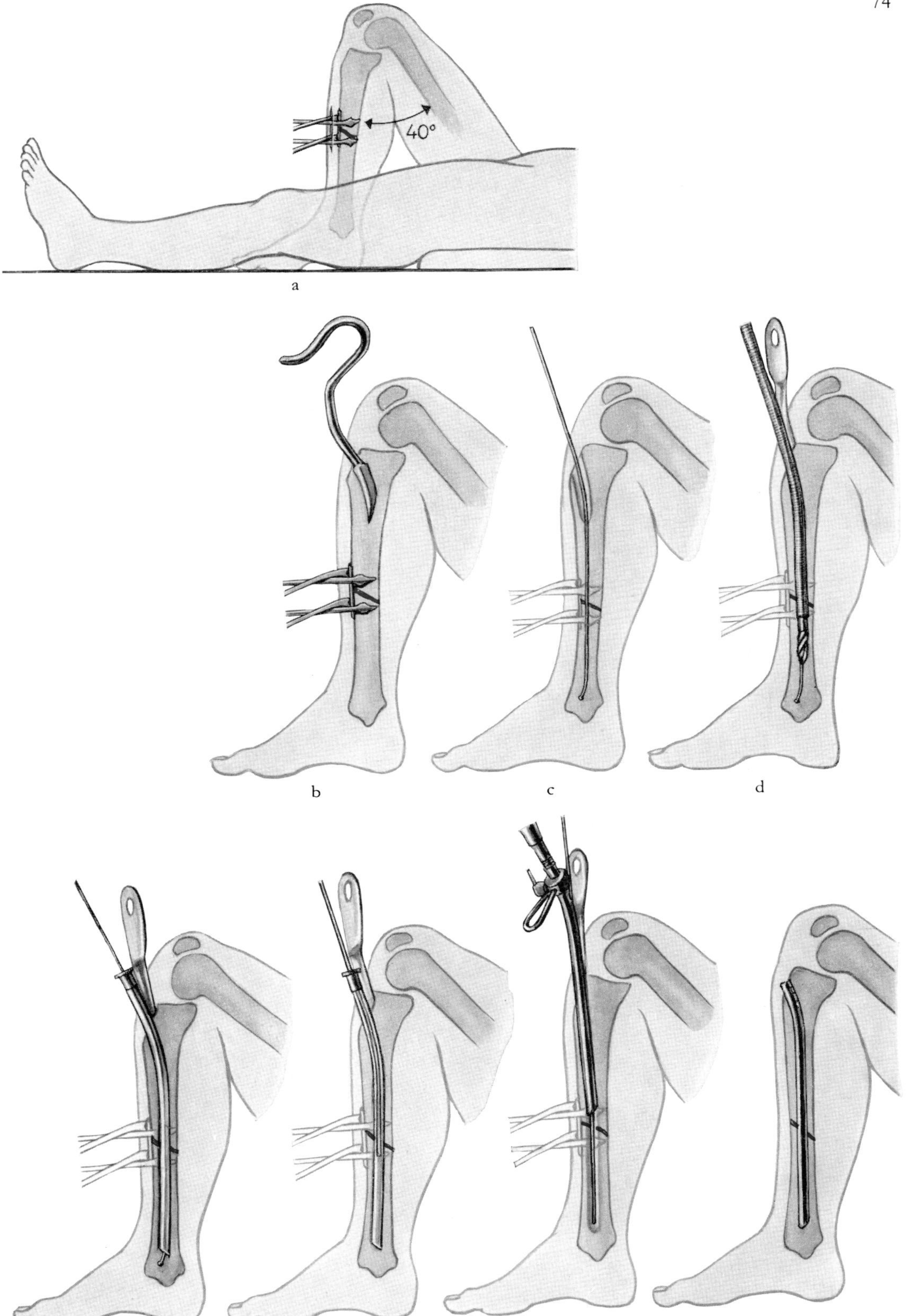

In the femur a medullary nail should not be introduced through the top of the greater trochanter but somewhat more laterally, so that neither the retinacular vessels nor the hip joint are damaged. The insertion of a guide rod in a retrograde manner from the fracture is to be condemned, because if the guide rod is introduced thus it often comes to lie too far medially and may damage the hip joint. The skin incision over the greater trochanter should be made longitudinally and the gluteal muscles split in the line of their fibres. The tip of the greater trochanter is exposed and is perforated with the awl downwards and medially to open the medullary canal.

The medullary canal is always reamed out 1 mm wider than the nail that is to be used.

N.B.:

1. In comminuted fractures of the middle third of the femur medullary nailing may be combined with cerclage wiring. Cerclage wires should be removed within two months. In the upper third of the femur we recommend using a condylar plate as the best method of internal fixation.

2. In adolescence, between 11 and 16 years, when there is an indication for medullary nailing of femoral shaft fractures, we have found the 10–12 mm tibial nail to be most useful. It should be introduced from the postero-lateral aspect just distal to the epiphyseal plate for the greater trochanter, so as to avoid damaging this.

Fig. 75   *The position of the patient for medullary nailing.*
The patient lies on his side with the hip and knee joints flexed.

Fig. 76   *The technique of open medullary nailing of the femur.*
The nail is introduced through the outer aspect of the greater trochanter. The groove in the nail should lie posteriorly so that the anterior bow of the nail will correspond with that of the femur.

Fig. 77   *The combination of medullary nailing with cerclage wiring in comminuted fractures.*
The cerclage wires must be removed after six to eight weeks.

Fig. 78   *Femoral nailing for children aged between 10 and 14.*
We usually use a tibial nail with the bent upper end and introduce it from behind just distal to the epiphyseal plate of the greater trochanter.

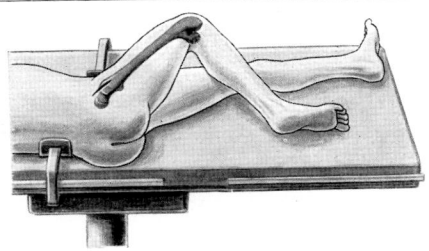

75

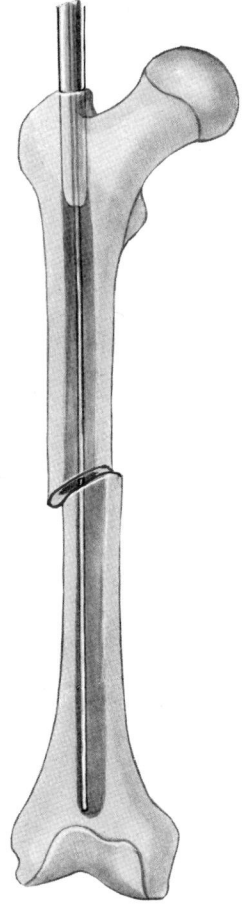

76

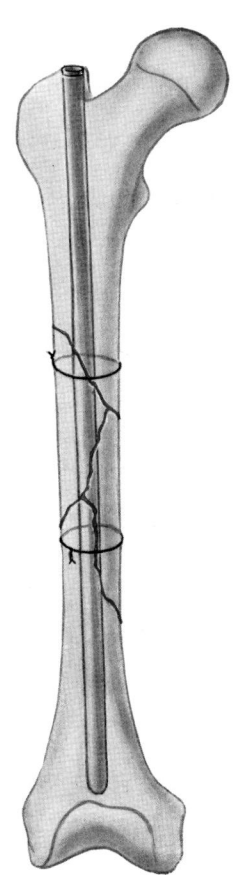

77

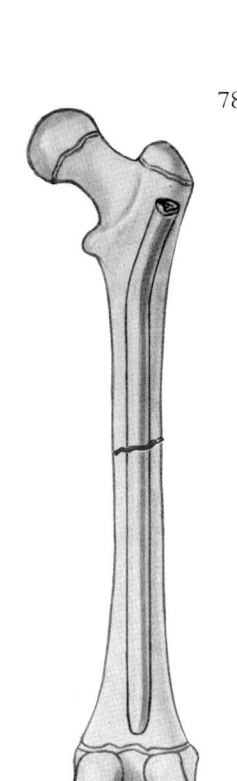

78

87

The Technique of Open Reduction of a Transverse Femoral Shaft Fracture, before Medullary Nailing

Fig. 79

a Insert the guide rod through the greater trochanter and advance it until it appears at the fracture. Increase the deformity until the fragments are almost at 90° to each other, and then introduce the tip of a small Hohmann retractor into the medullary canal of the lower fragment. Use this retractor as a lever to bring the fracture surfaces together. As soon as the guide rod enters the medullary canal of the distal fragment, the fracture can be temporarily stabilized with a semi-tubular plate

b The semi-tubular plate is held to the bone with two Verbrugge clamps and then the medullary canal can be reamed.

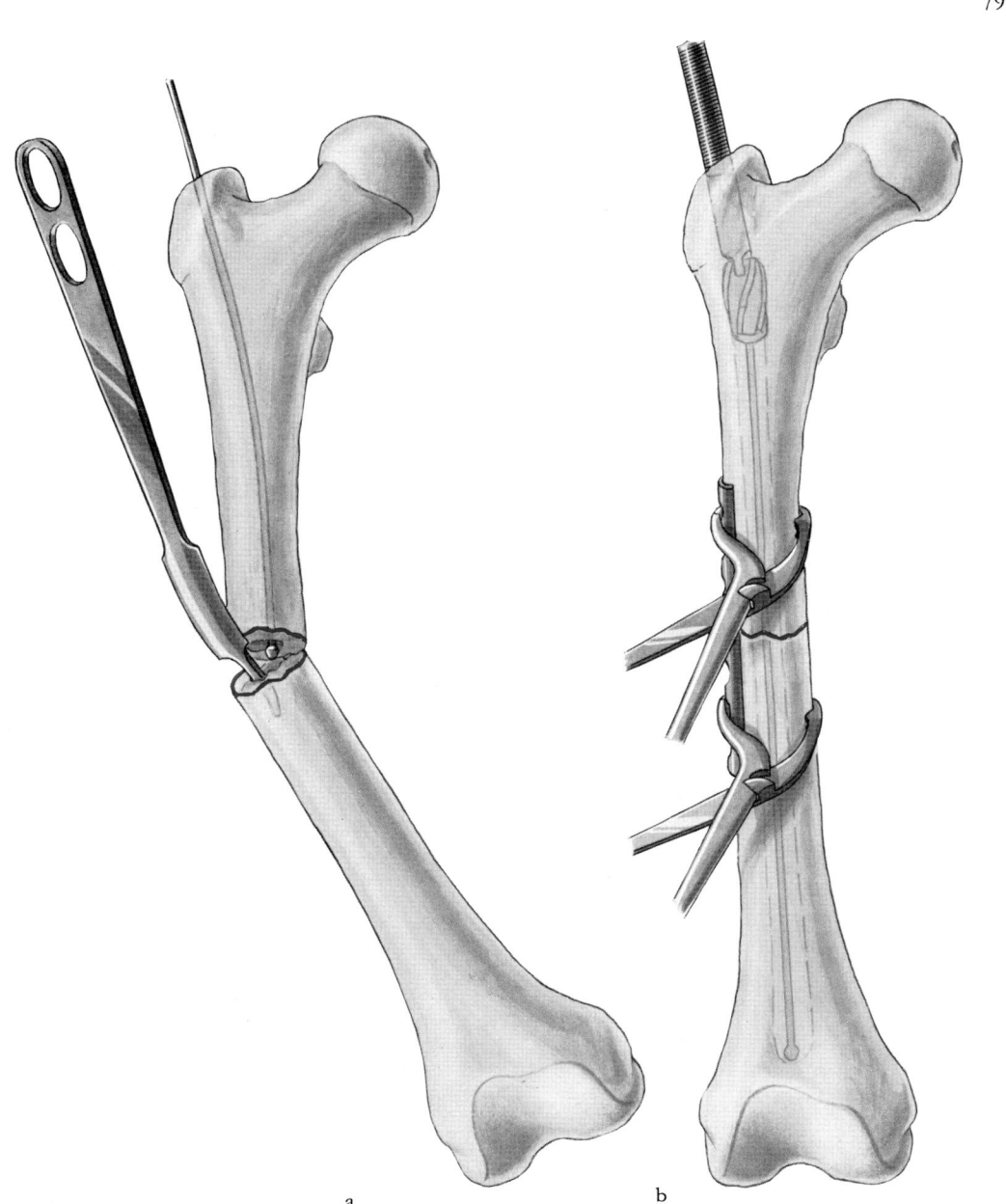

a

b

Closed nailing demands a special position and the use of an aseptically draped image intensifier with a TV screen. The surgeon can then check the important phases of the procedure. These include the reduction of the fracture after manipulation, introduction of the guide rod into the distal fragment, the distance of the end of the guide rod from the joint, the introduction of the reamer into the distal fragment, the length of the nail and finally the state of reduction at the end of the procedure.

Fig. 80   *The technique of medullary nailing of the tibia using the image intensifier.*
(a) The patient lies supine on the fracture table with the knee bent to at least 70–80°. Traction is applied either through a pin in the os calcis (b) or by means of a special leather shoe (c). Rotation is controlled by comparing the axis through the malleoli with that of the normal leg. The transmalleolar axis should be in 20–25° of external rotation (5–35°).

The medullary nailing itself is carried out following the above technique (page 84). Suction drainage of the fracture is recommended in closed medullary nailing also. A drain is introduced through a stab wound above the fracture line and brought out below.

Fig. 81   *Closed medullary nailing of the femur with image intensifier.*
(a) The patient lies on his side on the fracture table and traction is obtained either by a wire through the condyle (b) with the knee flexed which allows good rotational control, or by means of a leather shoe with the knee in extension (c).

The medullary nailing is carried out as described above for open nailing (page 86). Manipulation has often to be used to obtain a reduction. The slightly bent tip of the guide rod makes it easier to introduce it into the lower fragment, as well as to center it in the metaphysis.

N.B.: If the fracture is found to be distracted at the end of the procedure, it can usually be impacted by blows on the heel while the knee is held extended. If, in spite of this, reduction is not perfect, a small incision should be made over the fracture to make sure that the reduction is accurate and to carry out any corrective maneuver that may be necessary.

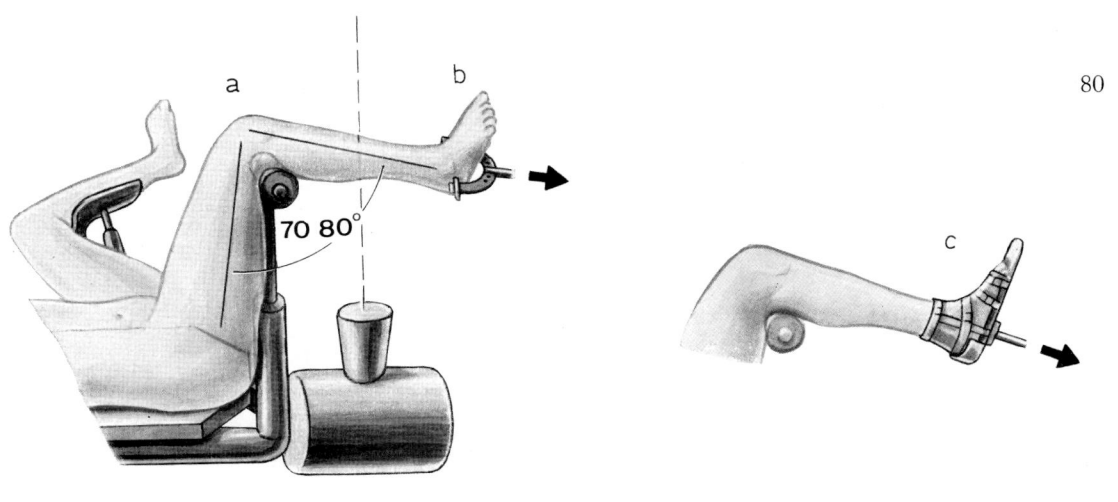

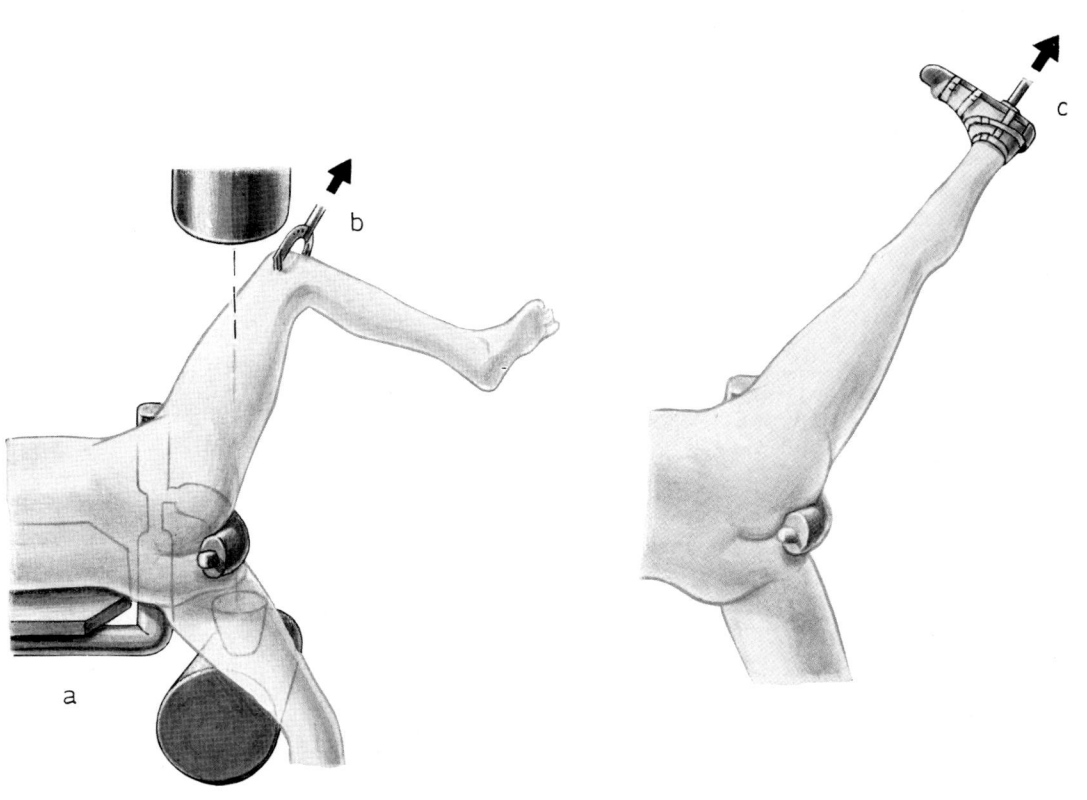

III. Pre-operative, Operative and Post-operative Guide-Lines

Bone surgery makes many demands on the surgical team, on the instruments used and on the implants. Perfect asepsis in this type of surgery is absolutely vital. Bone and joint surgery should only be carried out in specially constructed operating theatres and these should be of the highest aseptic standards.

To lower the infection rate we recommend the following practices: unnecessary moving about in the operating theatre should be avoided; thick masks should be used to cover both the nose and the mouth; the surgeons should wear cotton gloves over the normal rubber ones; regular bacteriological checks of the theatre personnel (air passages and hands) should be carried out; sources of pus such as boils, pimples and fistulae should be immediately detected.

The patient's skin must be carefully examined for sources of infection, and it should be disinfected and covered with a plastic film (Fig. 82). During operation we recommend frequent irrigation with Ringer's solution. Neomycin or Bacitracin may be added to this. Atraumatic surgery produces no tissue necrosis. Dead tissue provides a perfect nidus for infection. Electrocoagulation should only be applied to the minimum of tissue. Suction should be used sparingly, as it sucks air from the whole of the theatre into the wound. Use the least amount of foreign material such as catgut and avoid subcutaneous sutures. The skin should be closed atraumatically with thin synthetic material (Fig. 83). Prophylactic antibiotics are not recommended, for systematic antibiotic prophylaxis leads to a higher incidence of infection.

A full set of bone instruments should be available and a wide selection of *implants*. All implants must be made of the same metal and should be as corrosion resistant as possible and non-irritant to the tissues. One must not relax after just purchasing the AO instruments, but must keep up a regular and careful check to replace any faulty or worn out instruments, and all drills and other cutting instruments must be sharpened at regular intervals.

The timing of surgery depends to some extent on the organization of the department. There are three possibilities:

1. The patient may be operated upon before he comes into contact with other patients.

2. The patient is isolated for the night in an aseptic room and is operated upon the following day. This, of course, is only possible in simple fractures. The skin over the fracture must not be damaged. Do not operate if fracture blisters have formed.

3. The operation may be carried out between 4 and 14 days from the time of the fracture. The procedure may then be much easier, particularly in shaft fractures which have been maintained during this interval in traction. The danger of thrombophlebitis and of hospital infection, of course, rises. In comminuted fractures revascularization of the bone fragments may be better lessening the danger of avascular necrosis if the fracture is not interferred with during the first one to two weeks. No clear cut data are available on this point.

Before each operation the surgeon should have a *definite plan*. After a careful assessment of the X-rays, there may be more than one solution to the problem. We strongly urge that preoperative drawings should be made, to show the exact position of the screws and plates which are to be used in the internal fixation. At the same time it is wise to check that all the necessary implants are available, and that all drills and motors are working properly before operation. Opportunity should always be taken if necessary to survey the relevant literature and to review the anatomy of the part.

The manner in which exposures and reductions are often carried out in simple or comminuted fractures, is not what we would call "atraumatic surgery". The techniques of open reduction were described and illustrated when we dealt with screw fixation, plate fixation and medullary nailing. Brute force is never necessary. In the second part of the manual the exposures are fully described.

Post-operative Care

Physiotherapy is used to prevent thrombophlebitis in the form of breathing exercises, in general muscle exercises, in the control of any post-operative position, and for the general psychological well-being of the patient. Later in convalescence, physiotherapists train the patient in crutch walking, in further building up of the musculature and preventing passive oedema. Passive movements of the joints, mechanical therapy and massage are not indicated in any part of the AO method.

We shall now briefly discuss the *post-operative positioning*, the technique of *suction drainage*, which opposes soft tissues and eliminates dead space, and the technique of obtaining autogenous cancellous bone grafts which are the only bone grafts we recommend.

Fig. 82   The covering of the lower limb with plastic film.

Fig. 83

     a   The DONATI Skin Suture.

     b   ALLGÖWER's modification of the DONATI suture. The suture only goes through the dermis on one side. There are only two holes in the skin instead of four as in the usual mattress suture. This protects a poorly vascularized skin edge from further damage.

Fig. 84   Modified REDON suction drainage with disposable suction bag and outer spring.

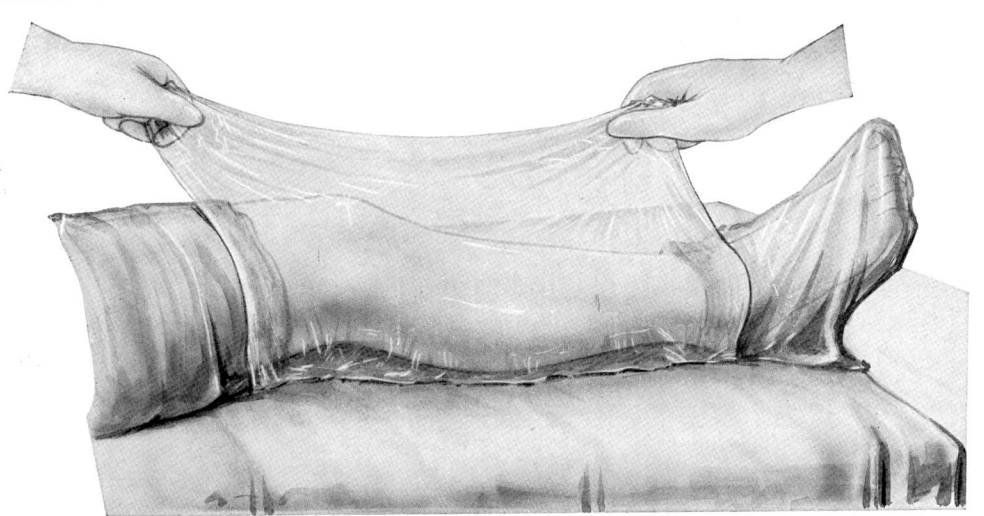

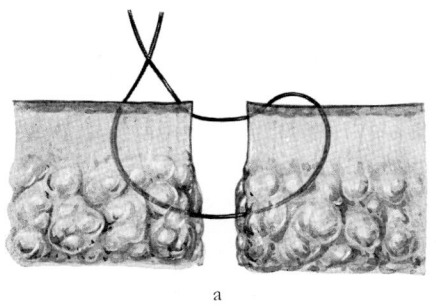

a

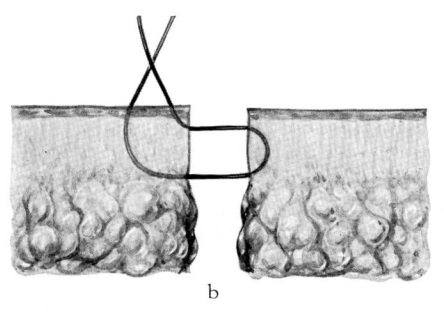

b

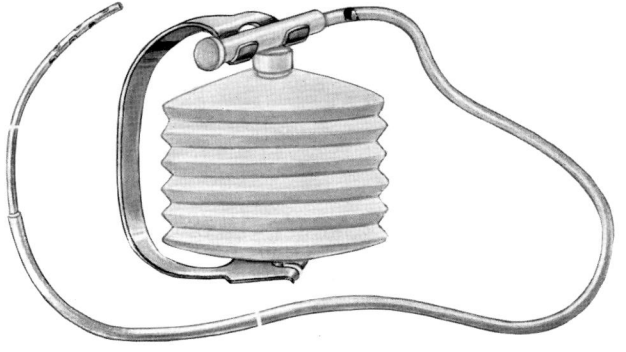

Post-operative Positioning

The position of the limb after open reduction and internal fixation is of the utmost importance. In intra-articular fractures active movement should be possible from the functional or neutral position. Small amounts of active movement do not interfere with healing, though the range of movement must be related to the stage of soft tissue healing. This is also true if much muscle stripping has been carried out, as may be necessary in exposing a femur.

After internal fixation of the lower tibia or after a malleolar fracture, the foot should be held at 90° for 4–7 days, though immediate active dorsiflexion exercises should be started. In any fracture of the elbow the position of the elbow should be 90°. All ftactures of the tibia are elevated on a Braun or Böhler splint padded with sponge rubber. Since we have been using this type of support, peroneal palsy from pressure has disappeared.

Every femoral shaft fracture is positioned with the hip and knee each flexed to 90°. After a week the patient may begin to sit, to dangle his feet over the edge of the bed and can begin to stand up. Using this method, recovery of knee flexion has never been a problem. It is also noticeable that as soon as the patient comes out of the frame, he can extend his knee. After internal fixation of both bones of the forearm we do not use compression dressings. The hand is held elevated for 48 hours to avoid post-operative edema and active movements may be begun on the 3rd day after operation.

Suction drainage is very useful in preventing post-operative hematomata and also helps in healing, as it draws the soft tissues together and aliminates dead space.

Fig. 85   *The three standard post-operative positions in bed.*

a   In *tibial fractures* the leg is supported on a Braun splint with the knee bent to 45°, the foot somewhat higher than the knee, the ankle at 90° and the sole of the foot supported in the splint.

b   *In fractures of the shaft or lower third of the femur*, the patient should have both the hip and the knee at 90° to regain an early range of movement in the knee. This is especially important after medullary nailing of the femur.

c   The elevation and support of the upper limb on a KEEL splint, after internal fixation of the humerus or both bones of the forearm.

Fig. 86   *Post-operative immobilization of malleolar fractures* (only necessary for 4–7 days).

a   The double U plaster splint for holding the foot at a right angle. This allows active dorsiflexion to be carried out.

b   Post-operative unpadded plaster. This must be immediately split and spread after its application.
     Both these methods of plaster support are highly recommended as an adjunct after open reduction and internal fixation of malleolar fractures. They should be used for one week.

85

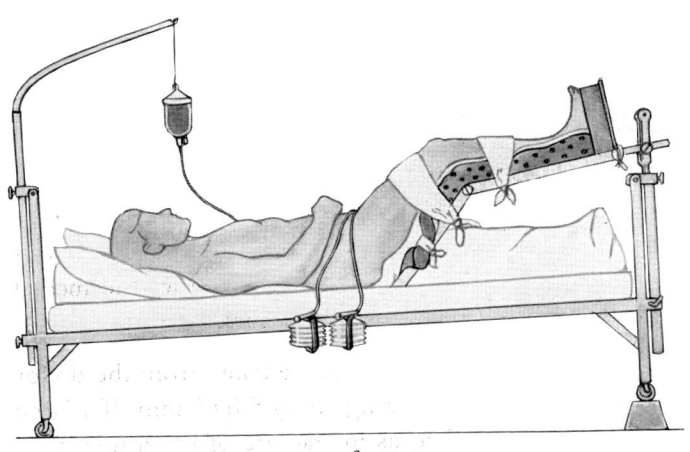

a

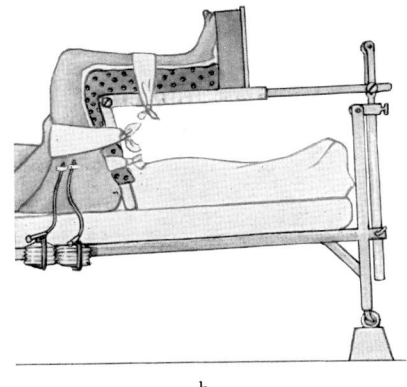

b

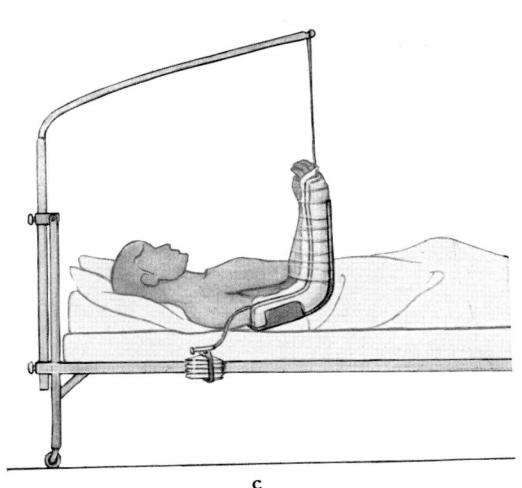

c

86

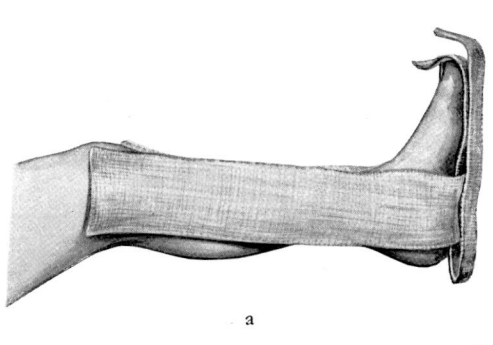

a

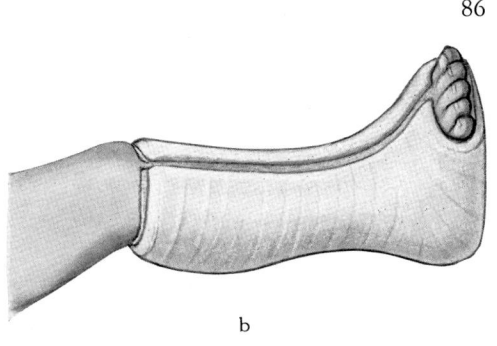

b

97

Autogenous Bone Grafts

In compression fracture of epiphyses or metaphyses, the defects have to be filled in with autogenous cortical or cancellous grafts. If bone grafting is carried out in the presence of infection, pure cancellous chips must be used.

In comminuted shaft fractures, especially of the femur fixed by a lateral plate, primary cancellous bone grafting should be carried out. This is particularly important when there is a defect of the medial cortex. If cancellous grafting is not used to reconstruct the medial cortex as soon as possible, fatigue fracture of the plate invariably occurs.

The bone is usually obtained from the ala of the ilium. The grafts are taken from the donor site with a curved osteotome and then cut into pieces measuring 15 by 5 by 5 mm. If a large amount of cancellous bone is needed to fill a large defect, as in fracture of the lower tibia, then this can be obtained from the greater trochanter. Cancellous bone can sometimes be obtained from other metaphyses as of the upper tibia, lower radius, etc.

N.B.: Pure cortical grafts are seldom used in bone surgery. A great drawback to autogenous cancellous grafts is the danger of post-operative hematoma at the donor site. To avoid this hemostasis must be secured before closure and this may be achieved by using a coagulating substance.

Fig. 87   *Donor sites for cancellous bone.*

a   The ala of the ilium is the common place for obtaining cancellous bone. Make a skin incision 2 cm over the iliac crest. Long sliver cancellous grafts may be obtained with a gouge or curved osteotome and are cut up to form chips 15 mm by 5 mm by 5 mm. We prefer the smaller chips to long corticocancellous strips, as the former are incorporated more quickly into a solid piece of bone. A coagulating substance is used for hemostasis.

b   In the prone position, obtain the bone from the outer ala of the ilium. Make the skin incision slightly lateral and below the iliac crest. After incising the fascia and elevation of the muscle, a wide exposure can be obtained so that strips of any thickness can be obtained.

Fig. 88

a   We have found the curved 1 cm osteotome most useful for taking bone grafts.

b   The greater trochanter is the best donor site for pure cancellous bone.

5-6 mm

15 mm

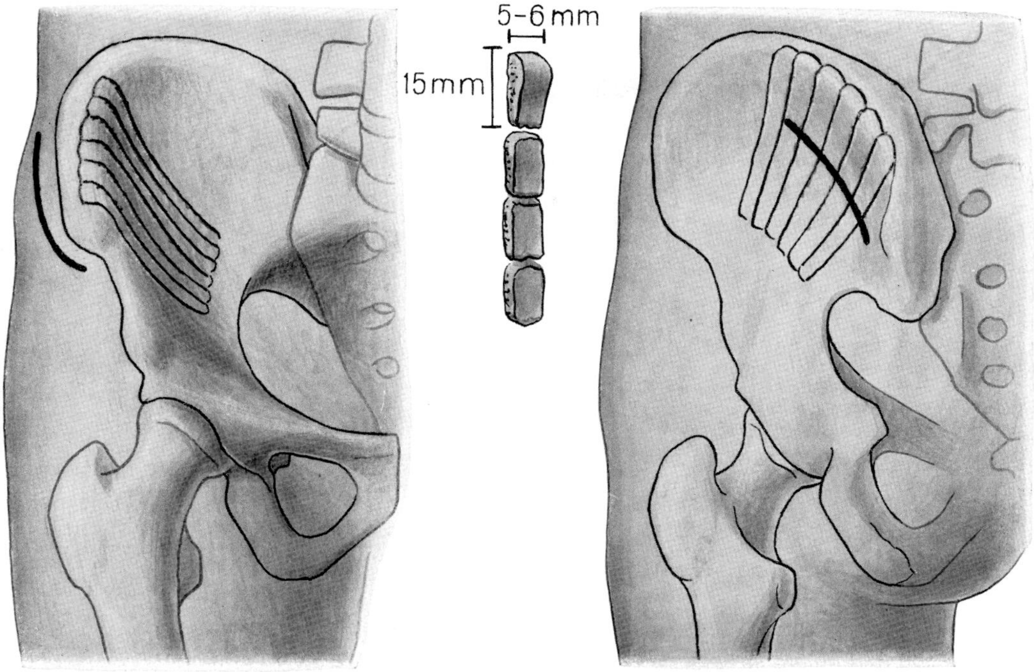

a   b

88

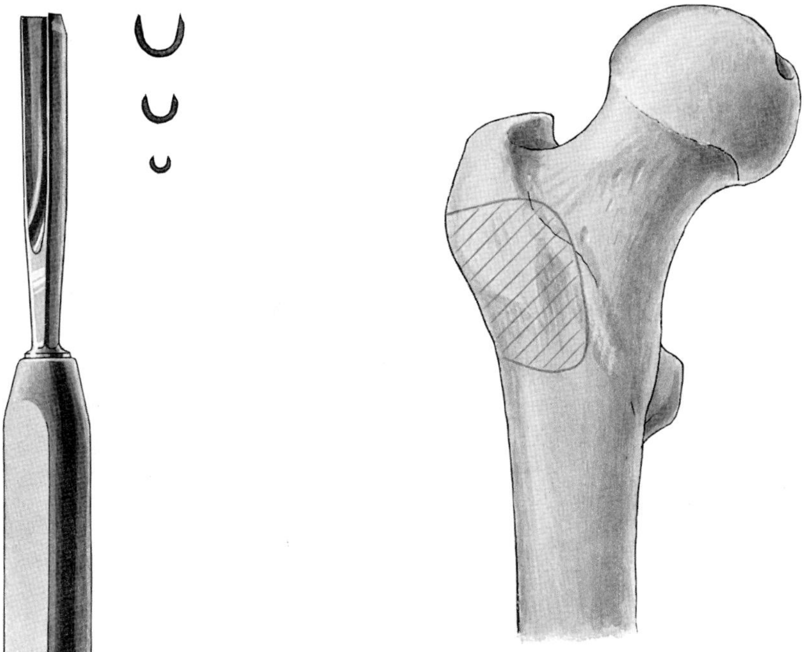

a   b

IV. Implants

A. The Removal

The removal of implants after bone union is necessary (between $1^1/_2$ and 2 years), not only because of possible corrosion of the metal but because implants are rigid and prevent the bone from responding to normal physiological stimuli. This is especially important in the lower limb, while implants seldom need to be removed from the humerus or forearm bones, unless they produce symptoms which is rarely the case.

To remove a plate from the medial surface of the tibia or to extract a medullary nail, only small skin incisions are needed. The patient seldom needs to be in hospital for more than four days.

Cerclage wire should be removed after $1^1/_2$–2 months, to prevent disturbance of the blood supply to the bone. Lag screws used to stabilize syndesmoses should be removed at 6 to 8 weeks.

Implants used for fractures of cancellous areas, as in malleolar fractures, can be removed after 3–6 months without any danger.

In children Kirschner wires are removed after 2–3 weeks.

Fig. 89   When a flexible column is fixed in its middle with a rigid plate, most of the column deep to the plate becomes rigid also. Even a single screw decreases the elasticity of bone because it alters the inner architecture.

Fig. 90   A plate removes the tensile or compressive stresses and this changes the inner architecture of the bone. *After double-plating of a fracture, the osteoporosis of the cortex is very marked*, and it looks like cancellous bone. Such internal fixation, therefore, should only be carried out in fresh fractures on clearly defined indications, as in a fracture of the upper tibia or upper femur. Otherwise the plates may completely neutralize the immobilized segment so that the cortex becomes thinner and thinner and may indeed vanish altogether. When two plates are removed simultaneously, the cortex is unable to withstand the physiological stresses of weightbearing, and fatigue fractures often happen after double-plate fixation.

N.B.: If for any reason double-plating is carried out, as in a femoral fracture when medullary nailing is not possible, then the plates should be removed only one at a time, with 4–6 months between them, and immediate cancellous bone grafting should be carried out on each occasion at the same time as a plate is removed.

Fig. 91   Removing a plate from the tibia may be done through few short incisions. In the illustrated case six screws are removed through three incisions 1.5 cm long.

a   After the screws are removed, the plate is lifted from the bone with a special plate lifter.

b   The plate extractor then easily slides the plate out.

Fig. 92   Removal of medullary nails has ceased to be a problem since we have introduced the conical threads within their ends. All tissue must be removed from the threads before the conical bolts can be screwed in, and the bolt must be tightened up after the first few hammer blows with an 11 mm open-end wrench.

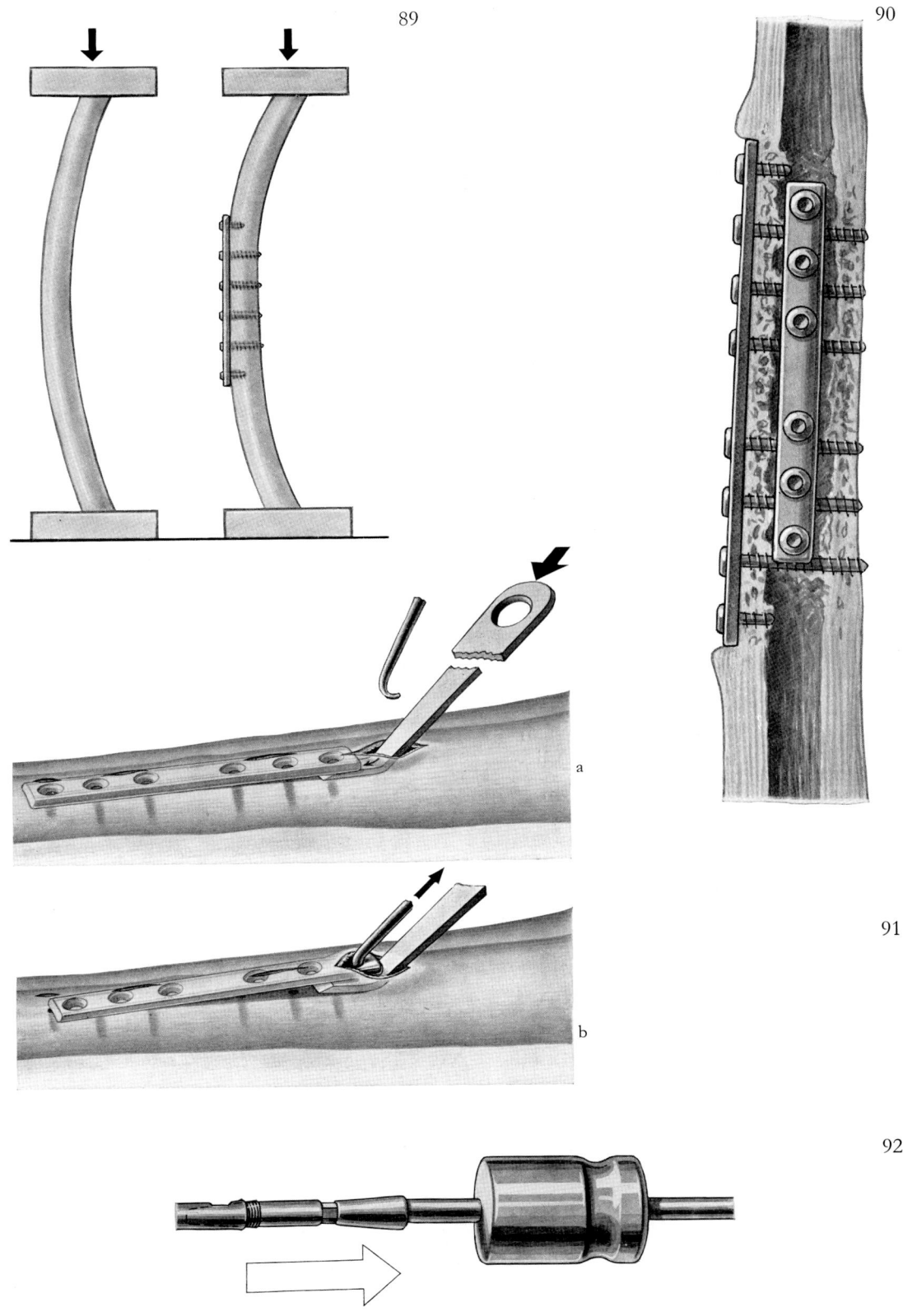

89

90

91

101

B. Fatigue Fractures

The Breaking of Plates

Plates are often submitted to us for metallurgical study and the relevant X-rays are sent with a request for an explanation as to why the implant has failed. In almost every case it was at once apparent from the biomechanical factors acting during the internal fixation, that implants were doomed to fatigue fractures. It was easily seen from post-operative X-rays, that the plates were being subjected to bending stresses instead of tension stresses. Under such circumstances even the most rigid and corrosion free implant must fatigue and break.

Most plate fractures occur in the femur, and we have therefore chosen this bone as our example.

A tension band plate is under tension when it neutralizes all tensile forces. Its loading is least when the fulcrum of movement is furthest from the plate. When the medial femoral cortex is intact the fulcrum of movement is 3–4 cm from the plate (Fig. 93a). If at the end of open reduction and internal fixation there is a medial defect, whether due to over-correction, as a result of the plate being under too great tension, or because a small fragment had to be sacrificed or could not be reduced, the plate will gradually bend until contact between the cortices on the medial side is again established (Fig. 93b).

Fig. 93

a	Diagram showing an eccentrically loaded column, with a tension band plate fixed to its lateral side. The fulcrum is on the medial side. The longer the distance (D) the smaller the bending moment. The bending moment determines the stresses that are exerted on the plate. The size of the bending stresses are in direct relationship with the required strength of the plate.
b	If there is a small defect on the medial side, the plate will bend slightly under the load. The defect will then close and the fulcrum will again come to lie medially as in a. The plate bends but does not break.

102

93

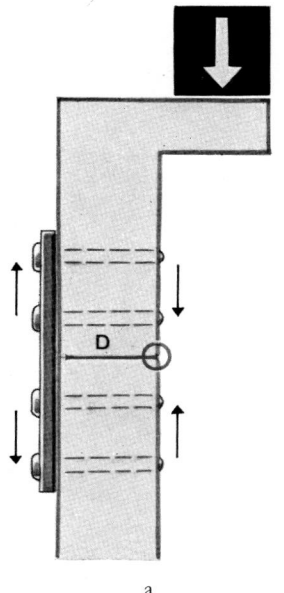

a

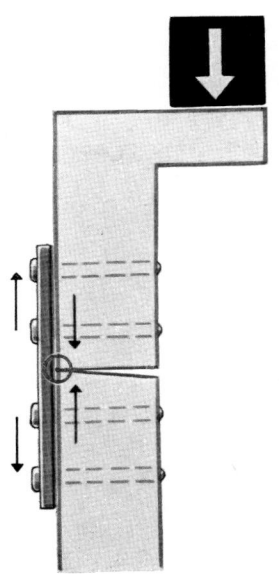

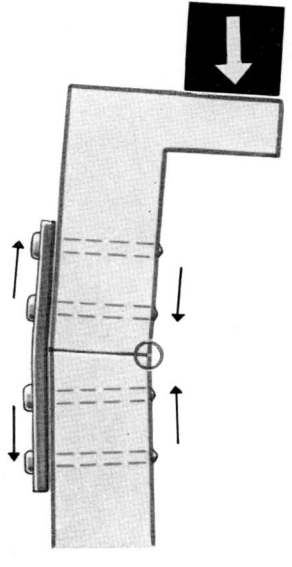

b

If, however, no resistance is possible on the medial side, then the situation results as shown in the diagram 94a or 94b. The fulcrum is no longer removed to a distance from the plate, but is lying within the plate itself. Bending stresses can then quickly lead to metal fatigue and the plate will break. Thus in clinical practice one should expect a plate to break if it is used to fix a femoral shaft fracture where there is a medial defect, as may result from severe comminution, loss of a medial fragment or slow resorption of a necrotic fragment (Fig. 94c to e).

How can one then overcome such bending stresses? The simplest way would be to apply a second plate immediately opposite the first one. The load acting on this one would be 20 to 100 times less than that acting on the single plate, and therefore a semi-tubular plate would be strong enough.

The insertion of a second plate immediately opposite the first one presents some technical difficulty and the potential for this type of fixation has not yet been fully explored. In trochanteric fractures therefore with loss of the medial buttress, we use other methods of internal fixation (page 158). In subtrochanteric fractures or fractures of the shaft with loss of the medial cortical buttress, we recommend extensive autogenous cancellous bone grafts (Fig. 95b). The patient should only start weight-bearing when there is radiological evidence of a medial bony bridge. This does not usually appear for at least six weeks. This also applies to comminuted fractures of the middle third of the femur, stabilized with open medullary nailing in combination with bone grafting or cerclage wiring, which are methods to be preferred to plate fixation.

Fig. 94

a	A broad medial defect. The fulcrum of movement lies close to the plate or within the plate itself.
b	The defect is in the column. The plate is subjected to bending stresses and a fatigue fracture is only a matter of time.
c	Pertrochanteric fracture with absence of a medial buttress.
d	Subtrochanteric, comminuted, partly irreducible fracture with a necrotic lateral fragment.
e	Comminuted fracture of the shaft. It can be said with certainty that in all these plates, fatigue fracture will occur within three months. This will result in a loss of fixation and non-union.

Fig. 95

a	To counteract bending stresses whenever there is a medial defect, an additional thin plate can be immediately applied. The stress in both plates is then reduced by a factor of 20–100, as compared with that falling on a single plate (Fig. 94b).
b	The same holds true if a large bone graft is applied medially. The resulting bony bridge is strong enough in 6–8 weeks to allow partial weight-bearing to be started.

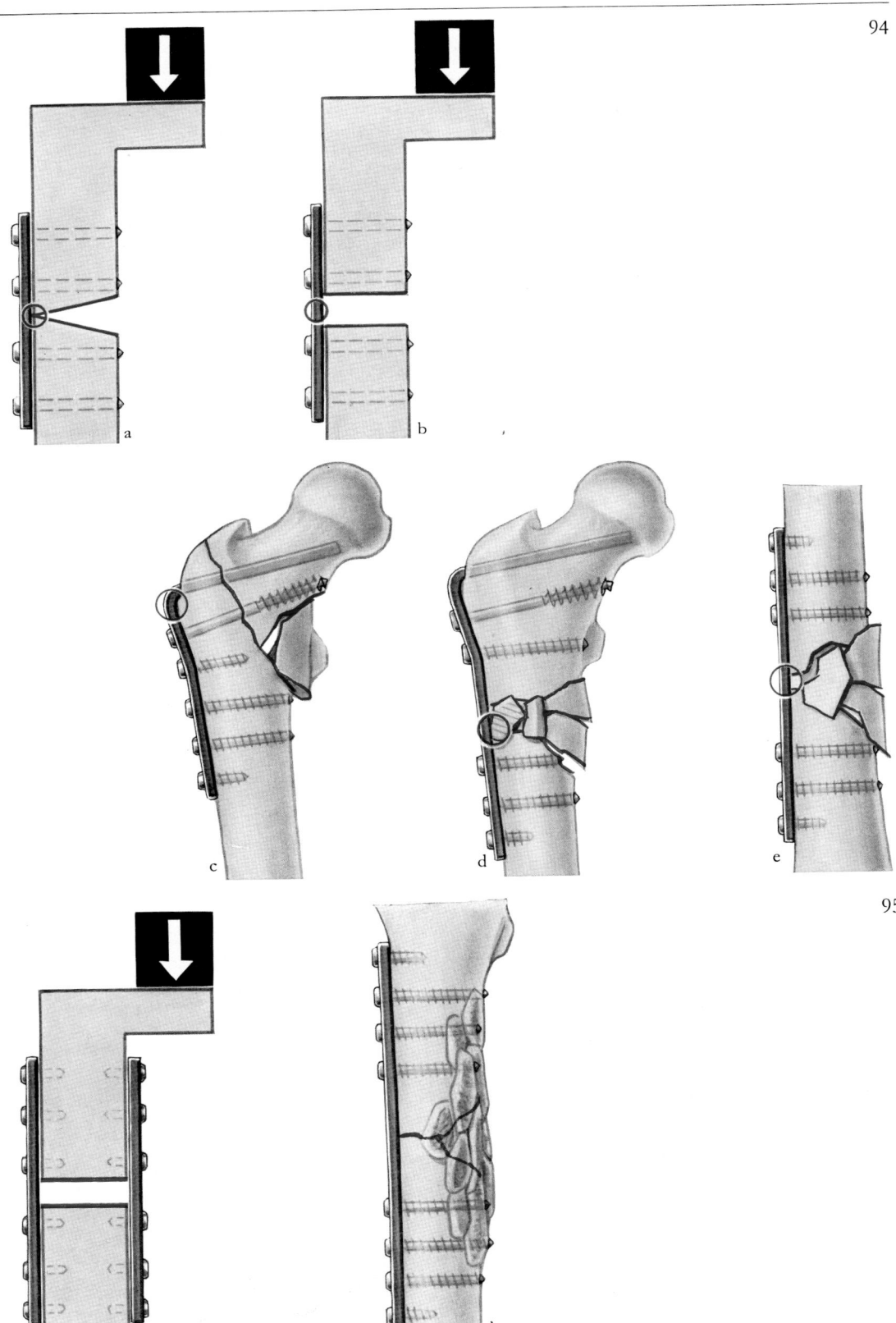

Special Part:

Internal Fixation of Fresh Fractures

Introduction

In this part we shall discuss proven methods of internal fixation for the most common fractures. These methods are all based on the principles of internal fixation discussed in part one.

At the same time we will take the opportunity to discuss special surgical techniques, the most reliable surgical approaches, and postoperative care. We have chosen as illustrative examples only those cases which have given a perfect result.

The Division of Long Bones into Segments

We divide long bones into five unequal segments: two joint segments, two metaphyseal segments and the shaft or diaphysis.

The shaft can be further subdivided into three segments: Shaft P (= proximal), Shaft D (= distal)—in both these the medullary canal flares out, and Shaft M (= middle), where the medullary canal remains the same diameter throughout.

Fig. 96   *Arrangement of the bone segments.*

a   *Humerus.*
1. Head; 2. Pertubercular; 3. Shaft; 4. Supracondylar; 5. Transcondylar.

b   *Forearm.*
1. Radial Head, Olecranon and Coronoid Process; 2. Subcapital and Subarticular; 3. Shaft; 4. Supraarticular; 5. Transarticular.

c   *Femur.*
1. Head; 2. Neck: Subcapital, Medial, Lateral, Pertrochanteric; 3. Shaft; 4. Supracondylar; 5. Transcondylar.

d   *Leg.*
1. Tibial Plateau and Fibular Head; 2. Subcondylar of the Tibia and Subcapital of the Fibula; 3. Shaft; 4. Supramalleolar; 5. Transmalleolar (Malleoli and Distal Tibial Plateau).

96

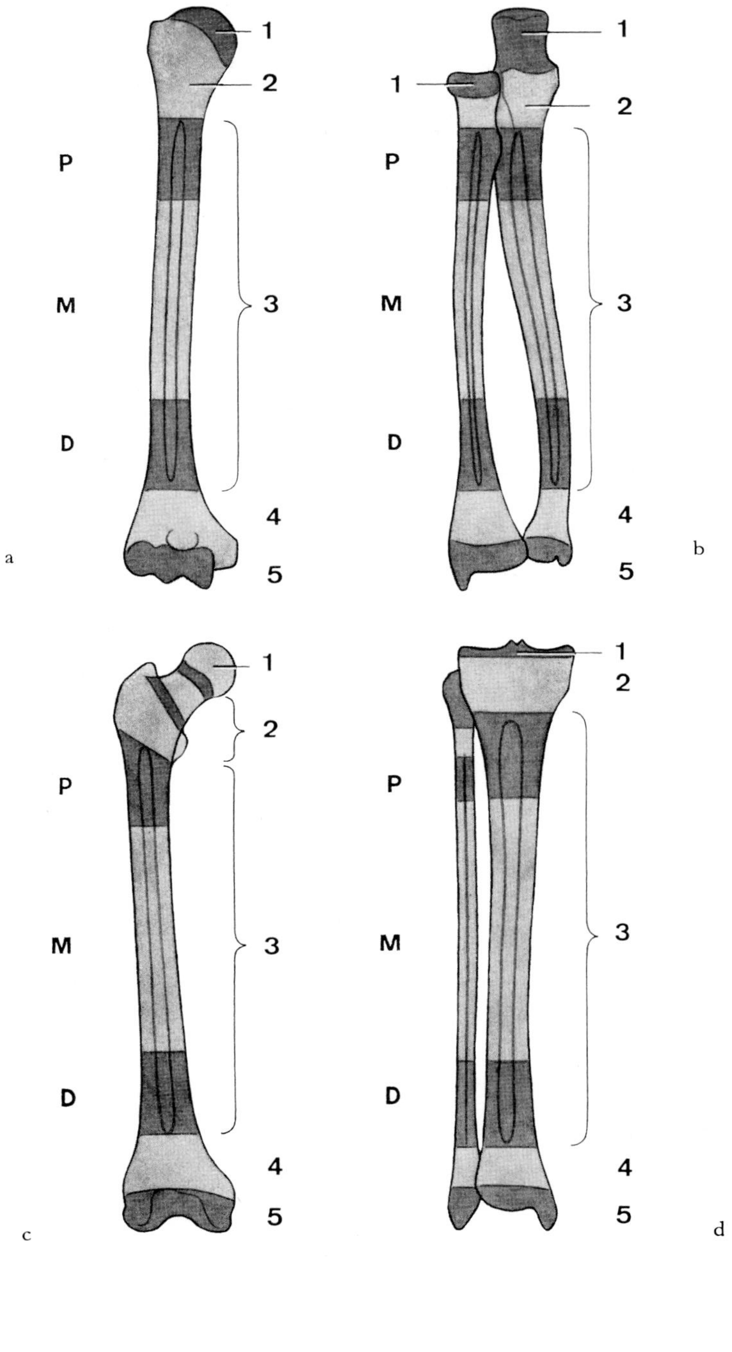

a
b
c
d

P
M
D

1
2
3
4
5

109

I. Closed Fractures in the Adult

A. Fractures of the Scapula

Intra-articular fractures, particularly in young patients, should be dealt with by means of an open reduction and internal fixation.

Surgical approach: See Fig. 102/6. The infraspinatus is reflected from its insertion as far as the axillary border of the scapula. The joint is opened from behind and *reduction is usually easy*. Internal fixation is achieved either with the small or the standard semitubular plate. Screws get an excellent purchase on the thick axillary border of the scapula.

Post-operative care: A Velpeau dressing is used until the wound is healed, followed by active mobilization. A fracture or an osteotomy of the acromion is stabilized by means of a tension band wire, a malleolar lag screw or, rarely, with a six hole small semitubular plate.

B. Fractures of the Clavicle

Shaft fractures of the clavicle heal with or without immobilization and for this reason do well with conservative therapy. Open reduction frequently results in unpleasant frequently painful scars, and pseudarthrosis is not uncommon after exposure of the fracture. Internal fixation becomes necessary if there is a step with a large gap in the fracture, if the fracture is badly comminuted, if one of the fragments has pierced the brachial plexus, or if there is delayed healing. When internal fixation does become necessary we employ the six hole semitubular plate or a very well contoured narrow plate. The small semitubular six hole plate is used only if the clavicle is very thin.

Internal fixation is frequently indicated for *fractures of the lateral end of the clavicle*. If the fracture involves the acromio-clavicular joint internal fixation is carried out with two Kirschner wires and a figure of eight tension band wire (Fig. 100). In transverse fractures just medial to the acromio-clavicular joint we like to combine the figure of eight tension band wire with a malleolar screw which is introduced across the acromio-clavicular joint (Fig. 101). The technique is, by and large, the same as for an acromio-clavicular dislocation where, in addition, the coraco-clavicular ligaments have to be repaired (as for example, with one half of the biceps tendon).

Surgical approach: Either through a curved incision one or two finger breadths below the clavicle or through the more cosmetic upper incision (Fig. 102/1b).

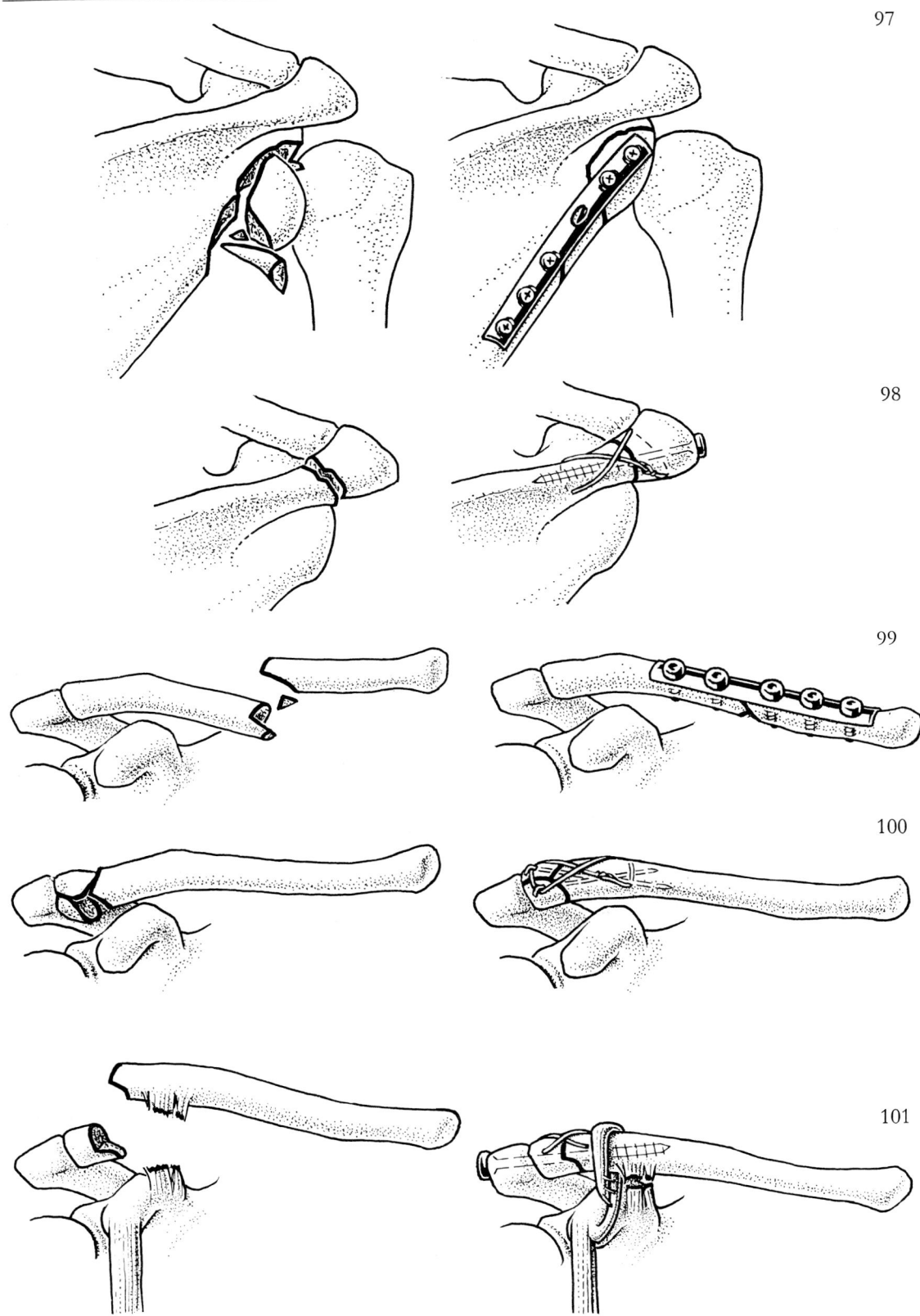

C. Fractures of the Humerus

Introduction

In fractures of the humerus the treatment is usually determined by the site of the fracture. Conservative treatment for proximal fractures is the best. In shaft fractures the problem is less simple. Slight axial or longitudinal malposition does not carry the same consequences as similar deformities in a weight bearing extremity. It is for these reasons that the prognosis of a conservatively treated fracture is much better, particularly if the fragments are allowed to overlap. On top of this, one must cope with the danger of an iatrogenic radial nerve lesion and the difficult surgical exposure. There are, however, from time to time, cases in the head and shaft region which can be treated successfully only by means of internal fixation, particularly when a conservative attempt has failed.

In fractures of the distal end of the humerus immobilization in the position of function is indicated. Intra-articular fractures or per-articular fractures of the humerus, particularly if unstable, and particularly if the congruence of the joint is disturbed, require, as do other intra-articular or peri-articular fractures, open reduction and internal fixation, to obtain the best functional result.

Fig. 102	*Skin incisions and surgical approaches in the region of the shoulder joint and the humerus.*
a	*Incision 1:* Exposure of the clavicle through a curved incision two to four cm below the clavicle (a). We have also found that the incision one finger breadth above the clavicle (b) in the supraclavicular fossa has been quite useful. It is, in any case, cosmetically better.
	Incision 2: A good cosmetic incision for exposure of the humeral head and the proximal third of the humeral shaft: The incision is begun at the tip of the acromion and is carried distally along the anterior axillary border until the lower border of pectoralis major is reached. From this point the incision is carried along an imaginary line joining the inferior border of the pectoralis major with the medial epicondyle, and is carried as far distally as necessary. The fascia over the biceps is opened medially, and exposure of the shaft is begun in the medial bicipital groove.
	In muscular patients the exposure is made easier if the incision is curved over the anterior border of the deltoid across the lateral bicipital groove and then extended distally as far as necessary along line 3. The subsequent scar always widens and is prone to frequent keloid formation. In incision 2 and extension of 3 one can aid exposure by osteotomizing the coracoid leaving the tendon insertion on the coracoid undisturbed.
	Incision 3: Midshaft of humerus. The incision is made along the lateral edge of the biceps and extended through the ventral substance of the brachialis. The radial nerve crosses the humerus in the distal segment of this exposure obliquely in a dorso-proximal direction.
b	In incision 2 the deltoid is divided 1 cm from its insertion on the clavicle to facilitate resuture, and is reflected laterally like a trap door, exposing the lateral subdeltoid region.
c	Exposure of the midshaft of the humerus: incision 3.
	Incision 4: Distal humerus, dorsal incision (see also Fig. 103c).
d	*Incision 5:* Dorsal exposure of the midshaft of the humerus: Through a dorsal incision (extension of incision 4 proximally) the long head and lateral head of the triceps are exposed and divided down the middle where they join. The radial nerve lies proximally and crosses the femoral shaft from a proximo-medial to a disto-lateral position.
	Incision 6: Incision for exposure of the scapula and the dorsal aspect of the shoulder joint after reflection of the infraspinatus from the scapula.

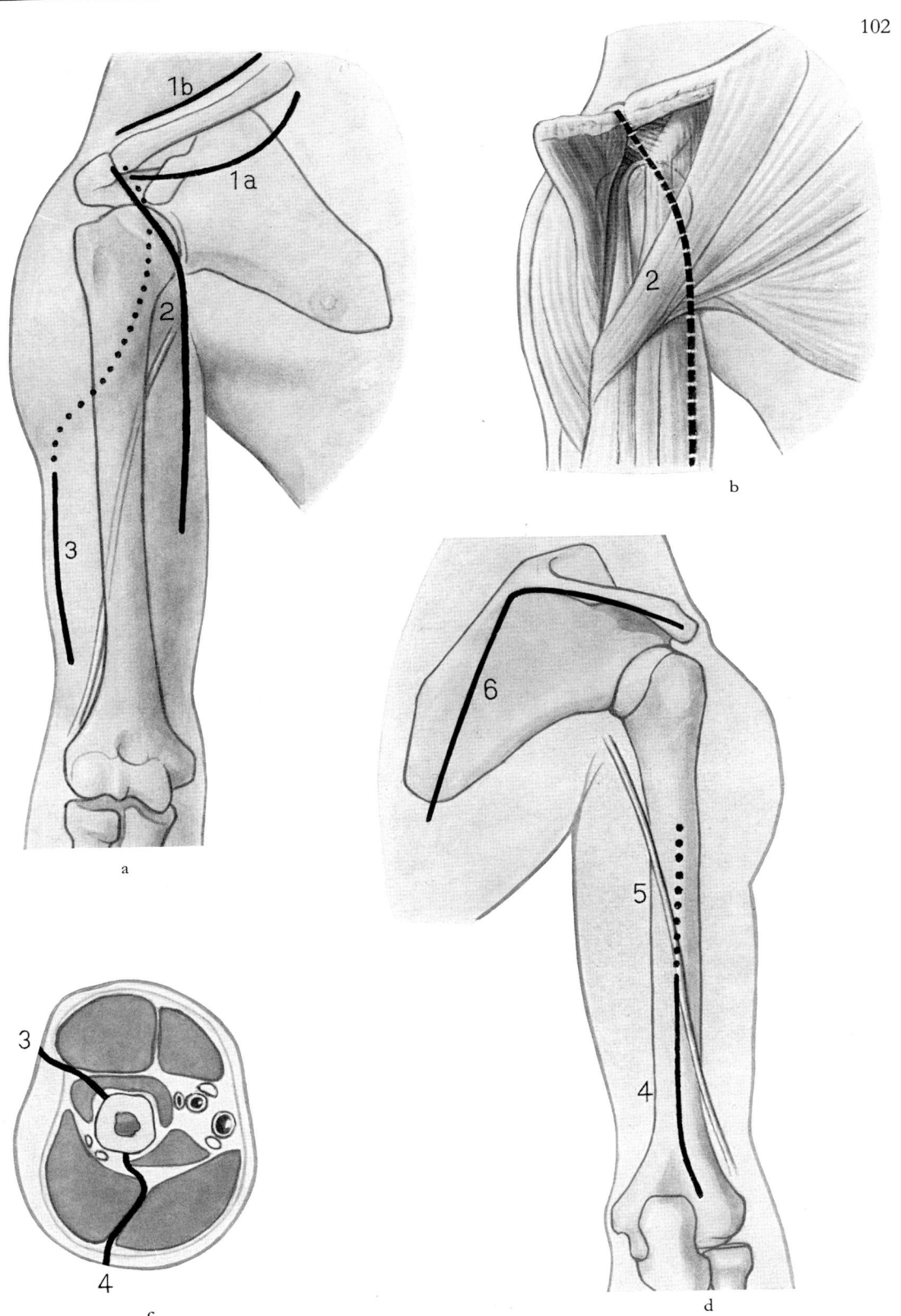

a

b

c

d

Fig. 103   *Standard exposure of the elbow joint without osteotomy of the olecranon.*

a   Use the prone position and position the patient so that the elbow is bent to 90° but further flexion to 40° is possible. In very obese patients one may be forced to operate in the supine position with the arm across the chest, but this will make reduction more difficult.

b   Cross-section through the elbow joint at the level of the base of the olecranon. The only structure of importance is the ulnar nerve which must be isolated at the start of the operation.

c   The incision is placed laterally in order to avoid the olecranon bursa.

d   Incise the triceps aponeurosis forming a tongue based distally, and turn this tongue down. This gives wide exposure of the elbow joint which is aided by Hohmann retractors which are inserted, one on each side of the shaft. As soon as the elbow is flexed to 40°, or if possible to 30°, the trochlea and the capitelum are completely exposed.

e   The radial nerve can be injured only in the upper part of the incision where it pierces the muscular septum.

Fig. 104   *Exposure of the elbow joint with osteotomy of the olecranon.*

a   Make the skin incision and then make a pilot hole in the olecranon with a 3.2 mm drill.

b   Transect the olecranon transversely with an oscillating saw.

c   The exposure of the joint is even more extensive than in the above approach (Fig. 103).

d   At the end of the procedure the olecranon is reduced and fixed with the longest malleolar screw. A tension band wire should be used to supplement the fixation in order to prevent the slightest displacement of the olecranon.

e   Approach without incising the articular surface. The olecranon is cut obliquely and turned up. Subsequently tension band fixation is not necessary since subsequent displacement is unimportant.

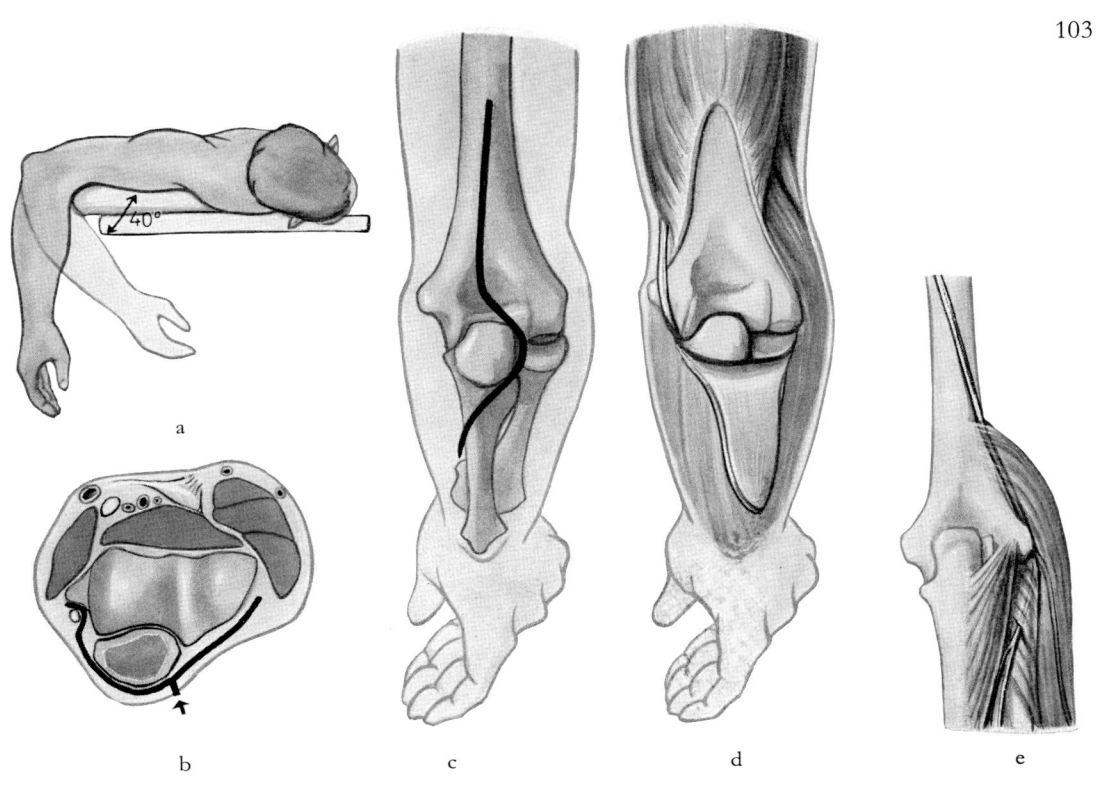

a

b

c

d

e

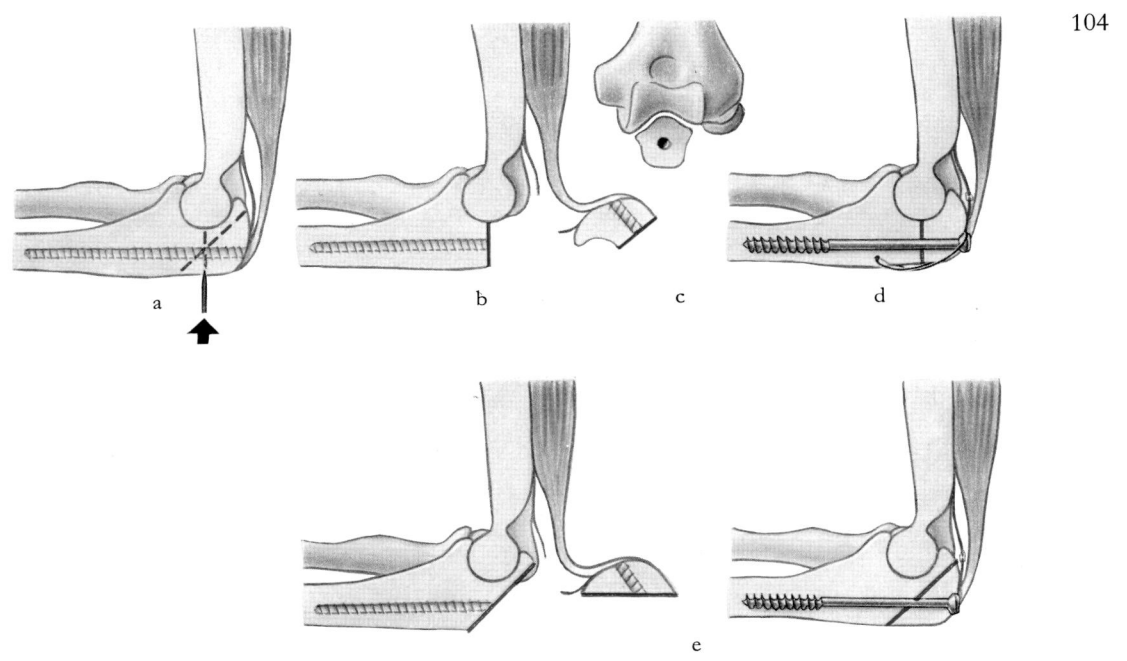

a

b

c

d

e

Head of the Humerus

Indications (seldom): Absolute indications for open reduction and internal fixation are irreducible fracture dislocation with the humeral head dislocated out of the glenoid, and irreducible subcapital fracture with no contact between the fracture surfaces.

A relative indication is a fracture of the greater tuberosity with the fracture fragment interposed between the humeral head and the acromion.

Exposure: See Fig. 102/2 or the extended exposure Fig. 102/3.

Internal fixation: In carrying out the open reduction particular attention must be paid to the correction of any rotational or varus displacement of the humeral head. The following measures may be necessary, depending on the particular case: fixation of fragments of the humeral head with 4.0 mm cancellous screws, reconstruction of the lost cancellous bone with fresh autologous bone and, after dislocation of the humeral head, re-attachment of the glenoid labrum with a screw. In adults internal fixation is usually carried out with the T-plate as described on page 46, Fig. 41. In young patients with very hard cancellous bone, simple fixation with 4.0 mm cancellous screws is often enough.

Postoperatively: Ambulation on the day of operation. Two to four days of immobilization in a sling. Subsequently, begin active mobilization: pendulum exercises, rotational exercises, sitting with the arm abducted. Passive support of active exercises, especially abduction and external rotation. In a patient who does not regain a satisfactory range of motion, particularly if he is anxious, a temporary abduction splint is recommended.

Fig. 105   *Fracture dislocation of the humeral head.*

Reduction and rigid internal fixation with the T-plate. Re-attachment of the glenoid labrum with two small cancellous screws.

Fig. 106   *Subcapital fracture with complete displacement of the shaft and dislocation of the long head of the biceps (L 467).*

Exact reduction and fixation with two 4.0 mm cancellous screws one on each side of the bicipital groove. The joint had to be opened to reduce the dislocated tendon of the long head of the biceps.

Fig. 107   *Trapping of the avulsed greater tuberosity fragment under the acromion obstructs movement.*
Reduction and internal fixation with a cancellous screw.

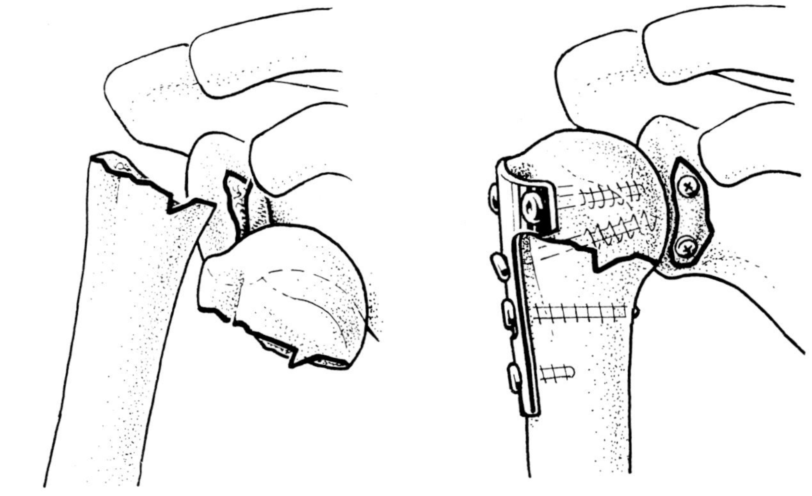

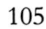

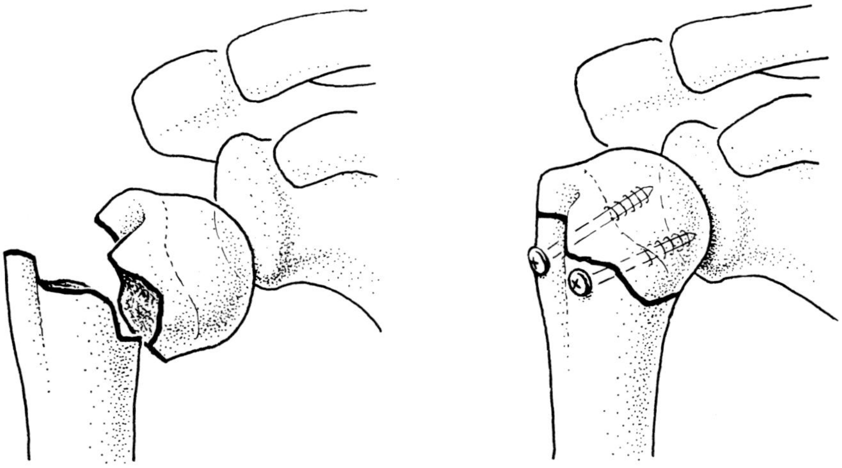

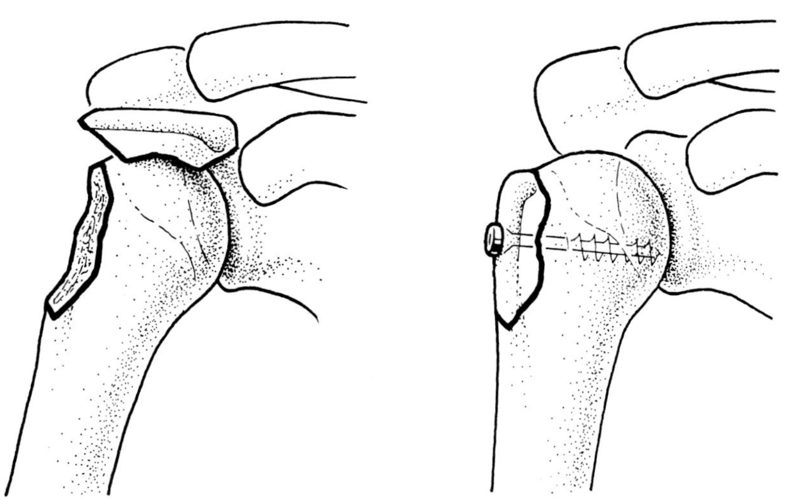

Humeral Shaft, P. M.

Indications: In dealing with torsional or comminuted fractures of the mid-shaft of the humerus, it usually suffices to immobilize the arm to the thorax for six weeks to obtain union in acceptable axial alignment.

Transverse fractures however heal very slowly, particularly when reduced end to end. Delayed healing of such a fracture is an indication for internal fixation. Furthermore, internal fixation would be indicated when a patient is anxious to return quickly to work.

It is difficult to lay down guidelines for the treatment of humeral fractures associated with radial nerve palsy. Since the type of nerve lesion (about $^5/_6$ are due to neuropraxia or neurotmesis, and $^1/_6$ due to axonotmesis) is usually unknown, we are inclined to carry out open reduction and internal fixation.

Further indications for open reduction and internal fixation are: rib fractures, double fractures of the humeral shaft, associated fractures through the elbow, compound fractures, Parkinson's disease or other neuro-muscular disturbances.

Approaches: For the proximal shaft incision 2 (page 115, Fig. 102), for the middle of the shaft incision 3 (page 115, Fig. 102), for stacked nailing a posterior approach with the patient in the prone position.

Internal fixation: Usually the six hole tension band plate (Fig. 111). If the radial nerve is exposed carefully there is no danger of damaging it. It is more difficult to prevent nerve damage at the time of plate removal. It is, however, rarely necessary to remove the plate from the humerus since it is a non-weight bearing bone and the plate lies under a good soft tissue covering. The stacked nailing method of HACKETHAL is advocated for a transverse fracture through the mid-shaft of the humerus. 2.5 to 3 mm thick Kirschner wires with blunt slightly bent ends, do just as well as Hackethal's original implants (Fig. 108). Enough stability can thus be achieved. The stacked nailing can be carried out blindly if no difficulties are encountered in reduction.

Fig. 108   *The stacked intra-medullary nailing (pinning) of* HACKETHAL.
The 3 mm thick wires which are slightly bent are introduced from behind and passed up the shaft. Because the wires are slightly bent, when they reach the humeral head, they separate. Distally, the wires must protrude slightly through the cortex to facilitate their subsequent removal.

Fig. 109   *Simple spiral fracture (34–2–13).*
Screw fixation alone is usually inadequate and, for this reason, is not recommended.

Fig. 110   *Spiral fracture with a butterfly fragment (WS 90).*
First fix the butterfly with two lag screws, then apply the neutralization plate.

Fig. 111   *Simple transverse fracture (BI 30–37).*
Stabilized with a tension band plate. The plate is slightly bent before application to prevent any malalignment once compression is applied with the tension device.

Fig. 112   *Transverse fracture of the humerus (34–2–8).*
Stabilized with a six hole compression plate without fixation of the small fragments. Primary autologous cancellous bone grafting is carried out to secure rapid consolidation.

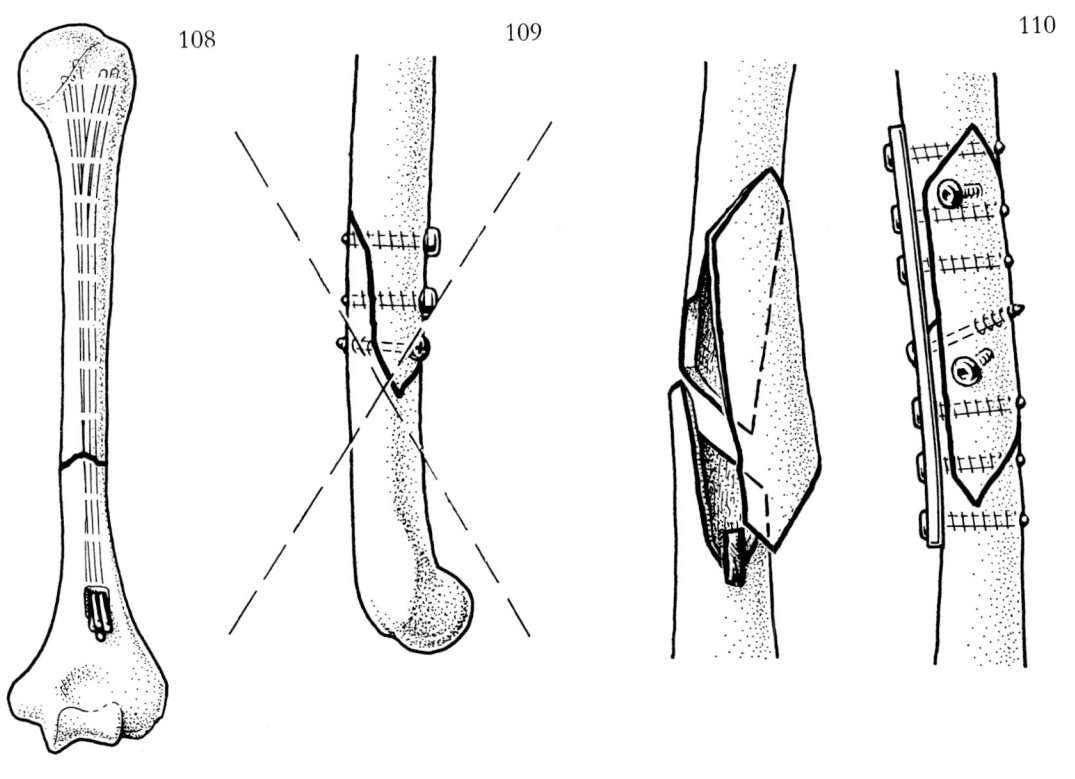

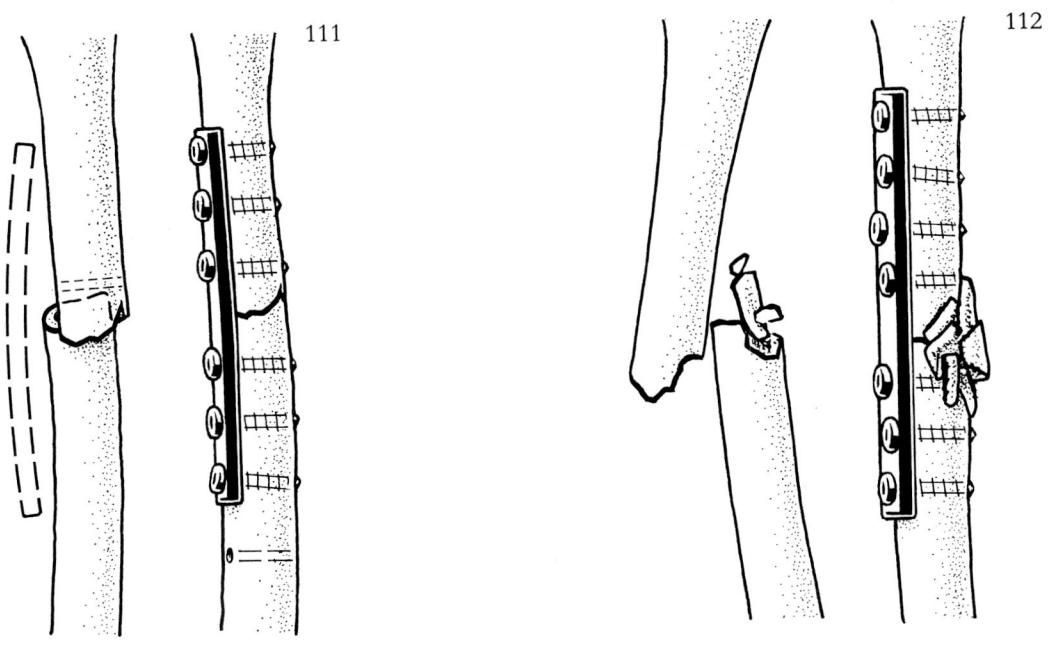

Distal End of the Humerus

Indications: In unstable fractures, and those involving joints. In compound fractures primary internal fixation is undertaken where possible.

In these fractures be particularly aware of concomitant vessel and nerve injuries, particularly of the ulnar nerve.

Approaches: Fig. 103 shows the standard approach for virtually all fractures of the distal humerus. In an isolated fracture of the medial or lateral epicondyle a medial or lateral approach is preferable. The first step in the medial approach is to identify and isolate the ulnar nerve.

Isolated fractures of the lateral or medial condyles. These do not present any particular problems and after anatomical reduction can be rigidly stabilized under compression with one, or better, with two malleolar screws. Rigid fixation is achieved only when the tips of the screws penetrate the contralateral cortex. Provisional fixation with Kirschner wires. If after the screw fixation there is still some doubt about rotational stability, one of the Kirschner wires can be left in place to supplement the fixation.

Isolated fractures of the medial epicondyle. The fragment is usually small and because of muscle pull is frequently interposed in the joint. Reduction and provisional fixation with a Kirschner wire or a hook can be quite difficult. All manipulations must be carried out with great care. A shattered, small fragment is almost impossible to fix. Dependable internal fixation in the adult of this fragment can be achieved only by means of screw fixation: 4.0 mm cancellous screws, malleolar screws (drill first a gliding hole in the fragment), and whenever possible, drive the screw through the opposite cortex.

Fig. 113   *Fracture of the medial condyle (AB 4/37).*

Fixation with two screws which penetrate the opposite cortex. The ulnar nerve must be identified and isolated during the procedure.

Fig. 114   *Fracture of the medial epicondyle.*

Fixation with one malleolar screw which penetrates the opposite cortex. The screw must never go through the olecranon fossa.

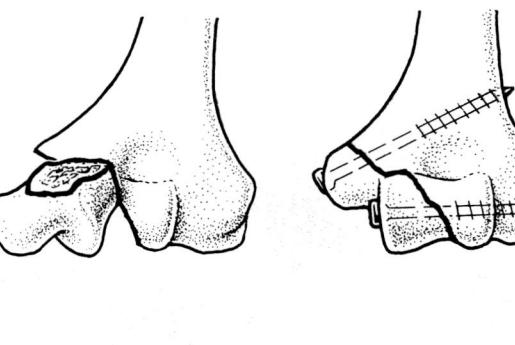

113

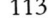

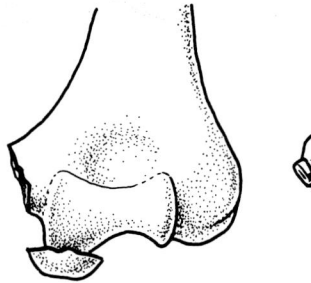

114

"Y" Fracture of the Distal Humerus

Approach with or without osteotomy of the olecranon.

Technique: See Fig. 103 and 104.

Fig. 115   *Technique of internal fixation of a "Y" fracture of the distal humerus.*

The first step is open reduction and provisional trans-condylar Kirschner wire fixation of the intra-articular fragments. The definitive fixation is carried out only after accurate reduction has been achieved and provisional fixation carried out. The definitive internal fixation employs a malleolar screw introduced parallel to the axis of the elbow joint and, whenever possible, *from the capitulum into the trochlea.*
There are now two ways of completing the internal fixation. One can carry out the fixation either with two crossed malleolar screws (a) introduced in such a way that they take a grip on the far cortex, or (b) by means of two small semi-tubular plates which are fixed proximally to the humerus with the same screw. With some practice the fracture can be compressed by means of the small semi-tubular plates.
If the first method is used, supplementary plaster fixation is necessary for the first three weeks; whereas in the second method movement can be begun at once.

Fig. 116   *An example of the "Y" fracture of the distal humerus which extends upwards (KZ 10/38).*

The intra-articular fragments are stabilized by means of one screw which is introduced in a radio-ulnar direction and as far distally as possible. The transverse component of the fracture is stabilized by means of a narrow plate. Simultaneously a cancellous bone graft is applied at the level of the transverse fracture.

a

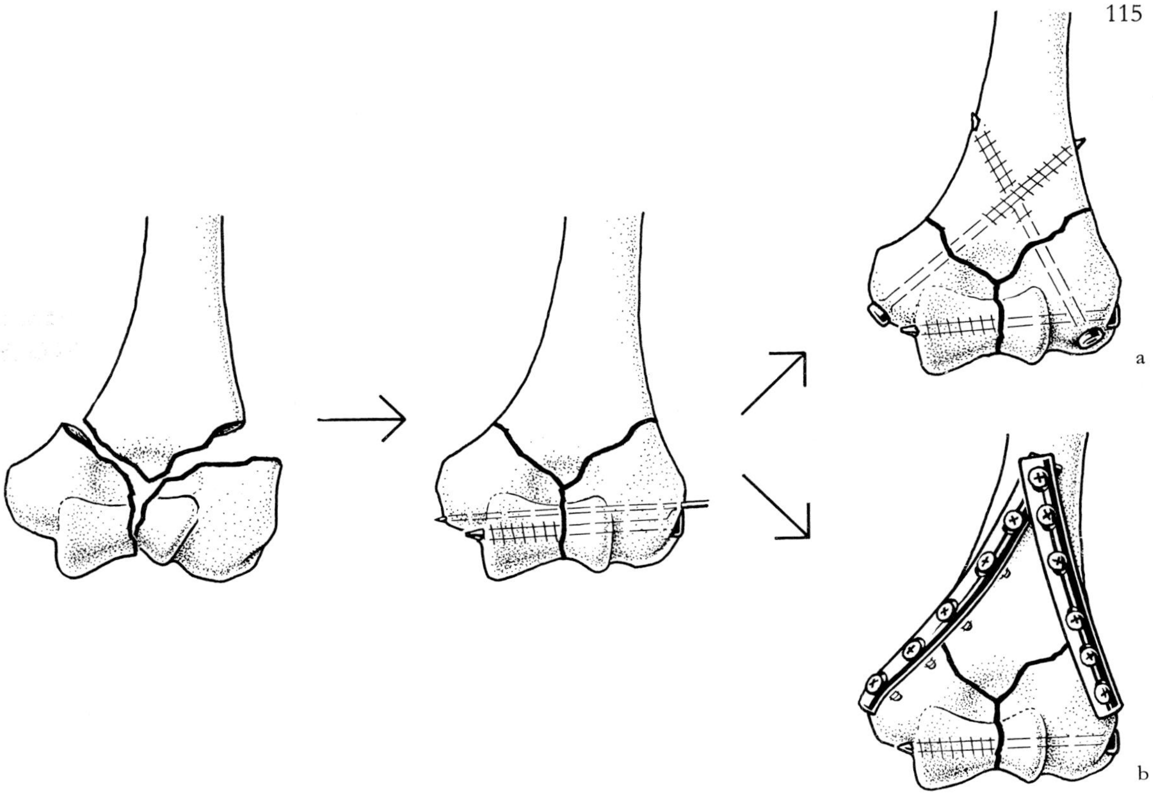

b

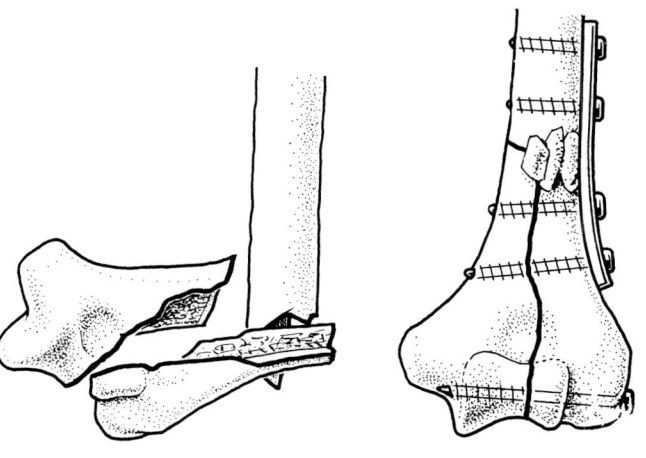

Comminuted Fractures of the Distal End of the Humerus

Best functional results are obtained only with operative treatment. The comminuted fractures are so varied that no definite rules can be layed down and one can speak about them only in general terms. The most important thing is to re-establish the trochlea as the hinge. It is often better to abandon the reduction of tiny fragments and do a primary autologous cancellous bone graft in order to reconstruct the trochlea. One must then pay particular attention to maintaining the normal width of the trochlea. Very rarely, reconstruction is impossible and a primary arthroplasty with sacrifice of both epicondyles is carried out.

The internal fixation consists of, first of all, stabilization of the reconstructed trochlea and then fixing the trochlea to the metaphysis respectively to the shaft. The type of internal fixation chosen depends on the type of the individual fracture.

General Comments about Fractures of the Distal End of the Humerus

In any internal fixation of the distal end of the humerus implants must be kept clear of the olecranon fossa and the coronoid fossa.

Postoperative regimen: Patients are to get up on the day of surgery. Immobilization for two to four days in a sling or cast, depending on the stability of the internal fixation. This stability will also determine the time to begin active and assisted exercises; it may be early or only after three to six weeks of immobilization. We have found the posterior half of a bi-valve plaster cylinder a most useful splint.

D. Fractures of the Forearm

Fracture of the radial shaft frequently result in varying loss of pronation and supination. Full return of rotation can be achieved only if the fracture of the radial shaft is reduced anatomically with preservation of its double curvature of the radial shaft. The healing of the fracture is achieved by means of rigid immobilization.

The medullary canal of the radius is narrow and curved. Intramedullary pinning does not prevent rotation. The intramedullary nail used with reaming results in lengthening of the radius. A plate which is not placed under tension results in delayed callus formation and frequently in pseudarthroses. The straight AO plate used as a tension band plate (see page 36) is a perfect method of rigid fixation of the fragments and allows early active mobilization. Furthermore, the fracture heals rapidly and good reduction is usually obtained. In order to prevent distraction of the fragments the plate must be slightly bent prior to its application and must be inserted on the postero-lateral aspect. As the middle of the radius is cylindrical we have found the semi-tubular plates most useful in the treatment of radial shaft fractures. They not only fit the contour of the bone, but also make it possible to place the fragments under compression without the use of the tension device which is a decided advantage in the radius because there may be difficulty in finding room for it. The screws must obtain a firm grip on at least four cortices on each side of the fracture.

On the straight ulna the straight tension band plate has stood the test of time. In fractures of the middle and upper third of the ulna, it is important that the screws have a full purchase on at least five cortices on each side of the fracture. It is for this reason that in these segments of the bone the four hole plate must not be used. A six hole plate should be used. In delayed union or a pseudarthrosis six hole or even longer plates are best. A four or five hole plate is only safe in fractures of the lower ulna.

In comminuted fractures it is often impossible to reduce devitalized fragments. A primary autologous cancellous bone graft should then be used at the time of internal fixation. The graft must never be placed on the interosseous membrane as this may result in cross-union. In comminuted fractures attention must be paid to the physiological curve of the radius and to achieving proper rotational alignment of the fragments. Restoration of the normal bone length will prevent later disturbance of the inferior radio-ulnar joint.

In fractures of both forearm bones, definitive fixation of one bone can only be achieved after the other has been carefully reduced and temporarily fixed.

Fractures of the upper radius are approached through a postero-medial incision (BOYD's approach). This protects the posterior interosseous nerve.

Fractures of the upper ulna are often comminuted and are best fixed with the semi-tubular plates as these can be easily fixed to the contour of the upper ulna.

Compression fixation has special advantages in forearm fractures especially if both bones are broken but the method is far from easy. Accurate anatomical reduction must be obtained and lengthy procedures may result in a higher infection rate. Operating time can only be shortened if one is fully familiar with the local anatomy and with the technique. Damage to motor and sensory nerves must be carefully avoided.

Postoperatively no pressure bandage is used but a light dressing only and reliance is placed on elevating the limb. If there is any suggestion of ischaemia resulting from edema (which is shown by loss of the radial pulse) all dressings must be removed and the arm raised up fully. If rapid improvement does not then occur, all sutures must be removed and the wound allowed to open*.

---

* Remark

As there is often difficulty in closing the wound open reduction should either be undertaken early before there is any post-traumatic oedema or after a delay of a few days when the swelling has subsided.

Fig. 117

a	To deal with both bones of the forearm or a Monteggia fracture first place the patient in the prone position with the chest and arms supported on sand bags as shown. If a solitary forearm bone is being approached then the patient can lie safely supine.
b 1	BOYD'S approach for a Monteggia fracture. The radio-humeral joint is usually approached from the ulnar side and it is seldom necessary to incise the anconeus (see also e 1).
b 2	For the exposure of the middle and distal third of the ulna see f 2.
b 3	Approach to the middle and lower third of the radius. This should not be used to expose the upper third of the radius because of the danger of damaging the posterior interosseous nerve which divides into four branches as it runs through the supinator muscle.
c	THOMPSON'S approach to expose both forearm bones, both proximally and distally. This is especially indicated in badly comminuted fractures.
d	THOMPSON'S approach: At the upper end this is the same as BOYD'S approach (b 1). Distally disection runs between the extensor carpi radialis brevies and the extensor digitorum communis.
e	Exposure of the proximal third and the placing of the plates (1).
f	Approaches through the middle third of the forearm (2 and 3). A semi-tubular plate was used on the radius and the ulna was fixed with a six hole tension band plate applied to its posterior surface.

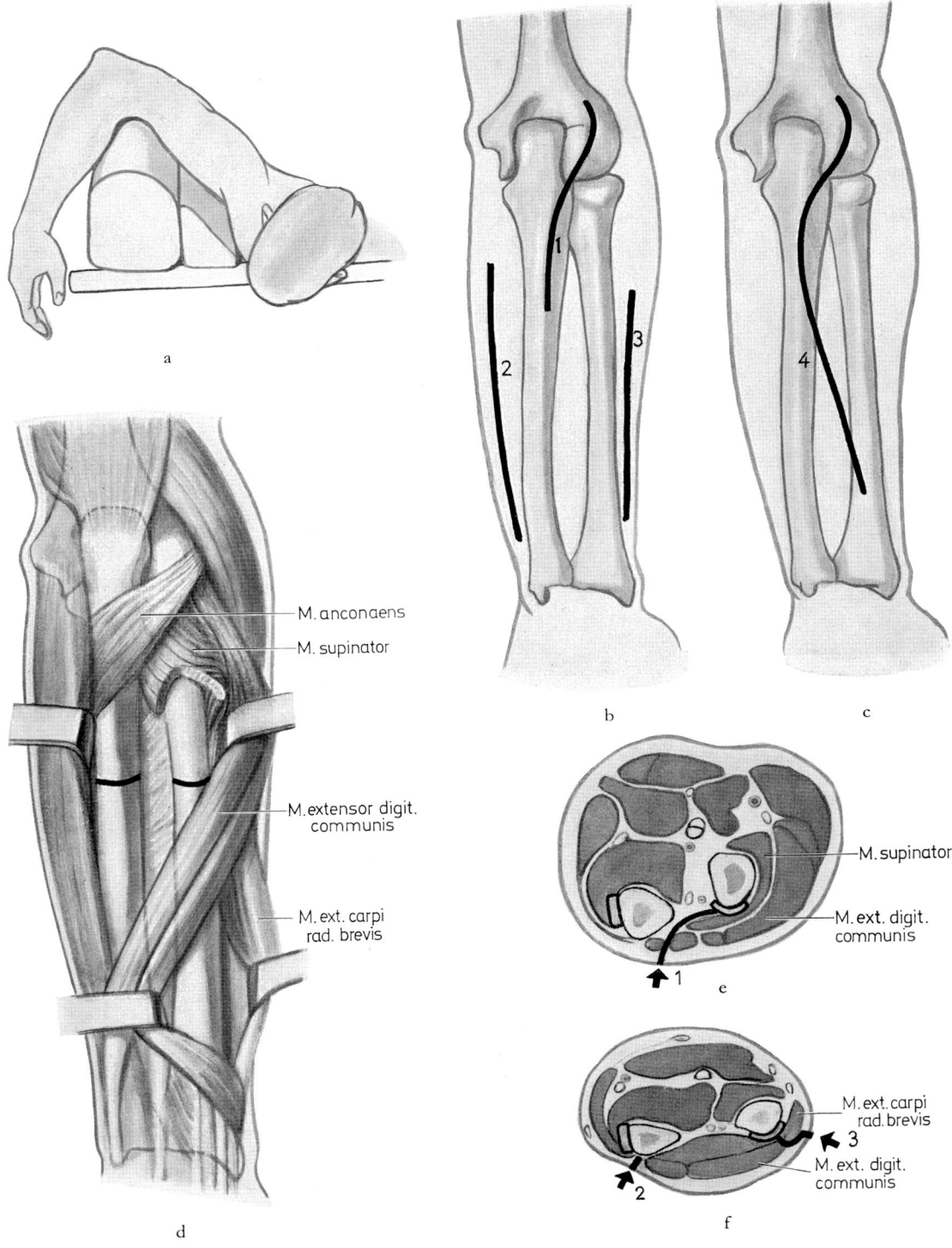

a

b

c

M. anconaens

M. supinator

M. extensor digit. communis

M. ext. carpi rad. brevis

M. supinator

M. ext. digit. communis

M. ext. carpi rad. brevis

M. ext. digit. communis

d

e

f

Fractures of the Olecranon

Transverse Fractures and Small Avulsion Fractures of the Tip of the Olecranon

Internal fixation using the tension band principle (after WEBER).

Technique: The fracture must be reduced as exactly as possible without devitalizing the fragments and provisionally stabilized with two to four Kirschner wires introduced parallel to each other and to the long axis of the ulna. A drill hole is now made transversally just distal to the fracture through the posterior cortex of the ulna. A 1.2 mm wire is then threaded through the drill hole. The wire is now crossed over and passed round the protruding ends of the Kirschner wires deep to the triceps tendon. The wire is then tightened and tied. This results in a figure of eight tension band wire with the cross over point lying over the fracture or just distal to it. The projecting ends of the Kirschner wire are then shortened, bent to form "u" shaped hooks which are then hammered into the bone, over the tension wire. This prevents the wire from slipping off the Kirschner wires and stops the latter from protruding through the skin (see Fig. 118).

Oblique Fracture of the Olecranon

After reduction temporary fixation is maintained with axial Kirschner wires or with a light bone-holding forceps. Internal fixation is performed with a lag screw which runs along the medullary canal as shown in Fig. 119 or with one inserted at 90° to the fracture line.

Comminuted Fractures of the Olecranon

If the coronoid process is broken off it must be reduced and fixed as a first step in the reduction and internal fixation (see Fig. 122). As in other articular fractures the reconstitution of joint congruence is important. Fixation is achieved either with Kirschner wires and the figure of eight tension band wire as for transverse fractures (see Fig. 120) or with the help of a semi-tubular plate.

Fig. 118   *Transverse fracture of the olecranon (HT 2/1).*
The combination of Kirschner wires and a figure of eight tension band wire. In such a simple case a plain figure of eight tension band wire would have been adequate without the addition of the Kirschner wires.

Fig. 119   *Oblique fracture of the olecranon (BG 10/40).*
In these, the proximal fragment is unlikely to become displaced. Fixation with an axial cancellous screw resulted in rigid immobilization and a perfect result. One must often apply a washer beneath the head of the cancellous screw.

Fig. 120   *Comminuted fractures of the olecranon (WL 47/17).*
Fixation with two or three Kirschner wires and a figure of eight tension band wire. Even if the initial reduction is not perfect, active movements result in small comminuted fragments fitting together to give a smooth joint surface.

Fig. 121   *Comminuted fractures of the olecranon (WS 13).*
For this type of fracture dislocation, we have found the semitubular plate to be most useful. A small middle fragment was fixed with a 4.0 mm cancellous screw.

130

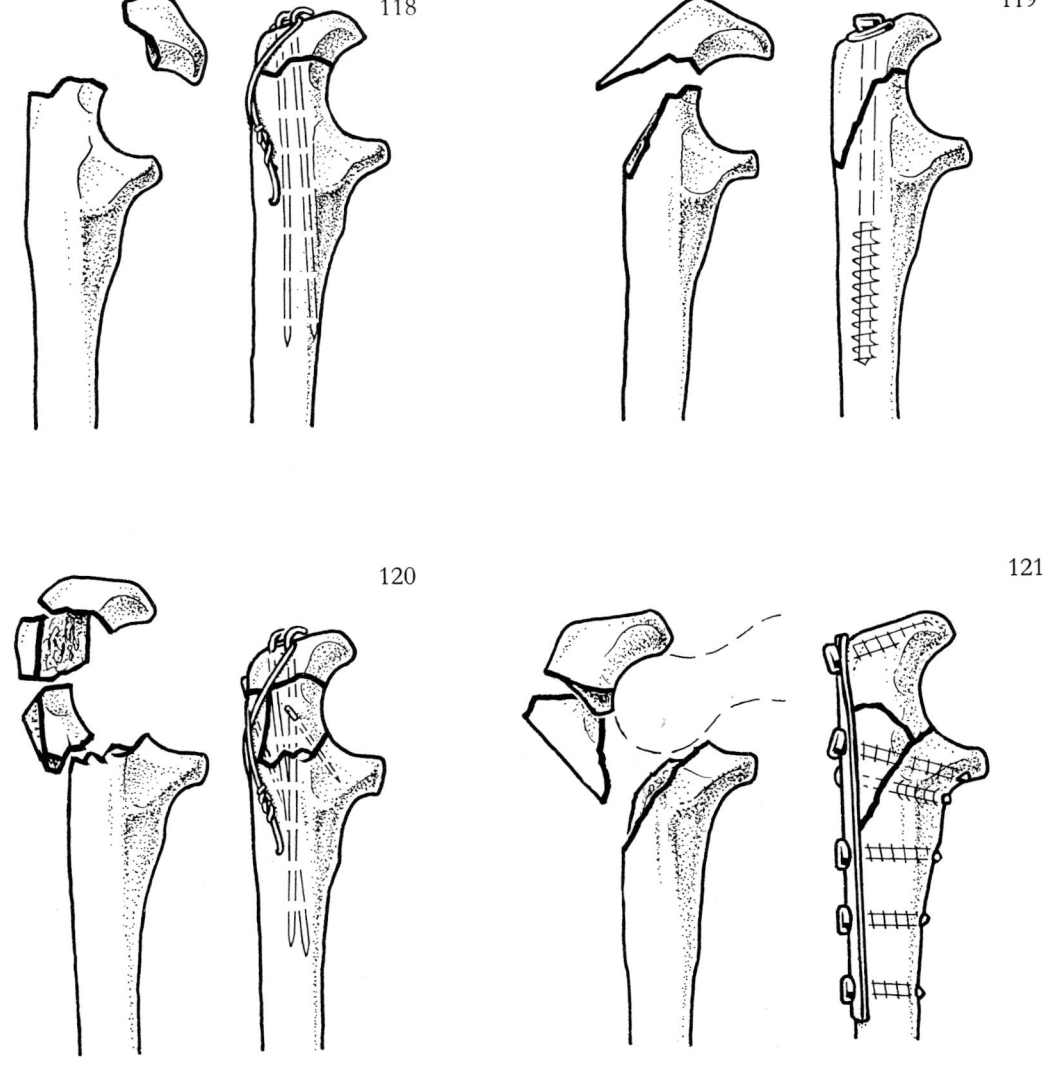

118

119

120

121

Fractures in the Upper Forearm

The object is to obtain perfect reconstitution of the joint surfaces. Reduction and fixation of a large fracture involving the coronoid process is very important as recurrent dislocation of the elbow may otherwise result.

The technique of open reduction and fixation of a Monteggia fracture: BOYD's approach is used (Fig. 117b-1). The periosteum over the ulna is incised and the bone exposed subperiosteally. The ulnar fragments are then carefully reduced and a narrow six hole tension band plate is applied posteriorly. When the ulna is well fixed the radial head is reduced. The annular ligament is repaired using chromic catgut. If the torn ends of the annular ligament cannot be sewn together a band from the triceps tendon should be cut leaving it attached laterally to the tip of the olecranon and the annular ligament reconstructed using this thin piece of tendon.

Fig. 122   *Fracture dislocation with avulsion of the coronoid process (WL 31/31).*

The coronoid process here was stabilized with a lag screw. The comminuted radial head was resected almost at the insertion of the biceps tendon.

Fig. 123   *Fracture of the radial head (WS 95).*

This fracture was fixed with a small cancellous screw inserted just below the annular ligament.

Fig. 124   *Monteggia fracture.*

Here the fracture of the ulna as well as the tear in the annular ligament were approached through the same incision (BOYD's approach, Fig. 117b–1). A narrow six hole plate was used on the ulna.

Fig. 125   *Comminuted fracture of the upper end of the ulna (ST 9/12).*

A lag screw was first used and then a semi-tubular plate. Where there was much comminution a primary autologous cancellous bone graft was applied to prevent a pseudarthrosis.

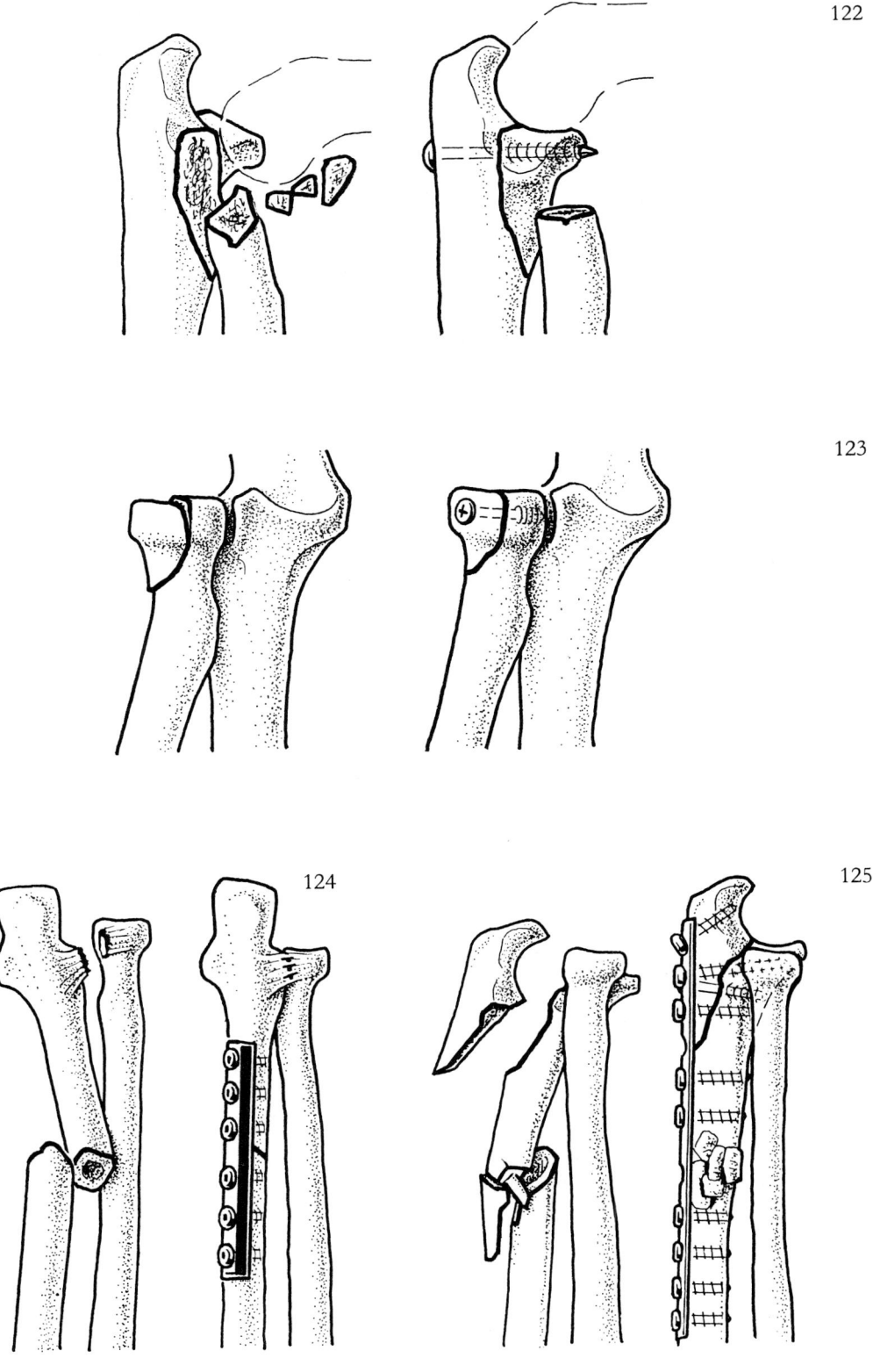

Fractures of the Shaft of Both Forearm Bones

The technique of open reduction and internal fixation of fractures through the middle thirds of both forearm bones or lower: The fractures may be approached either through two separate incisions (Fig. 117b2/3) or through a single incision (Fig. 117c4). Both fractures must be exposed and examined. The ulna is first reduced because it is easier. The plate should first be fixed to the shorter of the two main fragments and the fracture provisionally immobilized by holding the plate on with a clamp to the other fragment. Now attempts should be made to reduce the radius. To achieve this it is often necessary to release the clamp on the ulna until exact reduction and proper rotation of the radius is obtained in full supination. The radius may now be temporarily fixed with the semi-tubular plate and two screws. The fracture of the ulna is now again reduced, if necessary, and temporarily fixed by using the tension device. Supination and pronation are now tested and if full the plates may be screwed firmly home.

When rigid fixation and axial compression has been achieved active movements may be started forty-eight hours after surgery. If these conditions do not apply, as may be the case in a comminuted fracture where compression, if applied, might have resulted in shortening, a full arm plaster should be applied for three to four weeks to supplement the fixation.

Fig. 126   *A simple fracture through the shaft of the ulna (WL 41/8).*

A transverse or oblique fracture through the shaft of the ulna is rigidly fixed with a five hole tension band plate.

Fig. 127   *A simple fracture of the radius (WL 47/30).*

This spiral fracture was fixed using lag screws obtaining interfragmental compression between fragments. An additional semi-tubular plate was used to prevent displacement of the fragments. Here the plate acts as a neutralization plate through which further compression between fragments can be obtained.

Fig. 128   *Fracture of both bones of the forearm (BI 36/7).*

A transverse fracture of both bones rigidly fixed under compression using two five hole plates. A full range of movement was obtained at the end of the first week.

Fig. 129   *A comminuted fracture (HT 2/25).*

The simple transverse fracture of the ulna was stabilized with a six hole plate. The large comminuted fracture of the radius was fixed with a small cancellous screw. A six hole semi-tubular plate was then used to fix the main fragments. At the same time autologous cancellous bone was applied where the radial fragments had been devitalized.

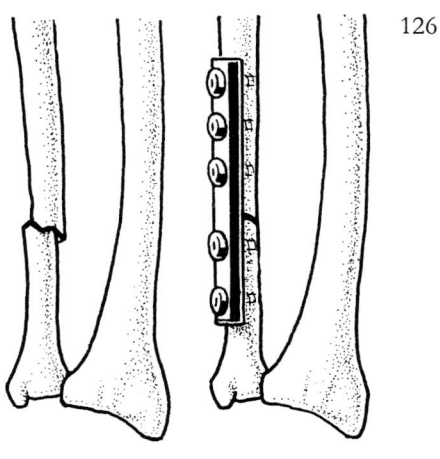

126

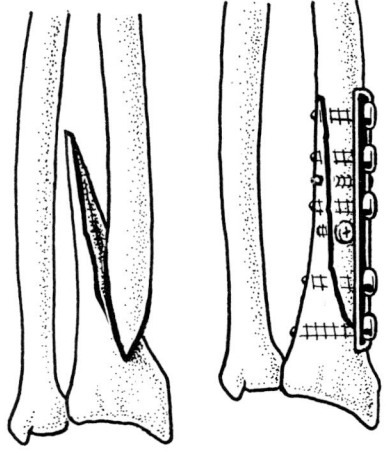

127

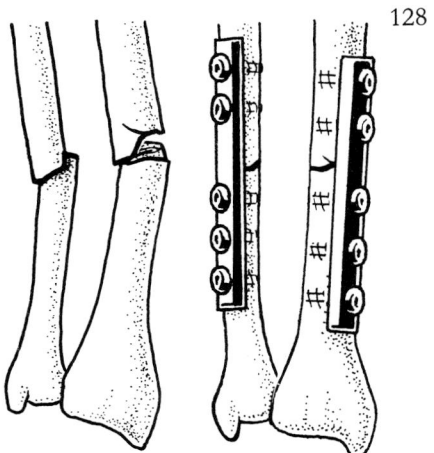

128

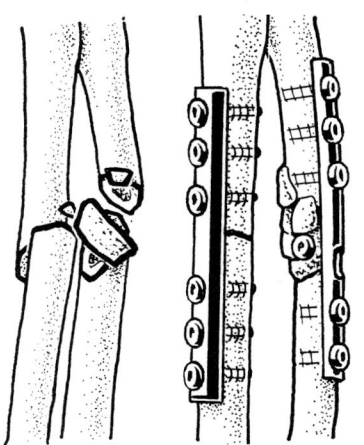

129

Fractures and Fracture Dislocations Round the Lower Radio-ulnar Joint

In GALEAZZI fractures the styloid process of the ulna is often avulsed and the fibro-cartilagenous disc is usually intact. This facilitates accurate reconstruction of the joint. We advocate internal fixation of the styloid process of the ulna because early movement may result in a pseudarthrosis.

Fractures of the distal end of the radius. We believe that these, especially in young patients, when closed reduction has not corrected deformity or shortening, should be openly reduced and internally fixed. This applies also to unstable and compound fractures of the radius.

The technique of dealing with comminuted and impacted fractures of the distal end of the radius: An axillary nerve block and tourniquet is used. A straight lateral incision six to seven cm long is made over the radius. The dorsal branch of the radial nerve is retracted backwards and the tendons of extensor pollicis brevis and abductor pollicis longus are retracted forwards. The fracture is exposed and examined. Reduction is achieved with the help of small elevators and a small sharp hook. WILLENEGGER's technique is used to fix the fracture with two or three Kirschner wires. Any defect in cancellous bone is filled immediately with an autologous cancellous bone graft. The wires are then shortened and bent over but in teenagers they may be left protruding through the skin. The limb is then held in a long arm plaster for four weeks. The cast is then removed, the Kirschner wires extracted and active movements are begun.

Comminuted fractures of the distal end of the radius with an intact cortex on the dorsum. These are unstable and provide absolute indication for open reduction and internal fixation.

Technique: Make a five to six cm cut over the flexor carpi radialis and extend it one finger breadth into the palm. The flexors and pronator quadratus are mobilized towards the ulna and the flexor carpi radialis and other radial tendons are retracted laterally. When an accurate reduction has been obtained internal fixation is performed with two small cancellous screws or sometimes with a small T-plate.

Fig. 130   GALEAZZI fracture dislocation *(ST 9/8)*.
The fracture of the radius is fixed with a six hole plate. The ulnar styloid is fixed with a small cancellous screw.

Fig. 131   *Irreducible fracture of the lower end of the radius (WL 43/38).*
The displaced fragment may be trapped between the tendons to the thumb and cannot be reduced by closed methods. Open reduction is then necessary. A Kirschner wire and a small cancellous screw are used for internal fixation here.

Fig. 132   *Comminuted fracture of the radius with impaction (WL 44/40).*
Reduction is achieved using a lateral exposure and the fracture is fixed with two Kirschner wires. Autologous cancellous bone is used to fill the defect.

Fig. 133   *Comminuted fracture of the radius with an intact dorsal cortex.*
Fix this with two volar cancellous screws.

Fig. 134   GOYRAND's *fracture of the radius.*
This is fixed with a small T-plate applied on the palmar surface using a palmar approach. The pronator quadratus is reflected and 4.0 mm cancellous and 3.5 mm cortex screws are used.

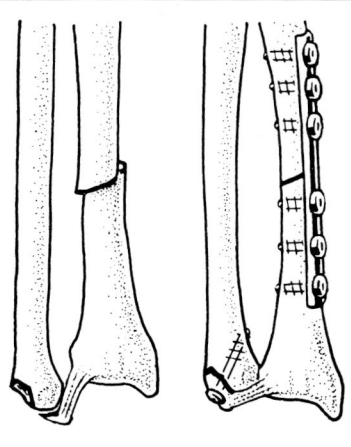

130

131 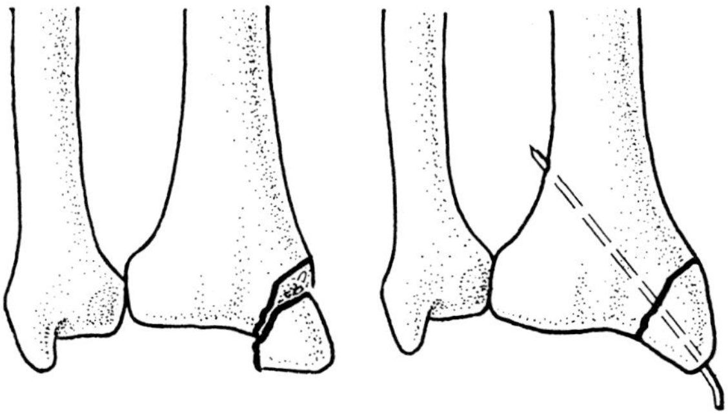　　　　　　　　　132

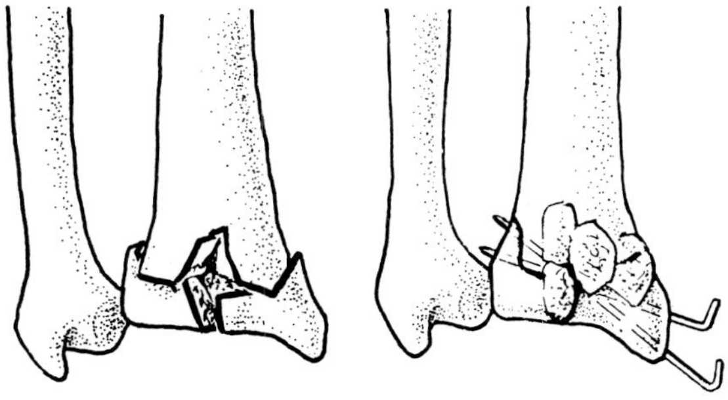

133

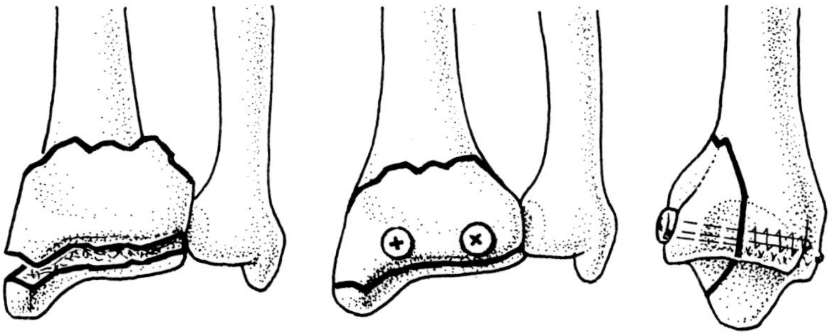

134

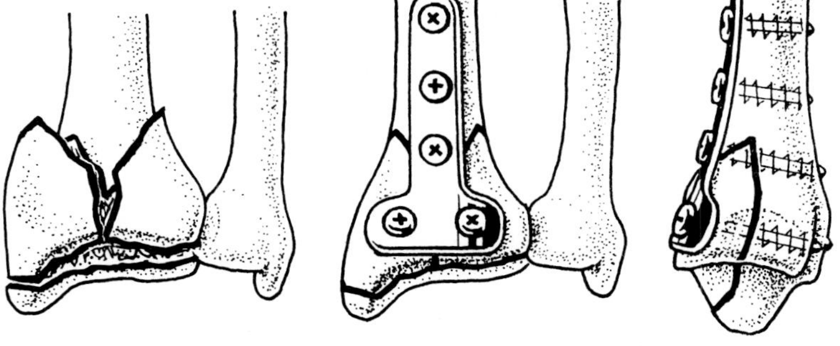

E. Fractures of the Acetabulum

Fractures of the acetabulum that unite with incongruity of the joint surface sooner or later result in post traumatic osteoarthritis. Any method of reduction that will restore joint congruity will improve the prognosis. To achieve this an anatomical open reduction is required followed by rigid fixation. One must appreciate fully the whole fracture complex as the type of fracture dictates the approach needed (JUDET, LETOURNEL). *Three special* x-*ray projections* will demonstrate almost all the important injuries.

Tactics of the Operative Treatment

Careful study of the three special x-rays will show the type of fracture involved, and thence which surgical approach should be chosen.

We have found it best to have the patient lying on his side as the leg can then be moved about to help in the reduction, and if necessary an anterior and posterior approach may be undertaken during the same operation.

Surgical approaches:

1. The postero-lateral approach of LANGENBECK-KOCHER. This gives the best exposure of the roof of the acetabulum, of the posterior lip of the acetabulum, and of the ilio-ischial column as far down as the ischial tuberosity (Fig. 141/5).

2. The ilio-crural approach of HUETER-SMITH-PETERSEN. This gives the best exposure for fractures of the iliopubic column, of the wing of the ilium, and of the anterior rim of the acetabulum as far as the iliopectineal eminence.

3. The ilioinguinal approach of JUDET-LETOURNEL. This gives the best exposure of the ventral column (the iliopubic column) both proximally and distally, of the floor of the acetabulum and of the inner aspect of the pelvis and the superior pubic ramus (Fig. 141/6).

For a better exposure of the acetabular roof and the adjacent ala of the ilium, osteotomy of the greater trochanter and upward reflection of the abductors is a most useful maneuver.

The Diagnosis of Fractures of the Acetabulum

In the center of the acetabulum we find the Y shaped intersection of three columns of bone (Fig. 135).

a) The ilium lies above and provides the roof of the acetabulum.
b) Posteriorly is the ischium forming the posterior lip of the acetabulum.
c) Below is the pubis providing the anterior lip of the acetabulum.

Three special X-ray projections ar eneeded to provide a pre-operative diagnosis (Fig. 136).

1. A standard a.p. projection of the pelvis.
2. Oblique views of the affected hip with the patient rolled over through 45°.
   a) Turning the patient to the affected side: This view spreads out the wing of the ilium demonstrating the posterior edge of the ilium, the sciatic notch, and the anterior lip of the acetabulum.
   b) Turning the patient away from the affected side: This view demonstrates the obturator foramen and shows up very clearly the medial border of the iliac fossa, the posterior lip of the acetabulum and the acetabular roof.

Fig. 135   *The three bony columns of the hip joint:*

A   The upper column = the ilium = the roof of the acetabulum.

B   The posterior column = the ischium = the posterior lip of the acetabulum.

C   The inferior column = the pubis = the anterior lip of the acetabulum.

Fig. 136   *The radiological diagnosis of fractures of the acetabulum.*

a   Normal a.p. projection.

b   45° rotation to the injured side. This is the so-called alar projection.

c   45° rotation of the patient away from the affected side. This is the so-called obturator foramen projection.
Each projection demonstrates important anatomical structures (see text).

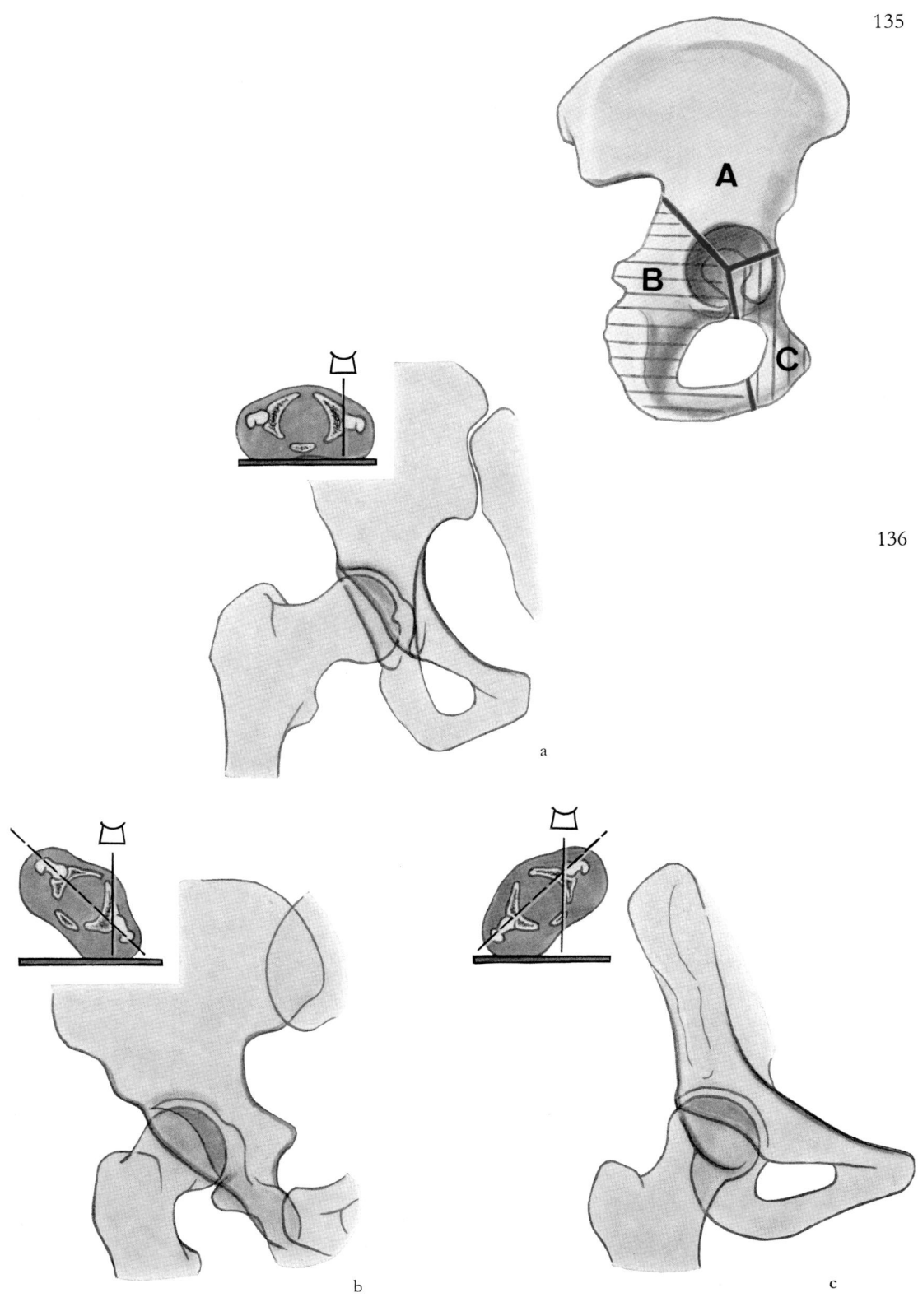

a

b

c

135

136

141

The Classification of Fractures of the Acetabulum (JUDET, LETOURNEL)

The four basic types of fractures of the acetabulum are determined by the direction and magnitude of the forces acting at the time of injury. They may occur in isolation or in combination.

The basic types of fractures of the acetabulum (Fig. 137):

A. The simple posterior lip fracture with postero-lateral subluxation or dislocation of the femoral head.

B. The simple posterior column fracture with postero-medial subluxation or dislocation of the head of the femur.

C. The simple anterior column fracture with antero-medial subluxation or dislocation of the femoral head.

D. The simple transverse fracture of the acetabulum with inward displacement of the femoral head.

Combination of fractures:

a) Transverse fracture with fracture of the upper and posterior acetabular rim.
b) Fracture of both columns.
c) Fracture of one column with a transverse fracture of the other.

In addition to the basic three fracture patterns there are two combined types of fracture which have elements of the basic three.

Fig. 137   *The basic types of acetabular fractures.*

A	Fracture of the posterior lip.
B	Fracture of the posterior column.
C	Fracture of the anterior column.
D	Transverse fracture of the acetabulum.

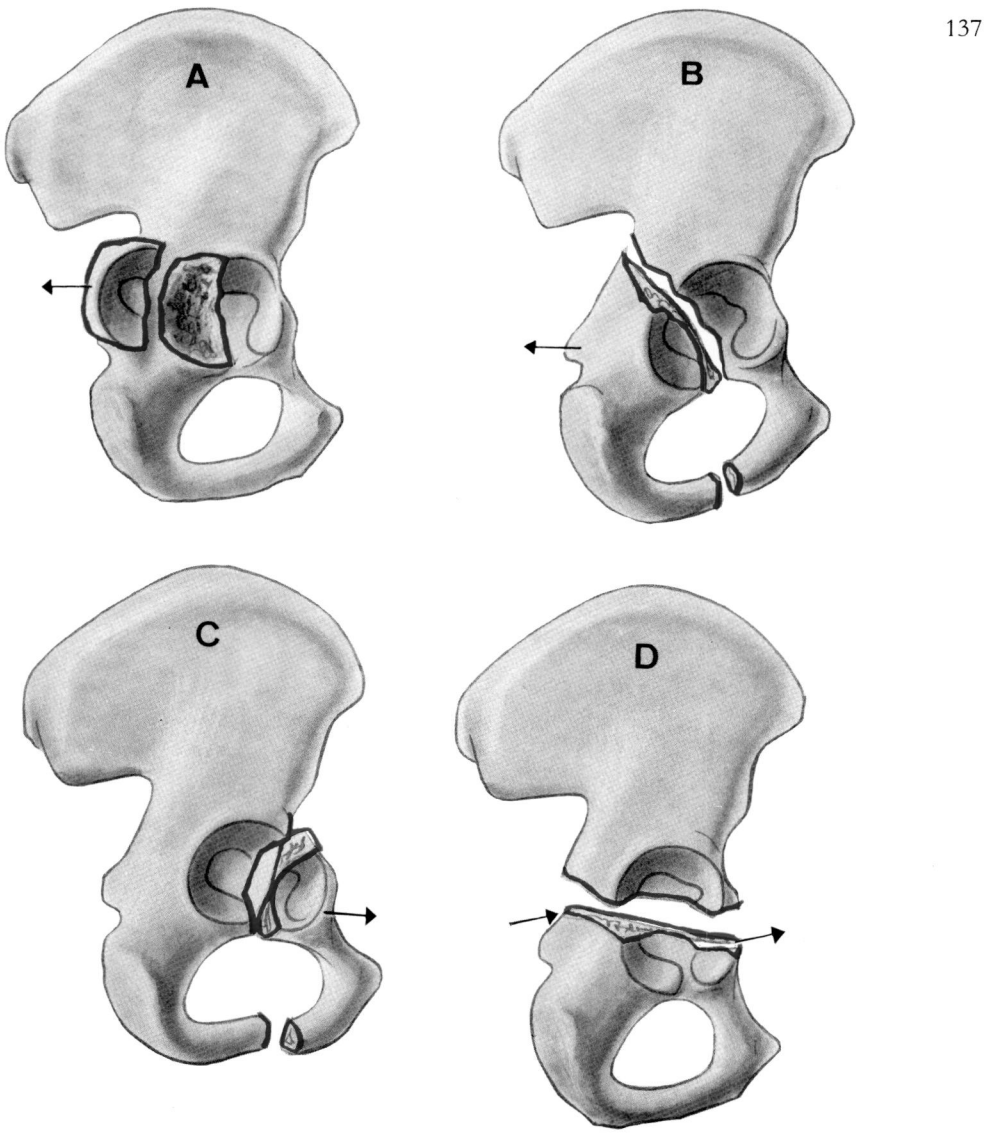

Operative Technique

Biomechanically the most important parts of the acetabulum to reconstruct are the roof and the dorsal lip and these are usually tackled first.

Fractures of the posterior lip which are greater than simple avulsions of the capsule are replaced and fixed with screws.

Fractures of the posterior column are most accurately reduced at the level of the acetabulum and are rigidly fixed with a contoured plate.

Transverse fractures of the acetabulum are fixed in the same way as column fractures.

Fractures of the anterior column are accurately reduced and fixed with a contoured plate applied to the medial border of the iliac fossa.

Combined fractures are carefully analyzed and then each component is reduced individually and fixed.

Post-operative Management

Suction drainage is used for forty-eight hours. The wound is closed in layers.

Three to four days after surgery active movements are begun in bed with the help of the physiotherapist.

Two to three weeks after operation non-weight bearing exercises are begun, best in a swimming pool.

Two to three months later the fractures are usually united and full weight-bearing is allowed.

Examples of surgically treated fractures.

Fig. 138   *Posterior fracture dislocation or posterior column fractures:*
Small to medium sized fragments are fixed with screws. Larger fragments must be fixed with a contoured plate.

Fig. 139   *Transverse fracture of the acetabulum.*
These are stabilized with a posterior plate, but occasionally it is necessary to use a supplementary anterior plate.

Fig. 140   *Anterior fracture dislocation with fracture of the anterior column.*
A contoured plate is applied anteriorly in this case.

144

138

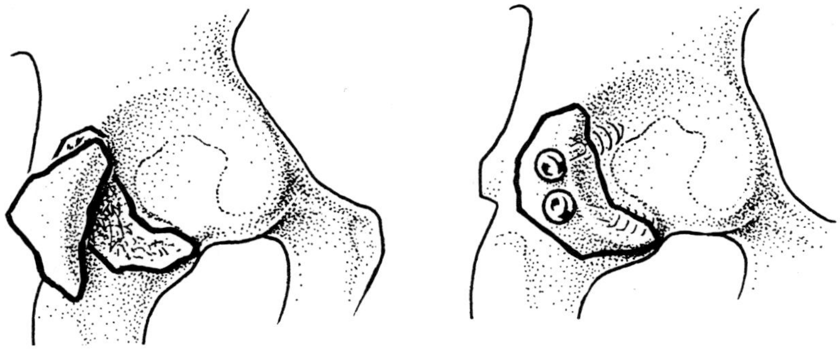

139

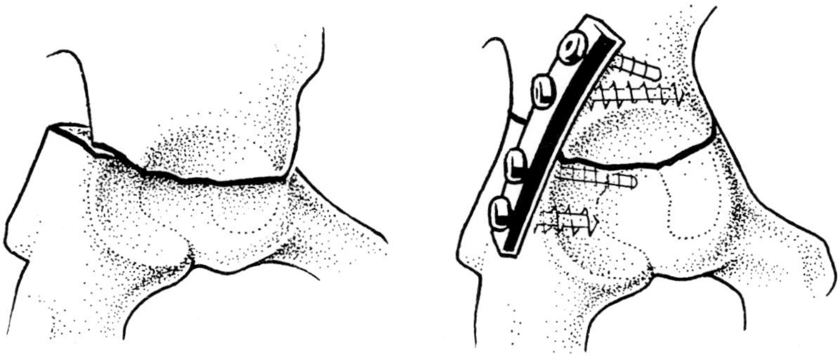

140

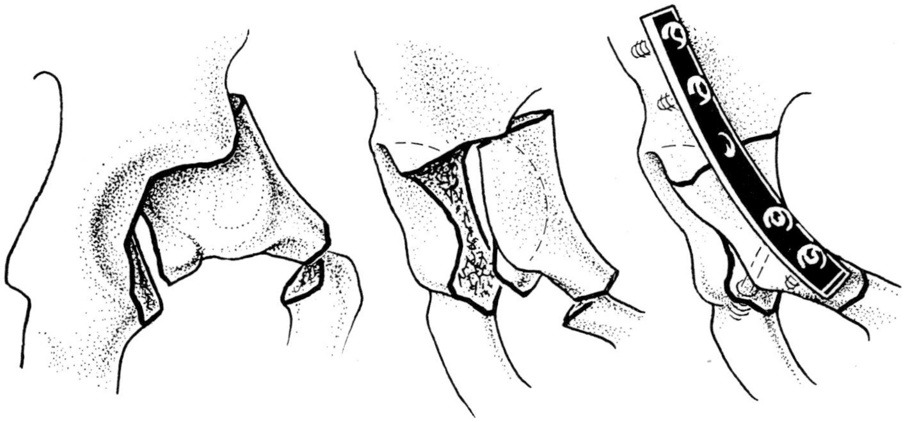

145

F. Fractures of the Femoral Neck

These fractures are divided into intra-articular fractures (the ab- and adduction fractures), base of neck fractures and trochanteric fractures. Fractures of the neck of the femur associated with the femoral shaft on the same side present special problems.

The average age of patients with intra-articular fractures of the femoral neck is between seventy and eighty, but trochanteric fractures occur in people between seventy-five and ninety. Base of neck fractures usually occur in patients under forty years of age.

1. *Subcapital and Medial Fractures of the Femoral Neck*

In these the main danger is avascular necrosis. The blood supply to the small femoral head fragment may be largely or completely disrupted resulting in partial or total *necrosis of the head*. Healing of these fractures, however, has absolutely nothing to do with avascular necrosis but depends entirely on the extent of the bony contact between the fracture surfaces and on the stability obtained by impacting the fragments with or without internal fixation.

Patients with *abduction fractures* may bear weight immediately and should only be operated on if the femoral head is retroverted through 30° or more or if there is evidence of instability shown for example by increasing displacement. In an open reduction we always impact the proximal fragment in full internal rotation and slightly increased anteversion. Internal fixation is then performed with the 130° blade plate as described on page 69.

Adduction fractures are always unstable and seldom unite without open reduction and internal fixation. In these fractures there is always impaction of the cancellous bone in the posterior part of the neck which results in a bone defect. This defect together with the posterior comminution makes it impossible to obtain an accurate reduction. Furthermore no reliable fixation of the reduced and shortened head fragment can be obtained. Internal fixation is used only to supplement the stability of a fracture that has been reduced and impacted in abduction. The aim is to convert every adduction fracture into an abduction fracture and to increase the anteversion. This can be expressed by the following analogy: The femoral head is hung on the cranial part of the femoral neck just as a hat is hung on a hook (WEBER). The fragments must be impacted and it is this impaction which makes the fracture stable and not the internal fixation itself. A blade plate is then used only as an additional safety factor. Though we have played down the importance of the internal fixation it is however vital to get the best hold for the blade plate in the femoral head. This part of the femoral head lies beneath the point where the compression and tension trabeculae cross.

In view of the danger of avascular necrosis and the difficulty of reducing the fracture, in patients who have a short life expectancy (meaning those of 70 and over) and in all so-called "pathological spontaneous fractures of the femoral neck" we advocate primary replacement arthroplasty. If the acetabulum is normal then simple endoprosthetic arthroplasty with a metallic (protasul) prosthesis is carried out. If there is any evidence of irregularity in the acetabulum or where there is osteoarthritis, the best procedure is a total hip replacement. All our prostheses are cemented in and the patients are allowed to walk on the third or fourth post-operative day to avoid complications of recumbency. All patients who are fit enough are operated on as emergencies.

The vertical type of neck fracture (PAUWELS type III) often cannot be converted into an abduction fracture. It is then better, especially when the bone is osteoporotic, to combine nailing with an intertrochanteric osteotomy (Fig. 148).

The timing of surgery: When nailing is decided upon it must be done within the first six hours to avoid the danger of thrombosis occurring in kinked retinacular vessels of the femoral neck. Immediate surgery also reduces post-operative mortality. If replacement arthroplasty is to be used there is less urgency and the patient can be more fully prepared.

The technique of nailing femoral neck fractures: The patient is placed on an ordinary operating table without traction. X-ray control is useful but not obligatory. Open reduction is carried out using an antero-lateral approach and full exposure is obtained by the correct positioning of three Hohmann retractors. The fragments are first dis-impacted by externally rotating, adducting and flexing the hip. The reduction should then be carried out very gently and carefully under direct vision using extension, internal rotation and abduction. For the criteria of successful reduction see Fig. 144. Temporary fixation is maintained with three Kirschner wires and reduction is checked by flexing the hip to 90° and examining the under surface of the femoral neck. The fracture should be over-reduced. At this point an X-ray may be taken if necessary. The temporary Kirschner wires are left in place and the special seating chisel is hammered in beginning at a point 2—3 cm distal to the prominence of the greater trochanter (Fig. 57). The chisel is then removed and the selected 130° pertrochanteric plate is hammered in. Impaction of the fragments is achieved by holding the slotted hammer against the greater trochanter and then hitting it firmly with a mallet. Now, if necessary, a further X-ray should be taken with the hip in full internal rotation and extension and another view with the hip at 40° abduction and 90° flexion to give an axial projection. Thus both an a.p. and lateral projection of the hip are obtained without moving the X-ray tube.

After operation the limb is supported on a sponge rubber splint and after four or five days, if wound healing is satisfactory, the patient is allowed out of bed.

Complications: Pseudarthrosis with a viable femoral head after an abduction fracture is treated by a repositioning osteotomy (Fig. 262—265). If there is collapse of a dead head then a total hip replacement should be undertaken. Arthrodesis should only be considered in young people.

2. Basal Adduction Fractures

These occur only if the cancellous bone of the neck is very hard which occurs only in young patients. Attempts to nail this type of fracture carries a danger of forcing the fragments apart with the seating chisel. We therefore advocate screw fixation using three large cancellous screws as in children (Fig. 231). Only after this type of screw fixation can an additional plate be considered (Fig. 147).

3. Pertrochanteric Fractures

There is no standard technique for internal fixation of trochanteric fractures though all should be reduced in varying degrees of valgus. When the lateral femoral cortex is intact trochanteric fractures are fixed with the 130° pertrochanteric plate (Fig. 153). When the lateral femoral cortex is weak then fixation with the condylar plate is used. For this to be successful, however, the medial cortex must be intact or must be reconstructed lest the blade plate break because of the constant bending stresses to which it is subjected (Fig. 154). When the medial cortex cannot be reconstructed the fracture should be reduced in marked valgus with slight medial displacement of the shaft, which may require osteotomy of the lateral cortex at the level of the lower edge of the fracture (Fig. 151). When the bones are very porotic and the patient has a short life expectancy, internal fixation is supplemented with methyl methacrylate cement (Fig. 152).

4. Fractures of the Femoral Neck Associated with Fractures of the Shaft on the Same Side

The femoral neck is dealt with first using the technique of reduction and fixation as described above. A high shaft fracture is fixed using the 130° pertrochanteric plate with an extra long shaft (Fig. 155). If the fracture is in the middle third of the shaft a long straight broad plate is used accompanied by autologous cancellous bone grafting. In a fracture of the distal third a condylar plate is used (Fig. 166).

Fig. 141

1   *The standard lateral incision:* This incision begins at the tip of the greater trochanter and runs distally. The fascia lata is incised longitudinally and the insertion of vastus lateralis is divided transversely and the muscle reflected forward. This exposure should be used for all trochanteric fractures and for inter-trochanteric osteotomies.

2   *The extended form of the standard incision:* The previous incision can extended 5–7 cm proximally and after incising the fascia lata the greater trochanter can be osteotomized. When the upper part of the hip joint capsule is excised, the abductors are retracted and the tip of a wide Hohmann retractor is hammered into the ala of the ilium just above the acetabulum.

Indications: Arthrodesis of the hip or total hip replacement when osteotomy of the greater trochanter is required.

3   *The modified* WATSON-JONES *incision:* This is used for the open reduction of subcapital fractures and for total hip replacement when osteotomy of the greater trochanter is not required.

4   *The* MOORE'S *approach (Southern):* The patient lies on his side, and the gluteus maximus is split in line with its fibres. The small external rotators are divided near their insertion.

Indications: Insertion of a simple femoral hip prosthesis or a total prosthesis after trauma when the acetabulum is normal.

5   *The extension of the* LANGENBECK-KOCHER-GIBSON: This approach runs between the gluteus maximus and minimus.

Indications: Central fracture dislocation of the hip with fracture of the ala of the ilium.

6   JUDET-LETOURNEL *incision:* This runs from the middle of the iliac crest along the upper ramus of the pubis and runs as near to the symphysis pubis as required.

Indications: To expose the anterior aspect of the hip joint in fractures of the anterior column.

N.B.: The SMITH-PETERSEN approach gives good exposure of the wing of the ilium, of the ischial spine and the hip joint. The skin incision runs from the middle of the iliac crest to the level of the iliac spine and is then extended distally along the line of the femur. This approach is most popular in the United States but we use it only for rare pelvic fractures (see Fig. 140).

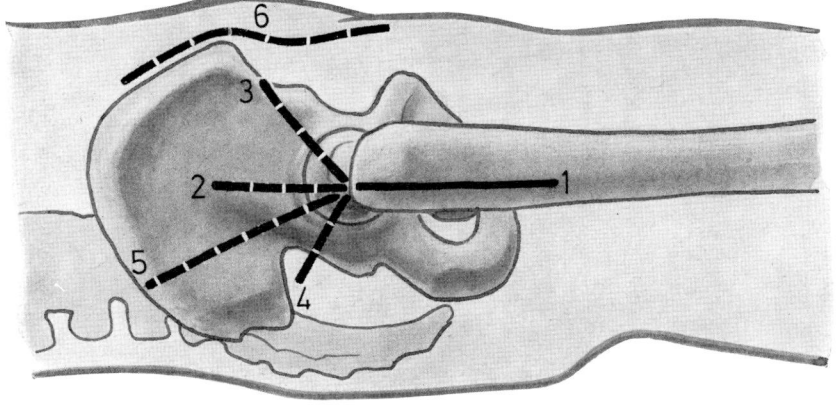

Fig. 142   *The exposure for open reduction of subcapital, transcervical and basal fractures of the femoral neck.*

a   The antero-lateral approach (modification of the WATSON-JONES approach) is used to expose the femoral neck. A curved incision is made (Fig. 141/3–1). The fascia lata is split anteriorly and the space between the tensor fascia lata and gluteus medius and minimus developed, making sure that the nerve to the tensor is not injured. The intertrochanteric area is exposed as in the standard lateral approach by reflecting the vastus lateralis downwards and forwards.

b   The capsule is now incised in line with the axis of the femoral neck. The tipe of one Hohmann retractor is now passed over the anterior rim of the pelvis. To preserve whatever vessels are still intact, the second Hohmann retractor should not be passed from above but should be inserted so that its sharp tip does not go any further back than the middle of the femoral neck. A third Hohmann retractor is passed below and medially around the femoral neck to expose its lower surface.
For the technique see page 68/70/160.

152

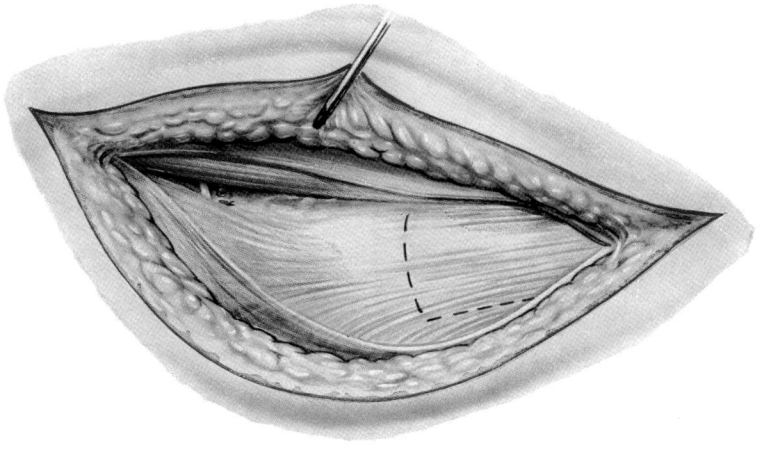

a

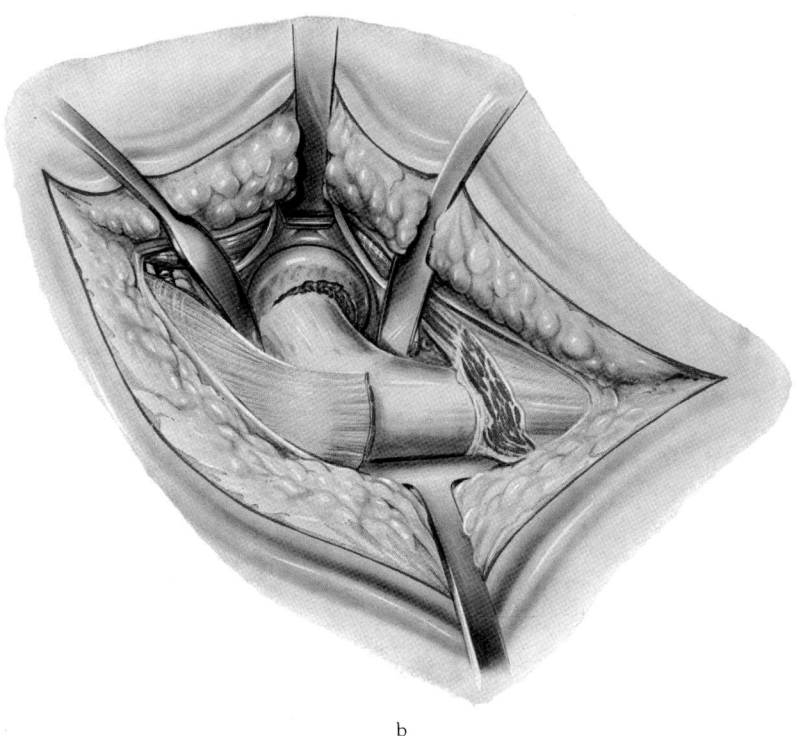

b

The technique of nailing an intra-articular fracture of the femoral neck.

Fig. 143   In a femoral neck fracture there is either impaction of the cancellous bone of the upper part of the neck (b) or severe comminution of the posterior cortex (a). Sufficiently broad contact at the fracture can only be achieved by impacting the fracture fragments.

Fig. 144   In an adduction fracture instability may occur in spite of reduction and nailing. (Compare the two displaced wooden frames, suggested by McElvenny).

a   If reduction is exact displacement may still occur because the cortex is hard and the cancellous bone soft. In addition to this comminution or impaction posteriorly may make exact reduction difficult.

b   Reduction is thus inadequate in both planes and internal fixation cannot prevent displacement.

c   The ideal reduction is in slight valgus. If the line of the cortex of the lower femoral neck is extended it comes to lie below the femoral head. In the axial projection the slight over-correction into anteversion is clear.

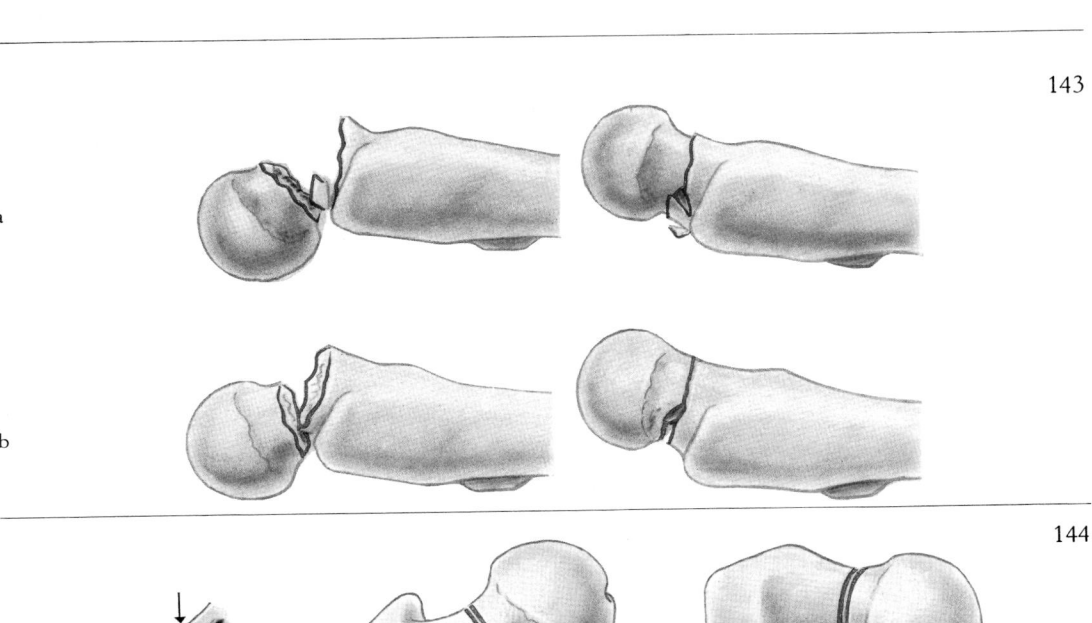

a

b

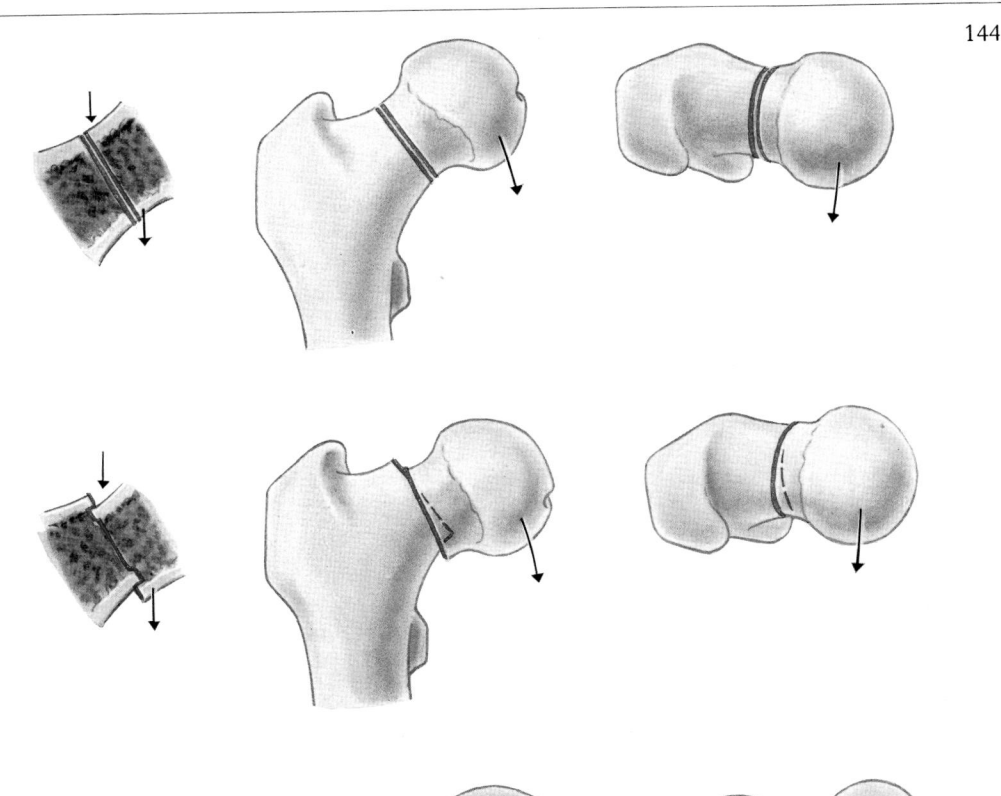

a

b

c

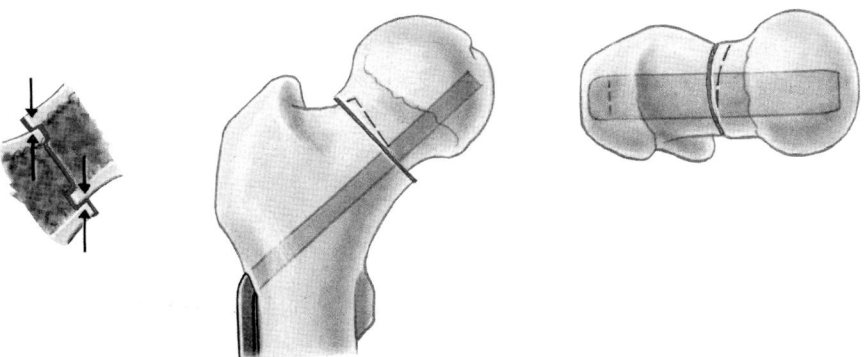

Examples of nailed intra-articular and basal femoral neck fractures.

Fig. 145   *Subcapital fracture of the femoral neck (MS 1686).*

Over-correction into valgus and anteversion. Fixation with a 130° blade plate. As the head was very large fixation was supplemented with a cancellous screw. The plate is supported by the calcar.

Fig. 146   *Mid-cervical fracture (MS 1413).*

Fixation is with the 130° angled blade plate. Because this plate was not adequately supported by the calcar a trochanteric plate was chosen. The head again was large and therefore a cancellous screw was used to supplement the fixation. This screw is not a lag screw because there is a tendency for it to back out showing that the neck does shorten. Because of this tendency it is important to place the screw parallel to the blade of the blade plate. The blade should not reach the bone under the articular cartilage but only to the inter-section between the tension and compression trabeculae.

Fig. 147   *Basal femoral neck fracture (MS 2015).*

Twenty-three year old patient. Fixation relying chiefly on lag screws. The pertro-chanteric plate was used to reinforce fixation because the patient was very stout.

Fig. 148   *A subcapital fracture with additional repositioning osteotomy (MS 1700).*

A sixty-seven year old patient with severe osteoporosis. A vertical neck fracture (PAUWELS type III). The head was elevated with the tip of the 120° blade plate and fixation was supplemented with two screws. At the same time a 30° trochanteric valgus osteotomy was performed and five years later there was no avascular necrosis and a completely normal hip joint.

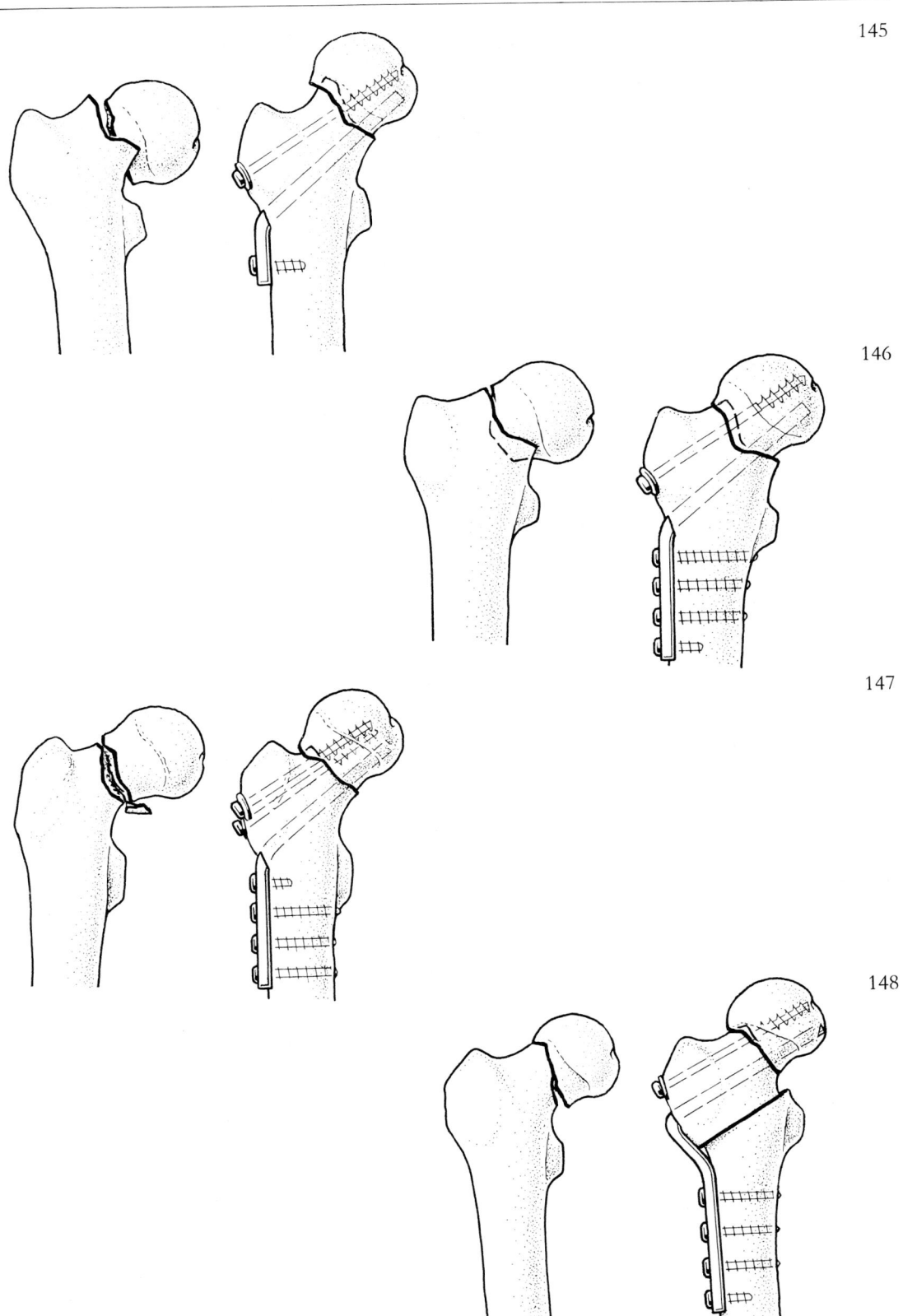

145

146

147

148

157

Pertrochanteric Fractures

There are four methods of internal fixation depending on the type of fracture:

a) The 130° pertrochanteric blade plate.
b) The condylar plate.
c) Valgus displacement of the head and neck fragment and medial displacement of the shaft using the 130° pertrochanteric blade plate.
d) The 130° pertrochanteric blade plate combined with bone cement.

Fig. 149   *The standard method of treating a simple pertrochanteric fracture with a 130° blade plate.*

The patient lies supine on the table and a lateral approach is used reflecting the vastus lateralis forward. The fragments are first dis-impacted using extension, external rotation and adduction. Next, the reduction is carried out again using extension but with full internal rotation and strong abduction.

a   Kirschner wires and a Verbrugge bone clamp are used to fix the fracture temporarily. A further Kirschner wire is passed along the front of the femoral neck into the head to serve as a guide to the anteversion of the femoral neck. A triangular positioning plate with a 50° angle is used to guide the 130° blade plate. A Kirschner wire is now introduced into the greater trochanter parallel to the upper edge of the metal triangle and also parallel in the sagittal plane to the Kirschner wire lying along the front of the femoral neck.

b   2.5 cm below the prominence of the greater trochanter, drill three holes with a 4.5 mm drill or triangular drill.

c   With a 7 mm router enlarge the holes and join them together. Use a flat chisel to cut an oblique part of the lower cortex to make a seat for the shoulder of the angled blade plate.

d   Hammer in the special chisel with its chisel guide parallel to the Kirschner wire in the greater trochanter.

e   Remove the chisel and drive in the angled blade plate.

f   Further fixation is provided by two cancellous screws which apply compression between fragments.

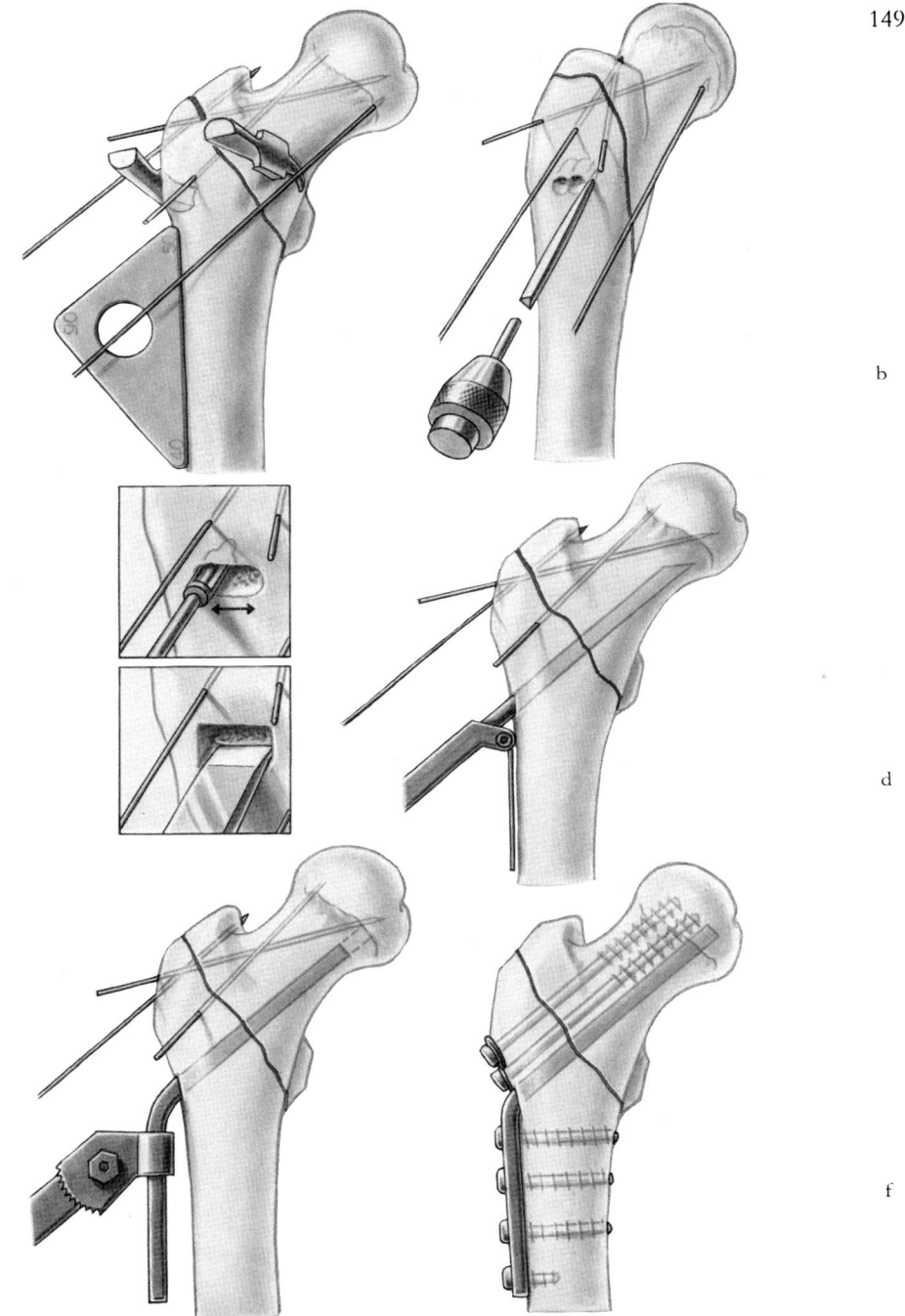

a

b

c

d

e

f

Fig. 150   *The fixation of a pertrochanteric fracture with an intact calcar femoralis using the condylar plate.*

a   Reduction and temporary fixation with Kirschner wires and a Verbrugge clamp. Using the condylar positioning plate, hammer in the special chisel into the greater trochanter as far proximally as possible. One should aim at slight over-correction and try to place the tip of the chisel in the postero-inferior quadrant of the femoral head.

b   Remove the chisel and drive the condylar plate into the precut channel. When the tension device is tightened up, the proximal fragment is put into slight valgus and the fragments become impacted. Give additional fixation to the proximal fragment with one or two cancellous screws which should obtain a grip on the calcar. Before the plate is screwed down, the reduction should be re-checked and if necessary, a further radiograph obtained.

Fig. 151   *Valgus displacement of the head and neck fragment and medial displacement of the shaft, using the 130° blade plate.*

If the outer femoral cortex is shattered or if the medial cortex cannot be reconstituted, valgus displacement of the proximal fragment with slight medial displacement of the shaft is carried out. This is begun by inserting the 130° blade plate just below the greater trochanter into the head and neck fragment, in approximately the same direction as the condylar plate. This plate should enter the neck through the fracture as far cranially as possible and should be aimed at the postero-inferior quadrant of the femoral head. After reduction, when the plate comes to lie against the femoral shaft, the proximal fragment should lie in a valgus position of 30–50° with the shaft, and the shaft itself should be displaced a little inwards. The displaced fragments of the greater trochanter to which the abductor muscles are attached, are reduced and fixed with a tension band wire to the femur.

Fig. 152   *The use of the angled blade plate together with cement.*

In old patients with a short life expectancy who are also osteoporotic, we use cement together with the angled blade plate to obtain rigid internal fixation. The first step is to gouge out all the cancellous bone from the femoral neck right up into the head and from the upper end of the lower fragment, replacing this with a plug of methyl methacrylate or similar cement. This is done in two steps, the first of which is to fill the hole with a thin layer of cement. Then a temporary reduction is obtained and all loose fragments are screwed to the thin layer of cement. Next, the holes in the shaft and the femoral neck are filled with cement, the blade of the plate is quickly driven into the soft cement, reduction is completed and while the position is maintained the plate is fixed to the shaft with screws. The tips of the screws which were first inserted into the loose fragments are now simply pressed into the still soft polymerizing mass of cement.

160

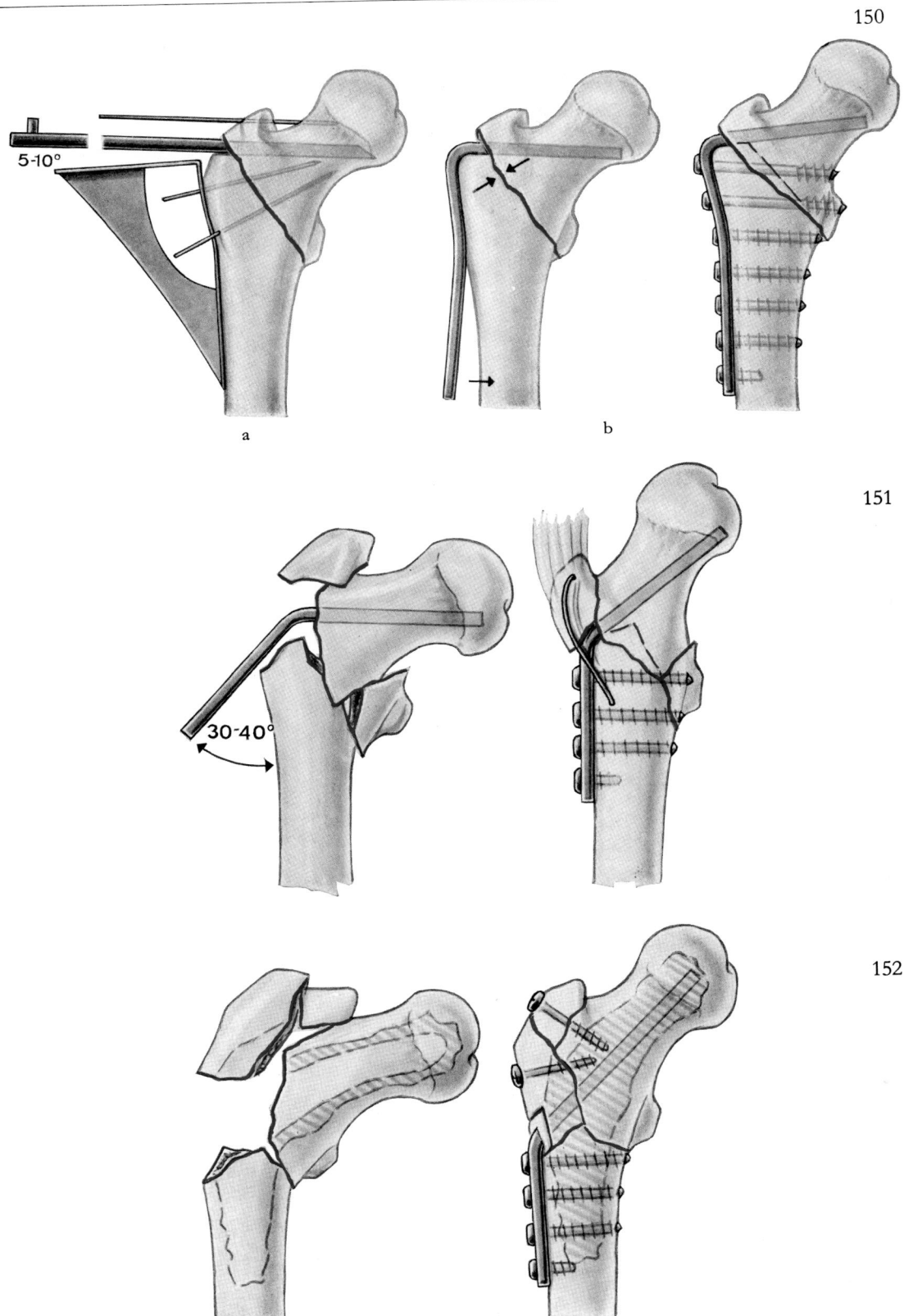

5-10°

30-40°

a

b

Post-operative Management

Early mobilization is of extreme importance in these old patients. Once they have been in bed for a few days, it is very difficult and time consuming to get them going again.

To require these old patients to start walking with two crutches without weight bearing is beyond their physical ability. Reduction and rigid internal fixation must be so efficient that early weight bearing can be undertaken. If there is any doubt about the rigidity of fixation, a primary repositioning osteotomy or a replacement arthroplasty should be undertaken. The time in hospital can be kept below four weeks in patients with femoral neck fractures only if these principles of treatment are adhered to.

Examples of trochanteric fractures.

Fig. 153   *Pertrochanteric fracture with an intact calcar (MS 1557).*

Over-reduce the fracture into a valgus position. Stabilize this with a 130° blade plate and two cancellous screws. These act as lag screws only for a short time and provide temporary compression between fragments. They serve no other function.

Fig. 154   *Trochanteric fracture with a thin weak outer cortex (MS 1990).*

Fixation with a condylar plate. For adequate fixation the condylar plate must be held to the proximal fragment with at least one cancellous screw which must gain a grip of the calcar. Over-correction of the fracture into slight valgus is also important.

Fig. 155   *Comminuted fracture of the upper femur (MS 1952).*

Fixation using a condylar plate with an extra long shaft. It is important to reconstitute the inner cortex and slight over-correction into valgus is much better than a varus position. Compression must be applied to the plate, and before it is inserted, the main fragments are fixed and placed under interfragmental compression by means of screws.

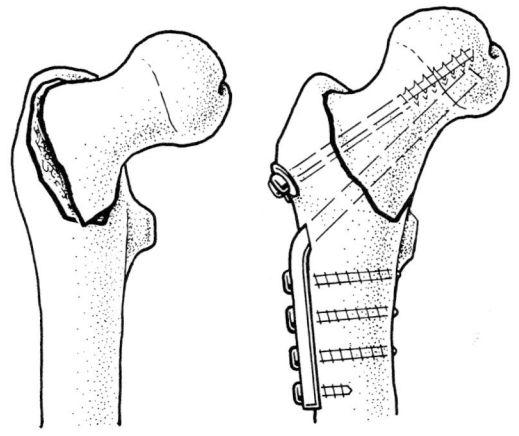

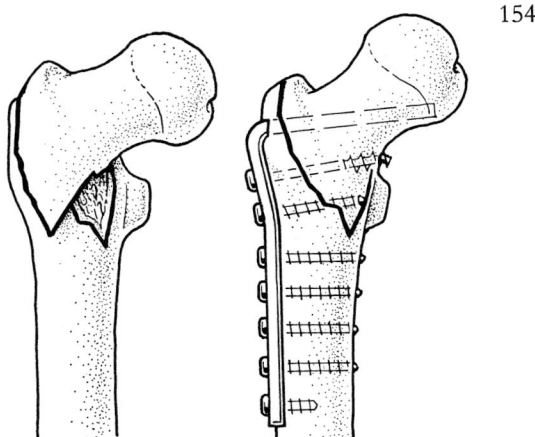

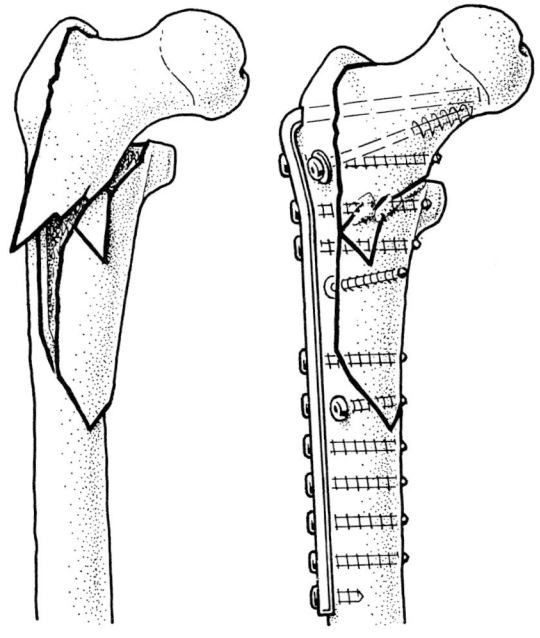

G. Fractures of the Femoral Shaft

The advantages of rigid internal fixation are most evident in fractures of the femoral shaft. Conservative treatment demands between two and three months of traction and after this long period, delayed union or malunion is not uncommon. To this must be added the many months required after union for restoration of function of the knee joint.

For these reasons we treat almost all fractures of the femur by operation. For the middle third we prefer intramedullary nailing with a thick medullary nail, after reaming. For the upper and lower thirds we use angled blade plates; for the upper third either the 130° blade plate or the condylar plate and for the lower third the condylar plate only. These plates are inserted postero-laterally and placed under tension so that they can exert a tension band effect. If the buttressing effect of the medial cortex is absent because of bone defect or comminution, a primary autologous cancellous bone graft must be performed.

In comminuted fractures it may be helpful to delay operation for one to two weeks, meanwhile applying a sixth of the body weight of traction via a Steinmann pin inserted into the tibial tubercle. This simplifies the reduction because of muscle atrophy, and diminishes the danger of avascular necrosis of small fragments because of post traumatic hyperemia.

Position of the patient: For medullary nailing, place the patient on his side (Fig. 81). For plating, the patient may be either supine or in the lateral position.

Fig. 156   *Surgical approaches to the femur.*

1.   For intramedullary nailing, make a longitudinal incision centered over the greater trochanter.

2.   For trochanteric fractures or for inter-trochanteric osteotomy, use the standard lateral incision. One must never incise through the belly of the vastus lateralis but should reflect it forwards and downwards.

3.   The so-called mail-box approach through the middle third of the thigh is carried out by going behind the vastus lateralis along the intermuscular septum, retracting the vastus lateralis forwards and separating it from the bone until the linea aspera is reached. The perforating vessels are ligated and divided in the lower part of the incision. Any other approach leads to adhesions or interference with the blood and nerve supply of the vastus lateralis. A plate is applied just anterior to the linea aspera but in middle third fractures of the femur intramedullary nailing is the treatment of choice under most circumstances.

4.   Approach to the lower femur. If the knee joint must be inspected, a counter-incision is made one finger-breadth medial to the patella (5).

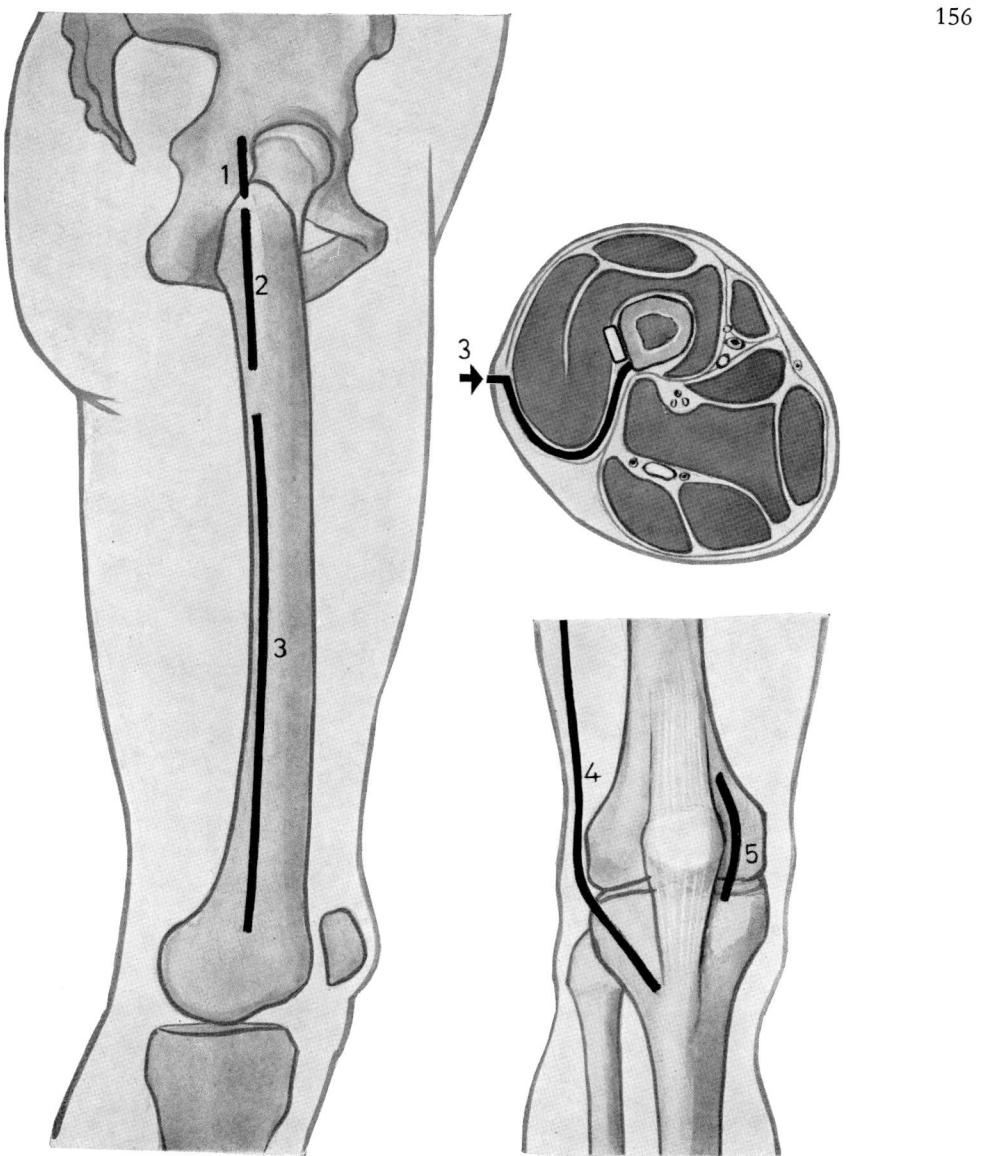

Subtrochanteric Fractures (Shaft P)

We have found the condylar plates most useful for upper subtrochanteric fractures and the long 130° blade plates for fractures lower down in the upper third. For rigid fixation it is not enough to have only the blade of the plate fixing the proximal fragment, but one or two screws passed through the plate into the upper fragment should be used as well. It is also important to place the plate under tension with the small tension device and thus compress the fracture. Where possible it is best to reduce the fracture and obtain compression between fragments before introducing the angled blade plate. In comminuted fractures it is sometimes necessary to reverse this procedure, as shown in Fig. 157.

The technique of internal fixation with an angled blade plate for simple subtrochanteric fractures: Make a 20 cm lateral incision, reflect the vastus lateralis anteriorly, insert three Hohmann retractors, expose the fracture and reduce it and apply inter-fragmental screw fixation, introducing the screws whenever possible from the front. The Hohmann retractors are placed so that one lies medially below the neck, one above and the third, narrower one along the front of the femoral neck and hooked round the brim of the pelvis. The blade plate is then hammered home as shown in Fig. 60 or 61. After introduction of the Kirschner wires, one showing the inclination of the femoral neck and the other the degree of anteversion, the seating chisel with its chisel guide is hammered in. Its position is checked and if it is correct, it is removed and the blade plate hammered into the slot, and is fixed with one screw to the calcar. The plate is then placed under tension with the small tension device and the reduction checked once more. Before the plate is screwed down, it must be confirmed that both the reduction and the position of the blade plate are perfect.

Examples:

Fig. 157   *A high subtrochanteric fracture (MS 1349).*

Stabilization with a condylar plate. The blade portion was accurately inserted in the neck. A cancellous screw fixes it to the proximal fragment. The second screw in this example is a lag screw and is therefore introduced after the plate has been placed under tension.

Fig. 158   *A subtrochanteric fracture with a butterfly fragment (BI 3202).*

At first rigid internal fixation with inter-fragmental compression was achieved using lag screws, after which the 130° blade plate was introduced. Some of the screws fixing the plate to the shaft are short ones; if long they would have gone through the fracture line or very close to it, possibly splitting the fragment. The other screws are long and wherever possible used as lag screws to provide interfragmental compression.

Fig. 159   *A comminuted subtrochanteric fracture with loss of the medial cortical buttress (MS 1959).*

Reduce and fix the main fragments, wherever possible with lag screws, providing interfragmental compression. Then insert the 130° blade plate. Roughen the cortex medially and apply autologous cancellous bone grafts. This cancellous bone is indispensable if an early fatigue fracture of the plate is to be avoided. After operation the patient must remain non-weight bearing for six to eight weeks to allow the bone graft to be incorporated and to form a medial bridge of bone.

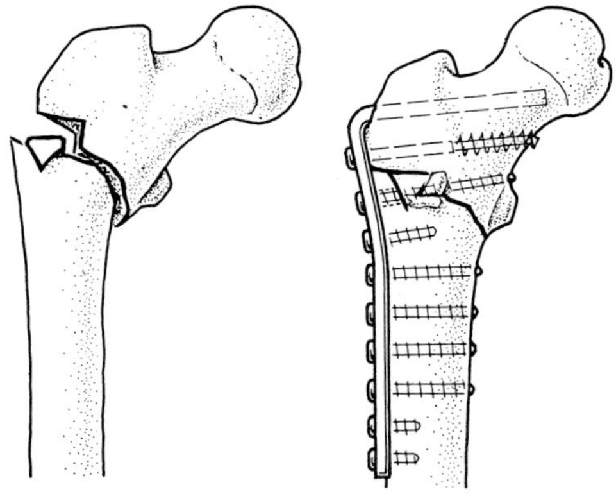

157

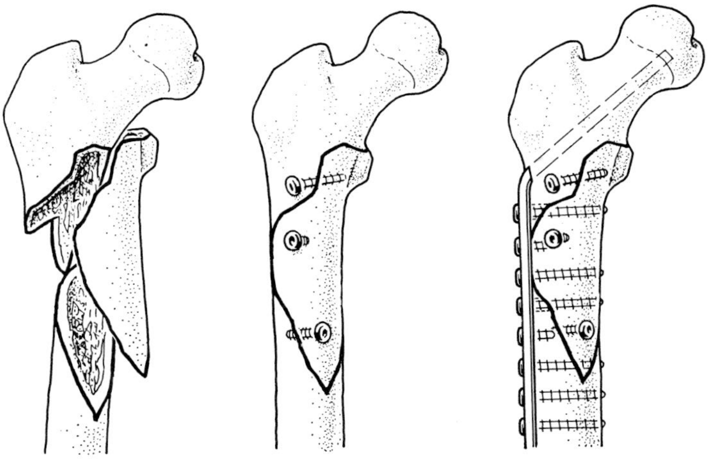

158

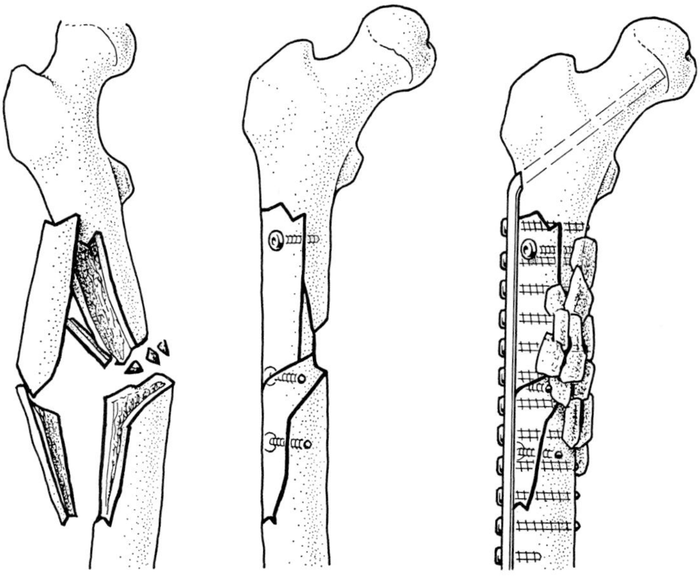

159

Fractures of the Femoral Shaft (M)

This segment of the femur is best fixed by a thick intramedullary nail, after reaming out the medullary canal. Sometimes cerclage wiring is used in combination with the medullary nail. A plate should be used only as a last resort in this area of the shaft, because it may lead to severe osteoporosis of the underlying cortex, increasing the danger of refracture. This is particularly so if two plates are used (Fig. 90). If cerclage wires are used (Fig. 161) they must be removed after six to eight weeks.

Position of the patient: See Fig. 75.

We usually do an open reduction and temporary fixation of the fracture with a semi-tubular plate and two Verbrugge bone clamps (Fig. 79). The approach is between the vastus lateralis and the inter-muscular septum. For access to the greater trochanter for intramedullary reaming and nailing, we extend the incision upwards or make a second longitudinal incision over the greater trochanter. If it is elected to undertake reduction as illustrated in Fig. 79, then it must be remembered that the proximal fragment must be considerably flexed and externally rotated. It is therefore best to reduce the fracture first before opening the greater trochanter with the awl. Otherwise the opening for the nail may be made too far anteriorly, which may split the anterior cortex of the femur during reaming or when the nail is introduced.

For the technique of intramedullary nailing see page 86.

Fig. 160   *Simple fracture of the femoral shaft (OR 6/35).*

Reaming to 15 mm and stabilization with a 14 mm nail, for men. In women a 12 or 13 mm nail is big enough.

Fig. 161   *Comminuted fracture (MS 1908).*

Temporary fixation with two cerclage wires and a semitubular plate and two Verbrugge clamps. The medullary canal was reamed to 15 mm and a 14 mm nail was used for fixation. The cerclage wires were removed after two months.

Fig. 162   *A double fracture (WL 37/21).*

Both fractures are in the middle third of the shaft. Open reduction and temporary fixation of the fractures with a long semi-tubular plate and three or four Verbrugge clamps. Ream only to 12–13 mm and use an 11–12 mm nail. Reaming must be done carefully to avoid rotational displacement of the middle segment.

Fig. 163   *A fracture at the junction of the middle and lower third (MS 1951).*

The medullary canal widens from this point down into the lower fragment and fixation with a medullary nail is often inadequate. Rigid fixation can be secured only with a laterally applied tension band plate. We add to this a cancellous bone graft on the medial side of the fracture, especially if there is any comminution of the medial cortex, destroying its buttress effect.

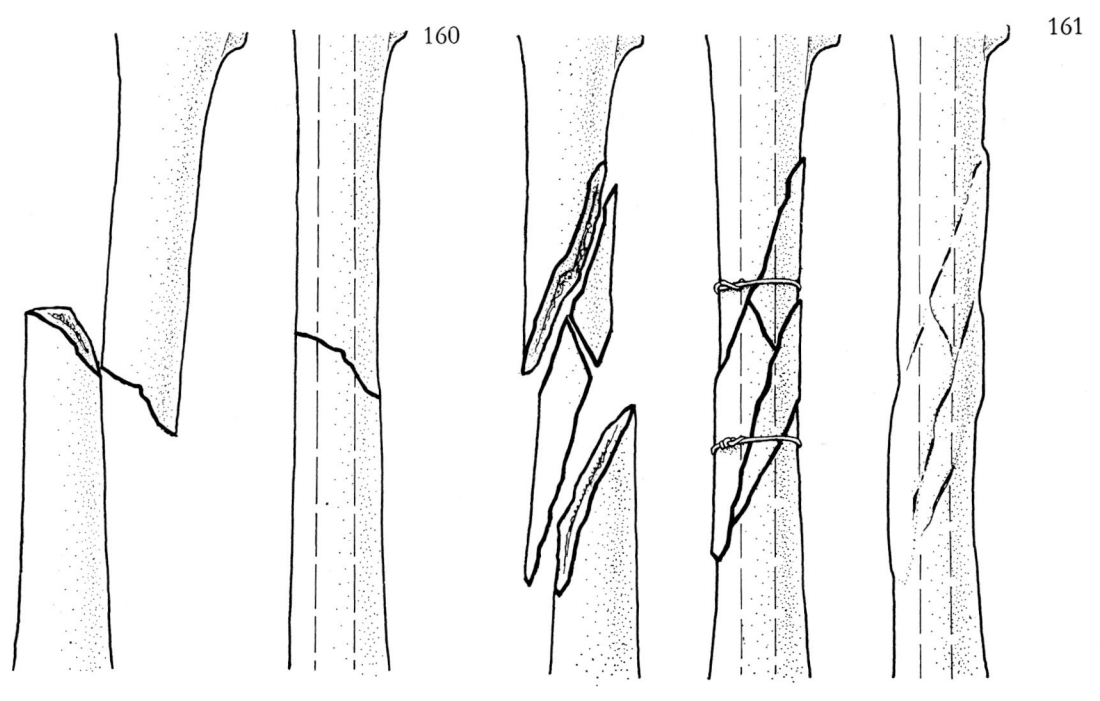

160   161

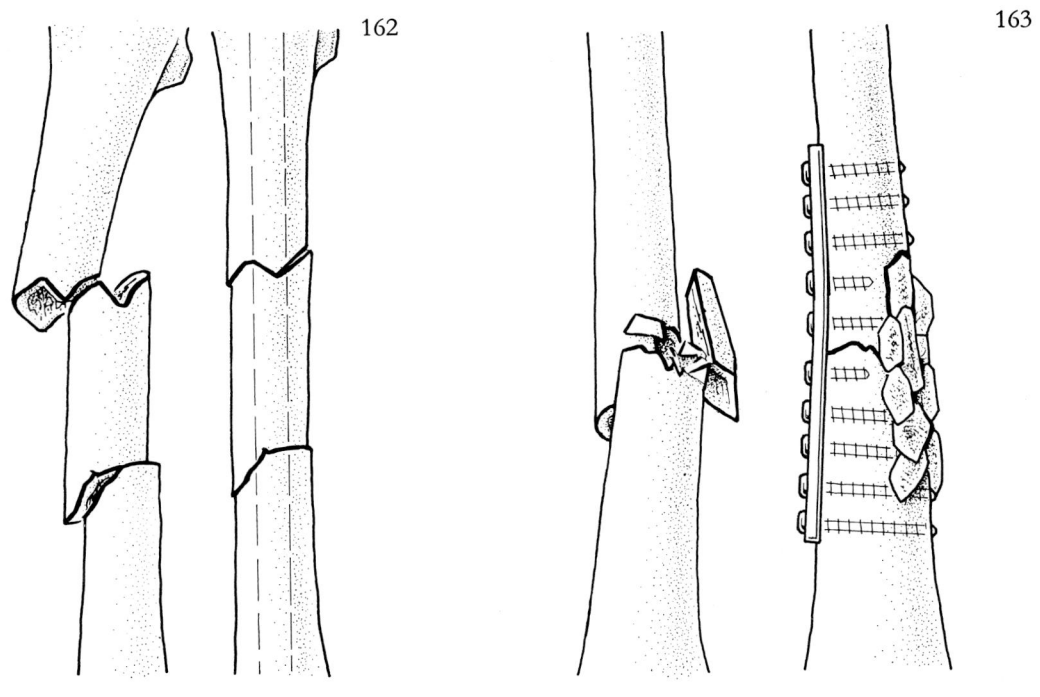

162   163

169

Fractures of the Lower Femur

These are stabilized with a condylar plate.

Fig. 164   *The technique of the reduction is made clearer by a diagram.*

a   *Incision:* Make a lateral incision at the level of the knee joint and extend it downwards and medially as far as the tibial tubercle. Open into the joint in front of the lateral ligament and gain a wide exposure of the joint so that the reduction of the joint surfaces can be carried out under direct vision. Temporary fixation can be obtained with a few Kirschner wires.

b   One Kirschner wire is then inserted transversely through the knee joint, parallel to the surfaces of the femoral condyles, to serve as a guide to the condylar articular surface. A second Kirschner wire is passed under the center of the patella. A third wire is passed through the middle of the femoral condyle as low as possible, which is 1 cm above the articular surface. It should lie parallel to both the first and second wires which indicate the plane of the articular surfaces of the femoral condyles. This third wire serves as a guide for the blade of the condylar plate. Its position should be checked, using the condylar positioning plate (Fig. 59 d). The vertical component of the "T" fracture should now be fixed with one or more cancellous screws. introduced 3–4 cm above the joint surface, somewhat anteriorly or, if not, as far backwards as possible. It is important to remember the projected position of the blade when placing these cancellous screws, so that they do not get in the way when the plate is introduced.

c   The special chisel with the chisel guide set parallel to the long axis of the femoral shaft, is now hammered in, so that the chisel travels parallel to the third or directional Kirschner wire. This ensures that the blade of the plate will lie parallel to the surface of the condyles and the plate will then be correctly aligned in both sagittal and coronal planes.

d   As seen from the side. The chisel guide is centered exactly over the middle of the femoral shaft. The head of the cancellous screw is clearly seen just in front of the chisel guide.

e   Remove the chisel and hammer in the condylar plate. Supplement the fixation of the plate in the distal fragment with a cancellous screw which must obtain a grip on the medial cortex. Now insert the tension device and place the plate under tension.

f   Check the reduction and the stability of the fixation. If both are satisfactory the plate is screwed home to the femoral shaft. If impaction of cancellous bone has occurred leaving a defect at the fracture site, this should be filled in at the end of the operation with autologous cancellous bone.

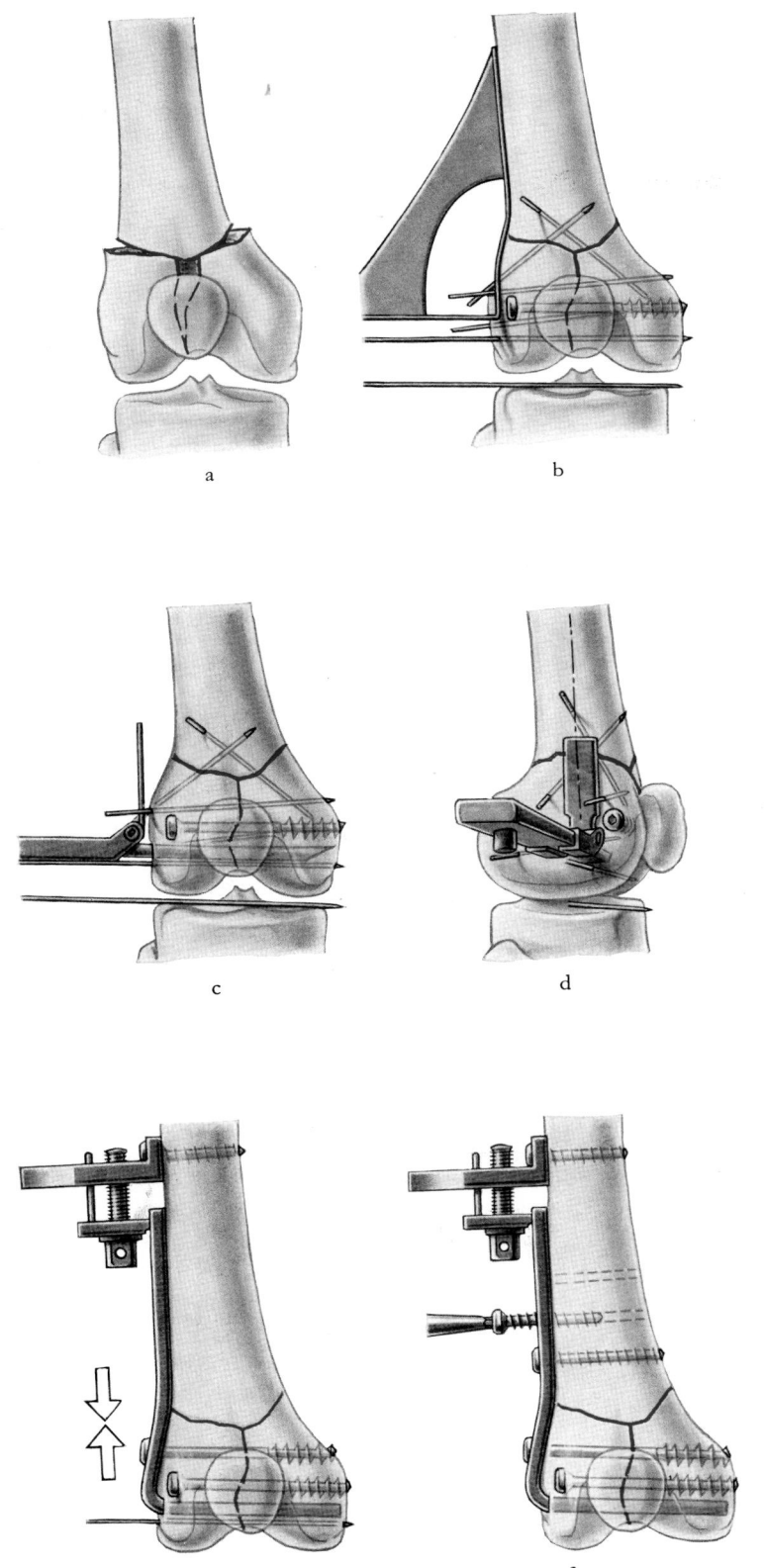

a

b

c

d

e

f

Post-operative Management of Femoral Shaft Fractures

After any open reduction and internal fixation of fractures of the middle or distal third of the femur, the limb must be held with the hip and knee flexed to 90° (Fig. 85 b). Immediate assisted active movements are begun. After six days the splint is discarded, the patient is encouraged to sit with his legs over the edge of the bed and to begin active unassisted movements. He is allowed out of bed on the eighth day after operation and may, after medullary nailing, bear weight within his tolerance. Progress is then so quick that within two to three weeks walking is usually possible with one stick. If plate fixation has been used, full weight bearing must be avoided for two to three months. In the interim partial weight bearing not exceeding 10—15 kilograms (which should be measured on a scale) is allowed with the aid of two crutches.

Plates are removed after eighteen months and intramedullary nails after two years. Before the metal is removed radiographs must show that the cortical structure is homogeneous throughout.

Examples:

Fig. 165   *A comminuted fracture between the upper and lower third (AC 30/8).*

The first step is to reduce the fragments and fix them with screws. The next is to apply a lateral plate and fix it to the shaft with screws. Note that some screws are omitted.

Fig. 166   *A comminuted fracture of the lower femur (FW 12/24).*

Here again the first step is to reduce the large major fragments and to fix them with screws to obtain interfragmental compression. The next step is to insert the condylar plate. Note that the blade of the condylar plate is inserted low down, which is necessary because the profile of the plate will only fit the lower femur.

Fig. 167   *Simple fracture of the condyle.*

In young patients screw fixation alone will usually suffice because the bone is not porotic and fractures are not comminuted. In older people, however, one has to compete with porotic bone and comminution. Therefore, besides screw fixation the buttress plate is employed just as in a plateau fracture of the tibia. A T-plate serves very well as a buttress plate in this situation.

Fig. 168   *Y-fracture (BS 1/3).*

Two incisions were used as shown in Fig. 156 4/5. The fracture was first stabilized with three lag screws inserted from both medial and lateral sides. The blade of the plate is a little too proximal.

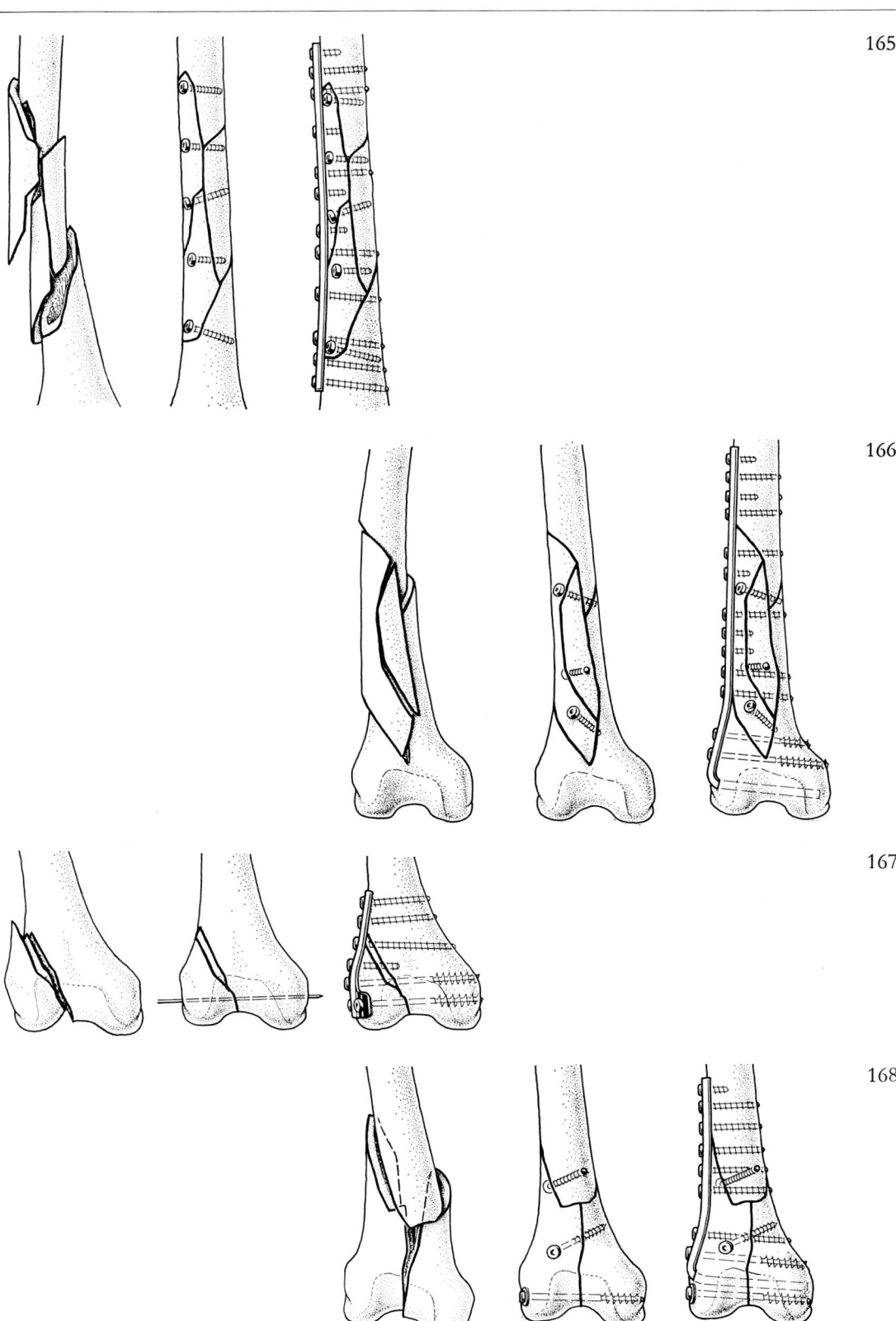

H. Fractures of the Patella

We have already described the pinciple of tension band wiring of the patella (Fig. 28). In simple fractures of the patella this is unquestionably the method of choice because, if done correctly, immediate active movements of the knee can begin. Early flexion of the knee joint is most desirable because in extension the patella does not articulate with the femur. In flexion, on the other hand, the articular surface of the patella lies against the articular surface of the femur.

A tension band wire applied anteriorly converts tensile forces into compressive forces. During the open reduction, the objective is to obtain slight over-correction (Fig. 28a). Comminuted fractures of the patella need rather more elaborate methods of internal fixation but the tension band wire principle still applies. Two tension band wires are needed, combined with either parallel or oblique Kirschner wires, to give the fracture some lateral stability.

PAUWELS showed that tension band wiring of comminuted fractures of the patella gives good results. Occasionally, however, patellectomy becomes necessary, after which immediate repair of the quadriceps and the patellar tendon should be carried out.

In avulsion fractures of the lower pole of the patella, this fragment may sometimes be reduced and fixed with a small cancellous screw before wiring (Fig. 171). The ruptured patellar tendon should be repaired and the suture line protected with a figure of eight wire which obtains a hold distally by passing round a screw in the tibial tubercle (Fig. 172).

Vertical fractures of the patella are treated conservatively. If they are very painful on movement, stability can be obtained with two transverse lag screws.

Tension Band Wiring of the Patella

Technique for a simple transverse fracture: Through a transverse skin incision, expose the fracture and examine the femoral condyles. Scrape back the tendon fibres 2—3 mm from the fracture line. Obtain an accurate reduction and hold it with two towel clips. The first wire is passed deep to the insertion of the quadriceps and patellar tendon. The second wire lies more superficially and passes through the Sharpey fibres. Slightly over-correct, tighten the wires and then tie them. On flexing the knee joint the over-correction vanishes and the fracture surfaces are squeezed together under compression. Repair the quadriceps expansion on either side of the patella, put in two suction drains, close the wound and immobilize the knee in a compression dressing for 48 hours. Quadriceps exercises immediately.

Post-operative Care

At first we were anxious about early active movement but are now convinced that this gives the best results. With secure tension band wire fixation, one need not fear loss of reduction. If there is any doubt about the fixation, after mobilization for eight to ten days a plaster cylinder is applied for four to six weeks.

Fig. 169   *Simple transverse fracture of the patella (MS 1575).*

Tension band wire and safety wire. Both are applied on the anterior surface of the patella.

Fig. 170   *Comminuted fracture of the patella (BI 32/6).*

Two Kirschner wires are introduced longitudinally to stabilize the small fragments. Fixation is then completed with two tension band wires.

Fig. 171   *Avulsion fracture of the lower pole of the patella (L 436).*

In avulsion fracture of the lower tip of the patella, tension band wiring alone tips the distal fragment. The lower fragment must therefore be stabilized with a small cancellous screw before applying the tension band wire.

Fig. 172   *Rupture of the patellar tendon (MS 1580).*

The tendon is repaired with chromic catgut. The suture line is protected with a figure of eight tension band wire passed proximally around the quadriceps insertion and distally around the transverse screw inserted in the tibia just distal to the attachment of the patellar tendon. Immediate movement can begin without fear of disrupting the repair. The wire and screw are removed after six months.

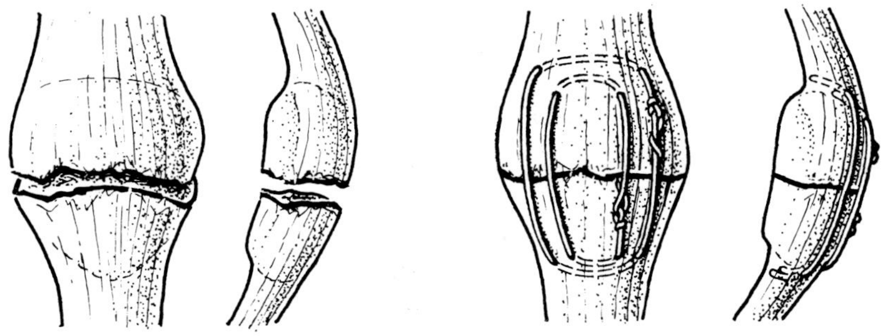

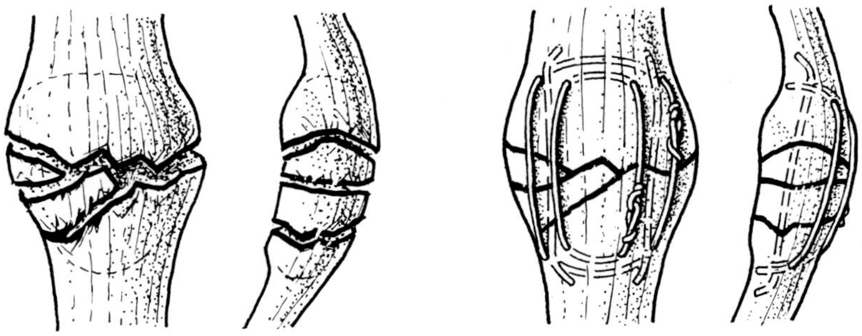

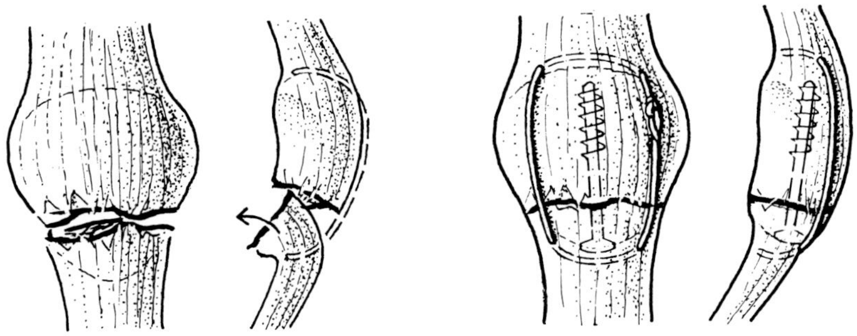

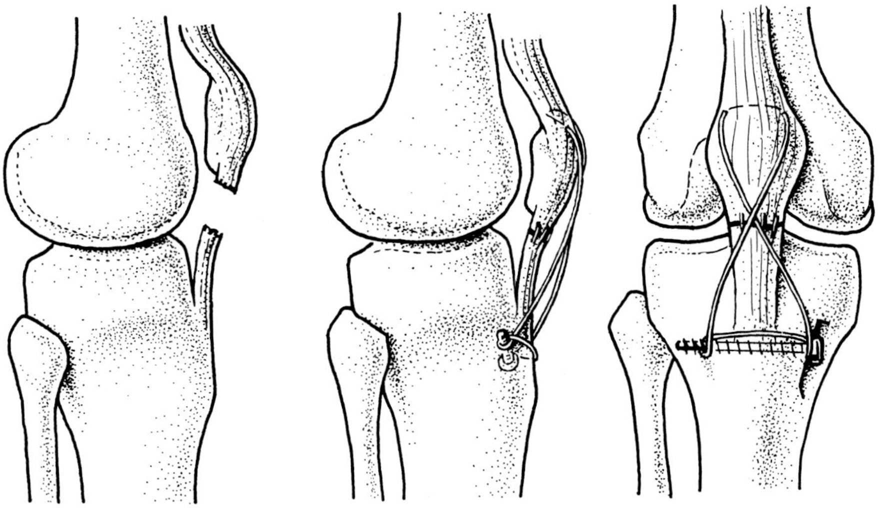

J. Fractures of the Tibia

Indications: The only absolute indication for open reduction is an irreducible intra-articular fracture. In all other fractures the indication for surgery is relative because BOEHLER has shown that patients with tibial shaft fractures, treated according to his principles, achieve good to excellent results, after a considerably longer period in hospital. Poor conservative treatment on the other hand, results in axial mal-alignment, shortening, chronic oedema, Sudeck's atrophy, joint stiffness and pseudarthrosis.

The choice of operation: The fracture type and location depend on the mechanism of the injury. Besides comminuted fractures, traffic accidents may result in short oblique or transverse fractures. Athletic injuries, especially in skiing, result in long spiral fractures. In a city hospital therefore, more tibial fractures are treated by medullary nailing; in a hospital which deals with athletic injuries chiefly, an equal number of fractures will be found treated with pure interfragmental compression methods. Most tibial fractures can be successfully treated by a combination of interfragmental compression and neutralization plating.

Surgical Approaches to the Tibia

The incision must be chosen so that the final scar does not lie over the metal implant, even a single screw head. The position of the plate must therefore be decided before making the incision.

Fig. 173		*Surgical approaches to the upper end of the tibia.*
	a	The approach for simple fracture of the medial plateau or of a lateral plateau when wider exposure of the joint is needed.
	b	A tri-radiate incision (120° between the incision) gives good access to both tibial plateau. The incision should not meet over the tibial tubercle but over the middle of the patellar tendon. To visualize the articular surface, one must go deep to the menisci. At the end, the insertion of the medial ligament must be carefully re-sutured.
	c	The transverse incision for medullary nailing of the tibia is made half way between the lower border of the patella and the tibial tubercle. The skin incision is transverse but the patellar tendon is split lengthwise and is held apart with a self-retaining retractor. Then bend the knee to 40° and open into the medullary canal with the awl, while the fracture is held with Verbrugge bone clamps (Fig. 74).
Fig. 174		*Surgical approach to the shaft of the tibia.*
	1	For fractures of the tibia, make the incision medial or lateral to the crest of the tibia. The incision should be made 1 cm from this border, more often on the lateral side. If screws are to be placed in the anterior tibial border or a semi-tubular plate is to be applied on top of it, then it is best to make the incision medially so that the neutralization plate can be applied further back.
	2	The incision is extended downwards and medially if a fracture of the medial malleolus has to be dealt with, or when the tibial fracture runs into the ankle joint.
	3	Incision over the fibula, as for a fibular osteotomy.
	4	The postero-medial approach to the tibia to expose its posterior surface. This approach is very similar to the mailbox exposure of the femur.

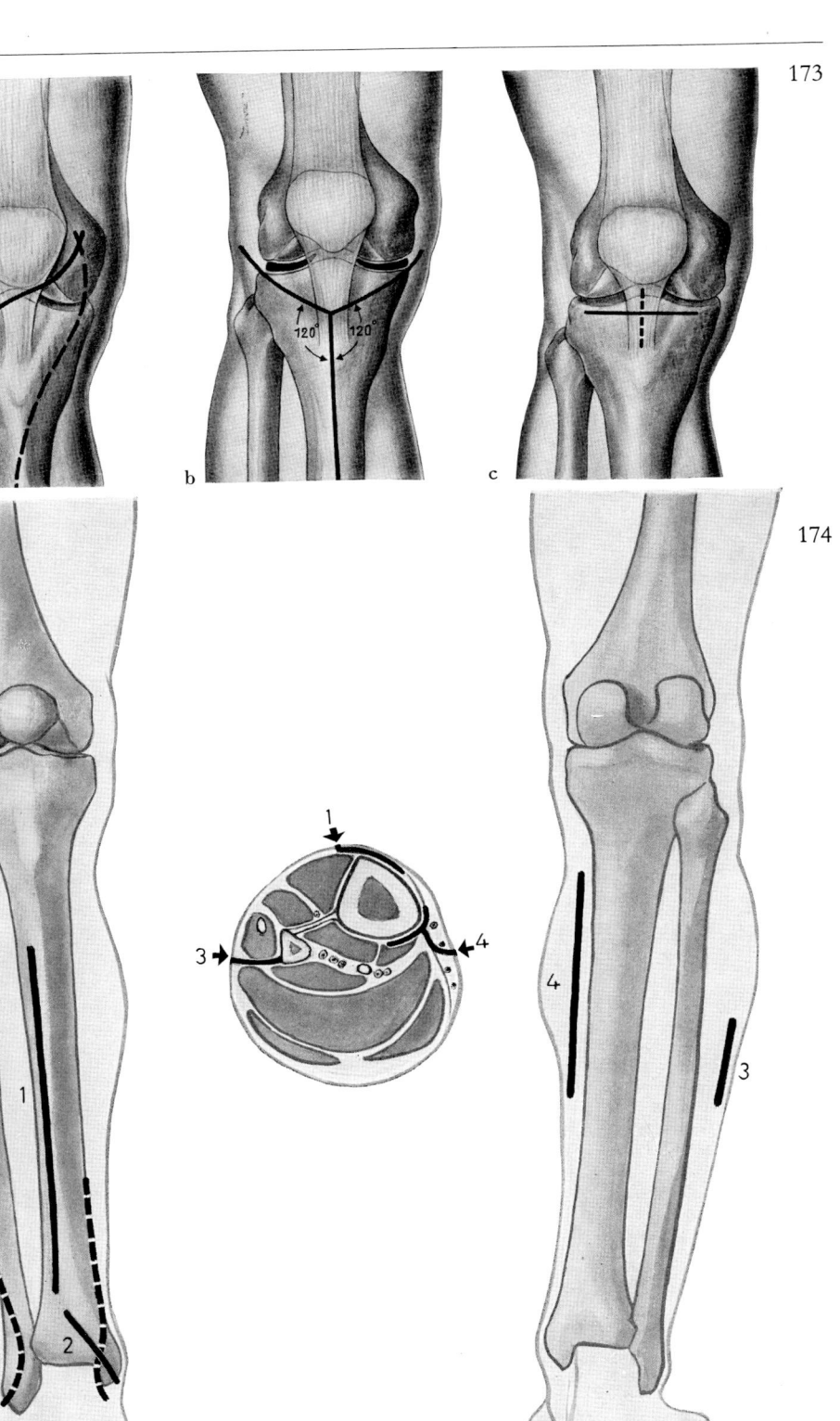

a

b

120° 120°

c

1

2

3

4

1

3

4

Fractures of the Tibial Condyles

We distinguish three types of tibial condyle fractures:

a) Cleavage fractures.
b) Impacted fractures.
c) Comminuted fractures.

For approaches see Fig. 173.

To examine the joint surfaces in (b) and (c) incise the capsule and go deep to the menisci.

a) Internal Fixation for a Cleavage Fracture

Cancellous screws with washers alone are adequate only in young patients with strong cancellous bone and no osteoporosis. In others, a buttress plate must be used in addition to screws.

b) Internal Fixation of an Impacted Fracture

Depressed fragments of the tibial plateaus should be elevated from below upwards. Sometimes it is best to drill a wide hole 5—6 cm below the joint surface of the tibia and then to punch up the fragments into place. The fragments should be over-reduced slightly, and the underlying defect should be filled with cancellous bone grafts. If the defect is large, this cancellous bone should be obtained from the greater trochanter. Compression is obtained with long cancellous screws, and the cortex buttressed with a T-plate.

c) Internal Fixation of a Comminuted Fracture

This is an extremely difficult procedure. Both sides of the joint must be exposed. It is often necessary to reflect the insertion of the patellar tendon to get a good view of the joint. Sometimes reduction is at first impossible, and only succeeds after one or more wires have been passed circumferentially around the upper end of the tibia, taking great care that they run between the bone and vessels and nerves at the back. Fixation is then with two T-plates, one on each side, sometimes supplemented with nuts and bolts (see Fig. 177).

Fig. 175   *Cleavage fracture (BI 31/22).*

In this case fixation with two screws was sufficient.

Fig. 176   *Impaction fracture (MS 1599).*

The T-plate used as a buttress and cancellous bone grafting.

Fig. 177   *Comminuted fracture of the tibial plateaux (MS 1815).*

If both condyles are broken then it is usually necessary to employ two T-plates. Reduction in this case was achieved with the help of a thick cerclage wire. No screws were inserted through the proximal holes of the plates but they were joined together with nuts and bolts. A massive cancellous bone graft was necessary.

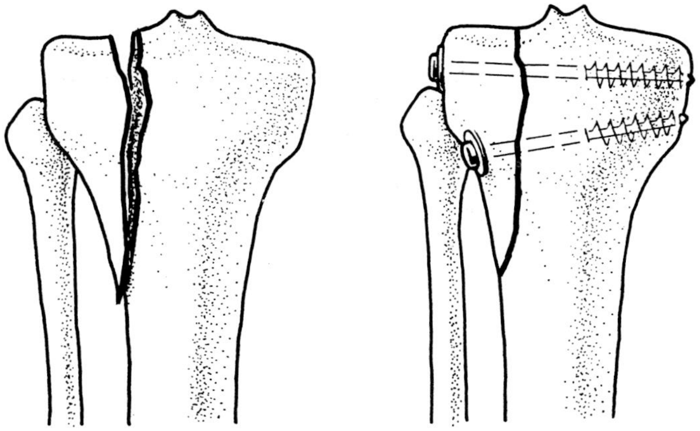

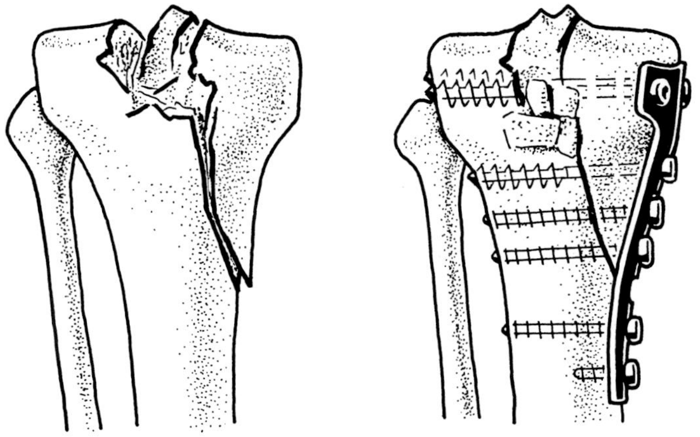

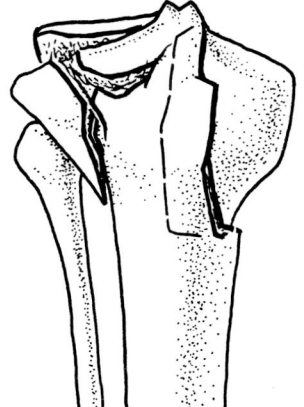
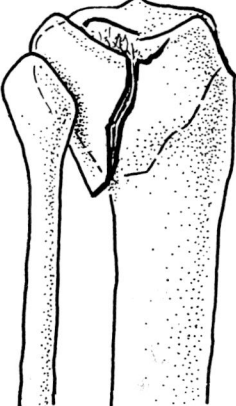
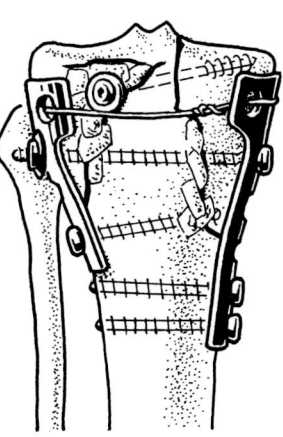

Short Oblique or Transverse Fractures of the Shaft

In the upper shaft short oblique or transverse fractures are best fixed with two plates. One may, for instance, apply a semi-tubular plate on the anterior border and another on the postero-medial border to fix the fracture under compression (Fig. 178). In fractures of the middle third, medullary nailing is the method of choice. In the lower third, a neutralization plate is the best method (Fig. 180b shows how this plate is used).

Spiral and Comminuted Fractures of the Shaft

Pure spiral fractures, in which the length of the fracture line is at least twice the diameter of the bone at that level, provide the chief indication for screw fixation alone to obtain compression between the fragments.

Spiral fractures with butterfly fragments comprise three types according to the location of the butterfly fragment: *anterior, postero-medial and postero-lateral* butterfly fragments. During open reduction and provisional fixation of these fractures, one must find the point where a bone clamp or cerclage wire will grip all three fragments to give temporary fixation. In fractures with an anterior butterfly, reduction forceps will suffice, but in postero-medial or postero-lateral butterflies, cerclage wires are better, as they devitalize the bone less seriously.

Fig. 178   *High, short oblique fractures.*

These can be well fixed with two semi-tubular plates. Excellent fixation is possible with short screws in the cortex of the crest of the tibia, but they cannot be inserted higher than the attachment of the patellar tendon. The anterior plate acts as a tension band. The incision for this is made on the medial surface of the tibia.

Fig. 179   *A simple spiral fracture.*

Reduction is easy with the help of reduction forceps. One must search carefully for incomplete butterfly fragments. (The dotted lines show where fissure lines of incomplete fragments may occur.)

Fig. 180   *Screw fixation of simple butterfly fragments.*

a   The screws are staggered and are inserted at right angles to the long axis of the shaft (see also Fig. 24).

b   *Oblique fractures without a spiral element.* In general, short oblique fractures are best fixed with an intramedullary nail (Fig. 74). If, however, an oblique fracture goes through the upper shaft, or is long or compound, then it is best fixed with a plate. The screw marked with an "X" acts as a lag screw (see also Fig. 52 and 53).

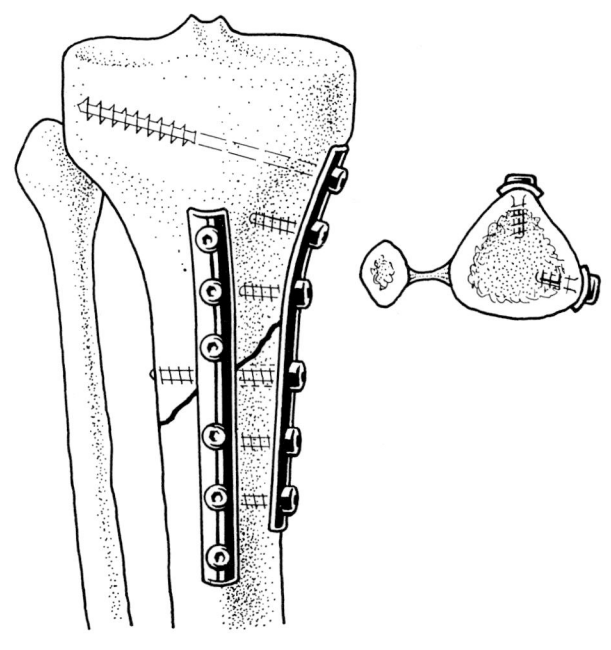

179　　　　　　　　　　　　　　180

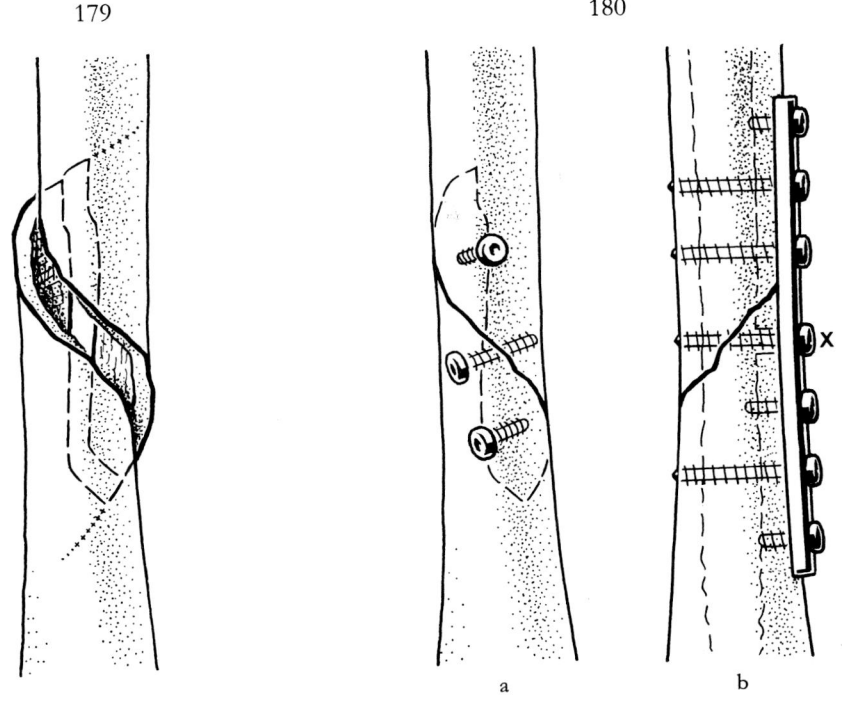

a　　　　　b

Spiral Fracture with Butterfly Fragments

The anterior or antero-lateral butterfly fragments are relatively easy to deal with. If the contact at the fracture between the two main fragments is longer than 3 cm, screws alone are enough. If it is shorter than 3 cm, then a screw between the main fragments will not give enough stability, and the fixation must be supplemented with a neutralization plate.

The posterior butterfly fragment. The most difficult butterfly fragments to deal with are the posterior and postero-lateral ones. The contact between the main fragments is often very slender and lies at the anterior border of the tibia. A compression screw under these circumstances would have to grasp the same cortex twice which is difficult to achieve and does not result in dependable fixation. It is therefore necessary to use a plate to obtain rigid fixation.

Fig. 181   *Screw fixation of an anterior butterfly fragment where there is good contact between the main fragments.*

a, b   The first step is to drill a 3.2 mm hole in the posterolateral cortex of the posterior main fragment. Next, reduce the fracture and hold it with a clamp. Insert the pointed drill guide in the thread hole of the posterior fragment and with its help drill a 4.5 mm gliding hole in the anterior main fragment. Now measure the length of the required screw with the depth gauge and tap the thread in the posterior main fragment. Then insert the screw to hold the two main fragments but do not tighten it. Place one lag screw each between the butterfly fragment and the distal and proximal main fragments using standard lag screw technique. Then tighten all three screws. All these screws are lag screws and when tightened will apply compression between the main fragments.

c   If there is a long area of contact between the two main fragments, more than one screw should be used to fix the main fragments together.

Fig. 182   *The anterior butterfly fragment with poor contact between the main fragments.*
Reduce the fracture and insert two lag screws through the butterfly fragment into the proximal and distal main fragments. Then join the two main fragments with a neutralization plate. (If the cortex of the butterfly fragment, as illustrated in (a) and (b) happens to be thin, use 3.5 mm cortex screws for its fixation.)

Fig. 183   *The postero-lateral butterfly fragment (LHDK).*
A neutralization plate applied to the medial surface of the tibia allows the two main fragments to be joined together, and two lag screws can be inserted through the plate into the postero-lateral butterfly, thus achieving compression between the butterfly and proximal and distal main fragments respectively.

Fig. 184   *The postero-medial butterfly fragment (MHDK).*
This is best fixed by screws inserted through the lateral surface of the tibia. The screws can be passed through the bone directly or through a plate applied to the lateral surface. The advantage of a lateral plate is that it need not be long and only two small screw holes need be made in the already badly devitalized butterfly without causing further damage.
In most cases the contact between the main fragments is so narrow that a neutralization plate is necessary. Lag screws can be inserted through the lateral plate to compress the butterfly against the proximal and distal main fragments.
Another good solution to this problem is to fix the butterfly with lateral lag screws and to apply the neutralization plate medially. Again any screw used to fix the plate that crosses a fracture line should be inserted as a lag screw to increase compression between the fragments. The disadvantage of this method, however, is that the gliding holes for the lag screws have to be made in the butterfly fragment and the butterfly is then more devitalized than in the technically more difficult lateral fixation.

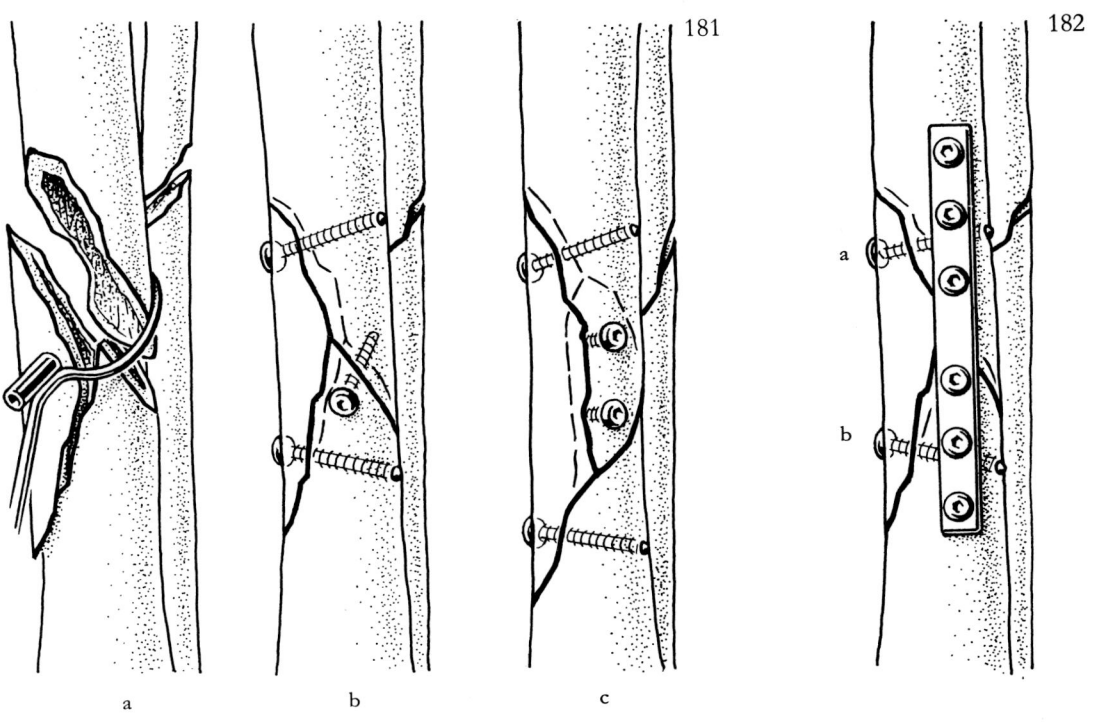

a   b   c

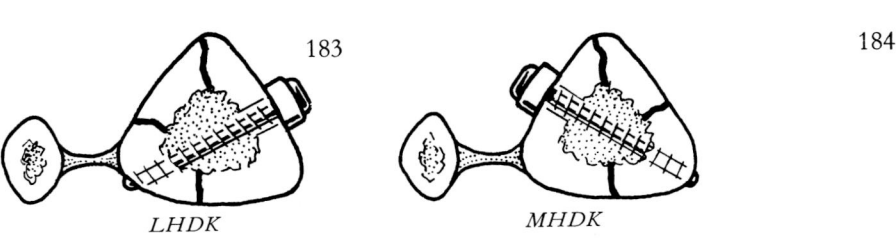

LHDK   MHDK

Comminuted Fractures

The general rule is that the more comminuted the fracture and the less the displacement of the fragments, the greater is the indication for conservative treatment. If, at the end of ten weeks, delayed union is apparent, it is usually found that only one fracture area is involved and this can often be successfully treated with a simple compression plate, leading to quick healing. If it is decided, however, to undertake open reduction and internal fixation in a comminuted fracture, then great care must be taken to operate as atraumatically as possible, which often means a longer incision. For technical details see Fig. 185.

Short Comminuted Fractures of the Shaft of the Tibia

These fractures usually result from high velocity injuries sustained in traffic accidents, and comminution is usually limited to one area of the tibial shaft. In these fractures a single plate will seldom give the required stability because there is a bony defect and the buttressing effect of the cortex opposite the plate is lost. This subjects the plate to bending stresses which are too great for it. It is then best to use two semi-tubular plates, applying one to the anterior and the other to the medial border of the tibia and to fill in the bony defect with autologous cancellous grafts (Fig. 186).

Fig. 185   *The technique of open reduction and internal fixation of a comminuted fracture.*

a–e   In the open reduction of these difficult fractures we have discontinued cerclage wiring for temporary fixation as it causes damage to the bony fragments. Posterior and lateral muscle attachments are preserved if possible. Beginning with the main fragments, the fracture is assembled like a jig-saw puzzle, drilling a thread hole here, a gliding hole there as indicated (see Fig. 49), until the whole fracture is reduced and held together with screws. Only at the end, when all the fragments have been reduced and the reduction is satisfactory, are all the screws tightened up. The procedure is completed by bridging the comminuted area with a neutralization plate.

There is often a long fragment bridging the comminuted segments. Reduction and temporary fixation is then much easier, because it is often only necessary to oppose this large fragment to the two main ones and secure temporary fixation with two reduction forceps, or one reduction forceps and a cerclage wire. When this is achieved, all that remains is to fix the fragments systematically with screws, and bridge the fracture with a neutralization plate.

Fig. 186   *Short, comminuted fractures of the shaft of the tibia.*

a, b   No fragment should be sacrificed when it is clear where it should fit. Small avascular cortical fragments, on the other hand, are best discarded and replaced with cancellous bone. This type of fracture area is then best bridged with two semi-tubular plates, one applied to the anterior and one to the medial border of the tibia. (A semi-tubular plate can also be combined with a narrow plate.)

186

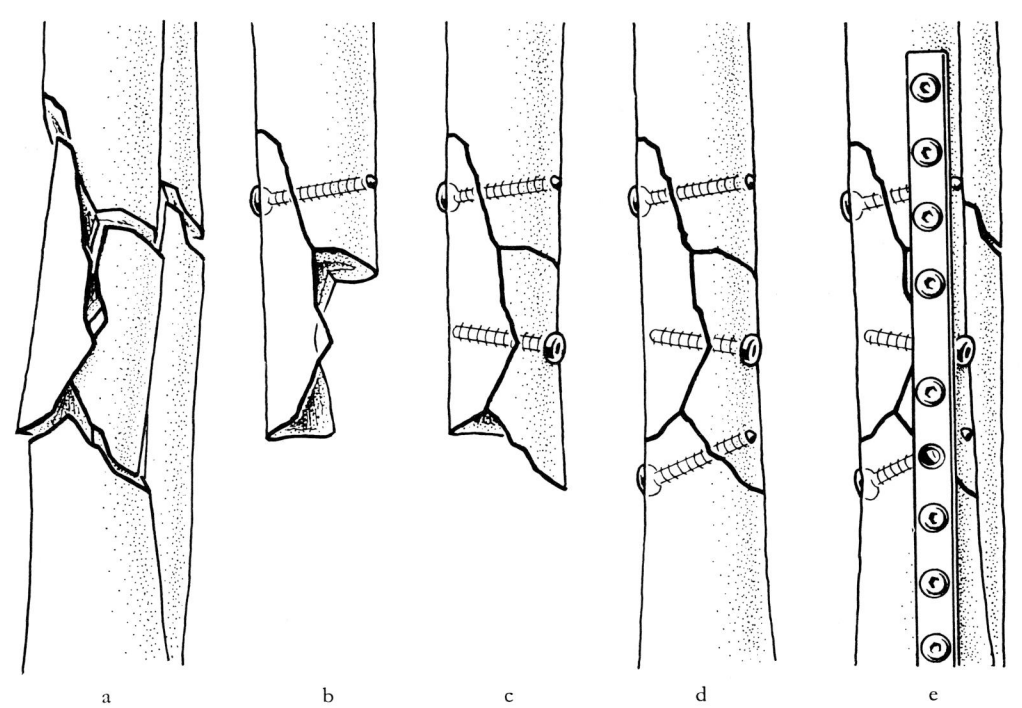

a   b   c   d   e

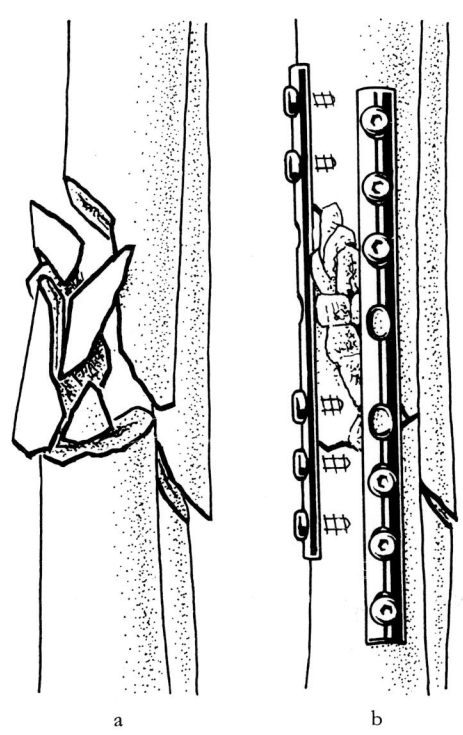

a   b

Fractures of the Lower Third of the Tibia

The general principles apply to these fractures as well. Long fracture lines can again be simply fixed with screws but in this region it is better to supplement fixation with a neutralization plate. It is important to remember that the contour of the tibia in this area is not uniform and the plate will often need to be bent and twisted (see p. 60). If this is done in such a way that a small space occurs between the plate and the bone, then, when the screws are tightened, axial compression of the fracture surfaces will result. This additional axial compression greatly increases the rigidity of the fixation.

Fractures of the Lower Tibia Involving the Ankle Joint

Approach: Both a medial and lateral incision are needed so that the articular surface of the tibia can be fully visualized (see Fig. 200). We have found the following four steps to be most helpful:

1. a) Most of these fractures are associated with a relatively simple fracture of the fibula. Reduction of the fibula often re-aligns the tibial fragments and indicates the correct length of the fibula and the tibia (Fig. 187a and b).

   b) When the lower end of the fibula is comminuted or in the rare cases where the fibula is intact but a tibio-fibular diastasis is present, there is usually a medial or lateral piece of the lower end of the tibia which is the key fragment. The reduction of this fragment will provide the correct length and the axial alignment and will allow the correct reduction of the remaining fragments.

2. Once the length and alignment of the tibia are restored, reconstruction of the articular surface of the tibia can be begun. It is important to obtain a good medial exposure so that the whole joint surface of the medial malleolus and the lower end of the tibia can

---

Fig. 187

a	The tubercle of Chaput usually remains attached to the fibula.
b	In eighty percent of cases reduction of the fibula results in reduction of the fracture of the tibia. A simple transverse or oblique fracture of the fibula should therefore be reduced as the first step of the whole manoeuvre. If the fracture of the fibula is comminuted or high up in the shaft, then the first step is to reconstruct the tibial component.
c	Reconstruction of the articular surface of the tibia is carried out, using the upper surface of the talus as a mould. Kirschner wires are used for temporary fixation of these fragments.
d	The medial cortex is buttressed with a contoured narrow plate or a T-plate to prevent secondary varus displacement. The impaction of the cancellous bone in the metaphysis leaves a defect which must be filled with cancellous bone grafts.
e	To help in the regeneration of articular cartilage of the joint, early mobilization must be begun but weight bearing delayed for at least five months. The patellar tendon weight bearing caliper is useful in these cases because, after a short period of training, the patient can walk without crutches.

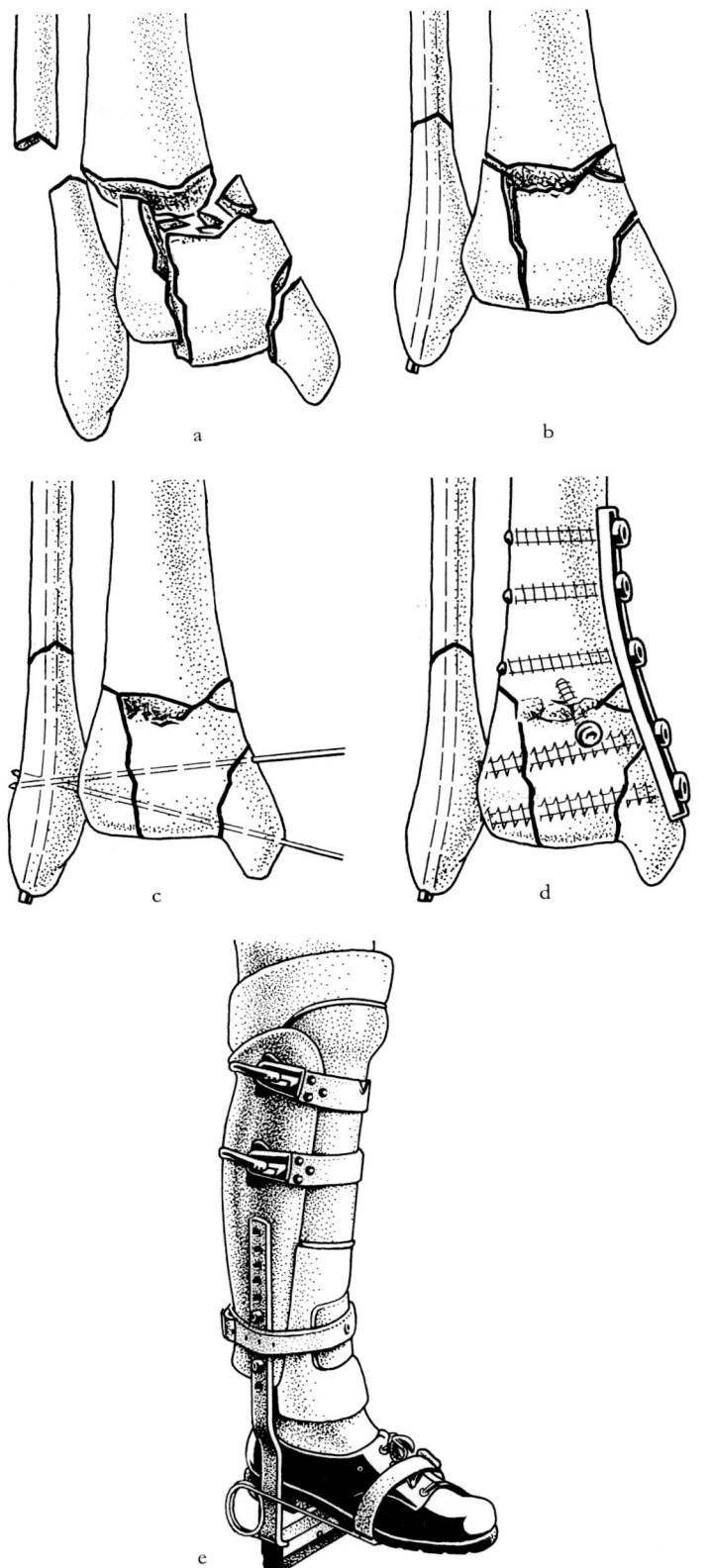

be seen. This enables one to assemble the small articular fragments and place them on top of the talus which can then act as a mould and they can then be trans-fixed with Kirschner wires for temporary stabilization (see Fig. 187c).

3.   Autologous cancellous bone is used to fill in the defect in the metaphysis, and this bone may be obtained from the greater trochanter on the same side. This cancellous graft not only fills in the defect, but buttresses the articular fragments while they rest on the upper surface of the talus (Fig. 187c).

4.   A medial plate must be used to act as a buttress to prevent the fracture from drifting into varus (Fig. 187b). The T-plate is useful for this.

The post-operative management of this type of fracture must involve early movement but weight bearing should not be allowed for at least five months. At the end of the operation the ankle is put up at 90° and held in position with a U-splint. In this position the patient can begin active dorsiflexion exercises. During the long period of non—weight bearing, the patellar tendon weight bearing caliper has been found most useful (Fig. 187e).

Double Fractures of the Tibia

Approach: In most cases a single long incision is required to expose both fractures. (If there is a very long middle fragment, two small incisions may be made, especially if one fracture requires only screw fixation.)

Basic rules for dealing with segmental fractures:

1. The middle fragment must never be allowed to lose its posterior and lateral soft tissue attachments, and there should be great care to avoid unnecessary stripping of bone.

2. Good results are almost always achieved with these fractures by using interfragmental compression screw fixation combined with a long neutralization plate to bridge the middle fragment. It is also helpful if axial compression can be obtained through the neutralization plate.

3. Only one or two long screws should transfix the middle fragment. The remaining screws should penetrate only one cortex.

4. Intramedullary nailing with reaming is definitely contra-indicated because the reamer can spin the middle fragment, shearing off all its soft tissue attachments. Intramedullary nailing with a thin nail can be considered, but this provides poor rotational stability in the upper fragment.

Fig. 188   *The procedures used in segmental fractures of the tibia.*

a   A fracture of the upper end should be fixed with two plates.

b   Showing two short or oblique fractures.

c   Short fracture combined with a spiral fracture.

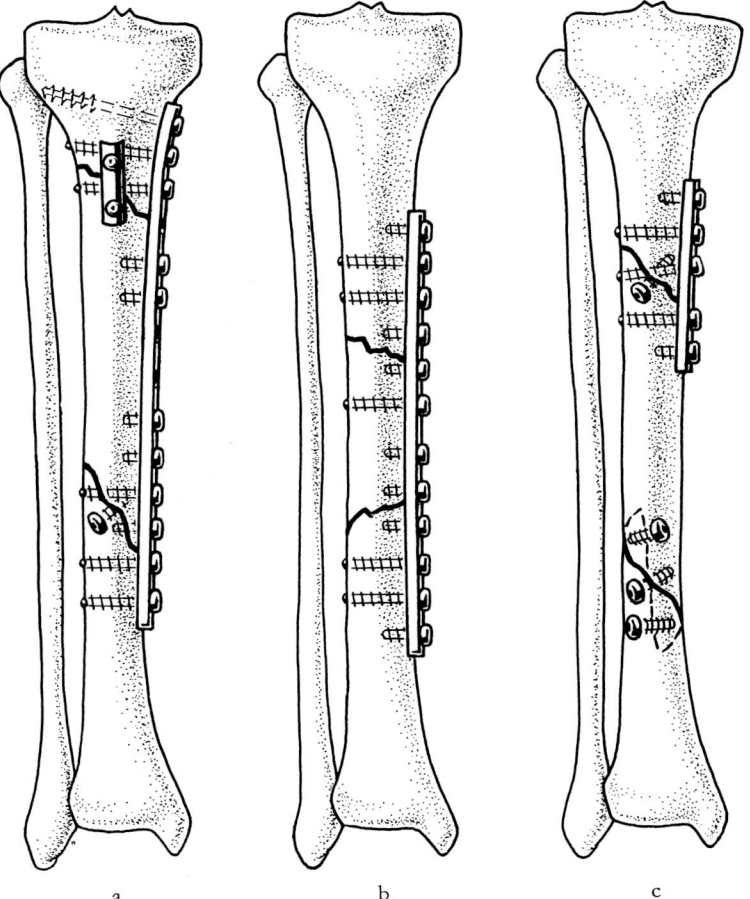

a   b   c

K. Malleolar Fractures

1. Malleolar fractures are intra-articular and result from subluxation or dislocation of the talus out of the ankle mortice.

2. The reconstruction of ankle mortice and the subsequent healing of all bony and ligamentous injuries in their correct functional position are the prerequisites of subsequent normal ankle function.

3. The ankle mortice depends on:
   a) The correct length of the fibula (Fig. 193).
   b) The integrity of the anterior and posterior tibio-fibular ligaments (Fig. 189).
   Thus, because of its biomechanical importance, the fibula, with its taut elastic attachment to the tibia via the ligaments of the syndesmosis and interosseous membrane, takes absolute priority over the medial malleolus.

4. By and large, perfect ankle mortice can only be achieved dependably by operative means. Therefore, as long as there are no general or local contra-indications in the shape of vascular insufficiency or fracture blisters etc., open reduction and internal fixation is almost always carried out.

5. To make a correct diagnosis in malleolar fractures, one must learn to recognize all the bony and ligamentous injuries. Damage to the tibio-fibular ligament can be deduced from the level of the fibular fracture. A fracture of the fibula at the level of the ankle joint or distal to this, is never associated with a lesion of the syndesmosis. By contrast, a fracture of the fibula above this level is always associated with a lesion of either the anterior or posterior tibio-fibular ligament. These facts have led to a logical classification of ankle fractures. DANIS classified them into four groups. WEBER has listed three separate groups: named A, B, C (Fig. 192), and the last group includes both numbers three and four of DANIS.

6. To make the diagnosis in malleolar fractures two X-rays are needed, an a.p. and a lateral projection centered on the ankle joint. The a.p. must be taken with the leg in 20° of internal rotation, to compensate for the 20° of external rotation of the ankle joint axis. If a lesion of the tubercle of Chaput is suspected, then a 45° oblique projection must be taken. Stress films are needed to demonstrate ligamentous injuries.

7. Besides lesions to the malleoli and ligaments, one must remember the avulsion or shear osteochondral or chondral fractures of the talus. These must always be sought on the X-ray films and when examining the ankle joint at operation, since loose fragments inside the joint may lead to very early post-traumatic arthritis.

Anatomical Aspects

The skeleton and ligaments of the ankle joint form a functional unit. A thorough knowledge of the ligamentous apparatus is of utmost importance, and there are two groups of ligaments that must be distinguished.

A. The tibio-fibular ligaments which maintain the taut elasticity of the ankle mortice.

    a) Those at the level of the ankle joint (inferior tibio-fibular ligament). Anteriorly the ligament is slender and runs from the tubercle of Tillaux-Chaput on the tibia to the fibula.
    Posteriorly the ligament is strong.
    b) Proximal to the syndesmosis lies the interosseous membrane.

B. The collateral ligaments which control the talus.

    The medial collateral ligament: The double layered triangular deltoid ligament. The lateral collateral ligament. It is composed of three parts: the anterior fibulo-talar ligament, the fibulo-calcaneal ligament, and the posterior fibulo-talar ligament.

Fig. 189   *The anatomy of the collateral ligaments as seen from in front and behind.*

    a   The anterior ligament of the syndesmosis = the anterior tibio-fibular ligament.

    b   The posterior ligament of the syndesmosis = the posterior tibio-fibular ligament.

    c   The interosseous membrane.

Fig. 190   *The collateral ligaments of the ankle joint.*

    a   The three parts of the lateral ligament.

    b   The three bands of the medial collateral ligament (the deltoid ligament).

Fig. 191   *A cross section through the syndesmosis.*
                  The fibula fits exactly into the fibular notch of the tibia and is held in place by means of the syndesmotic ligaments.

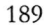

189

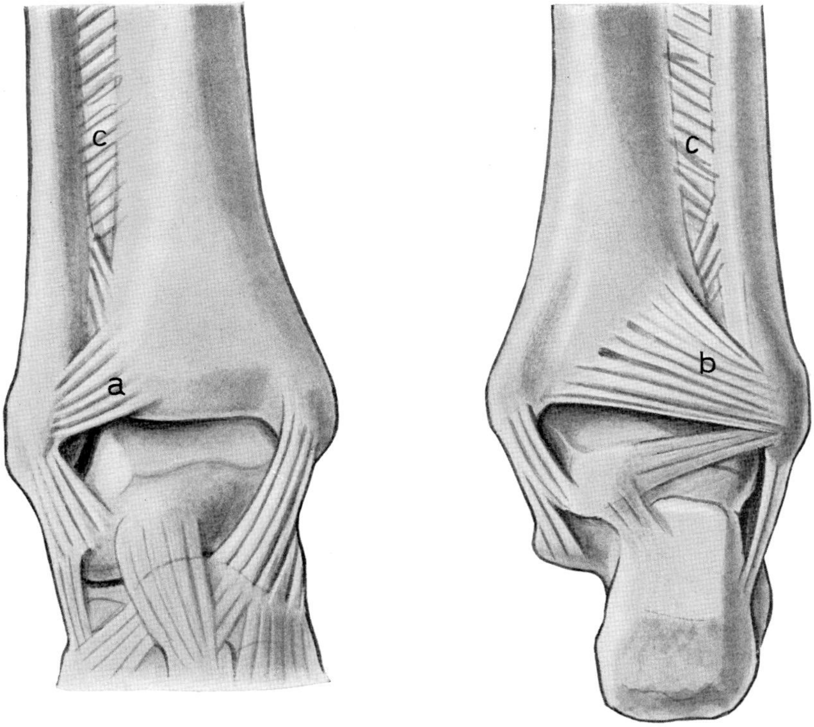

190

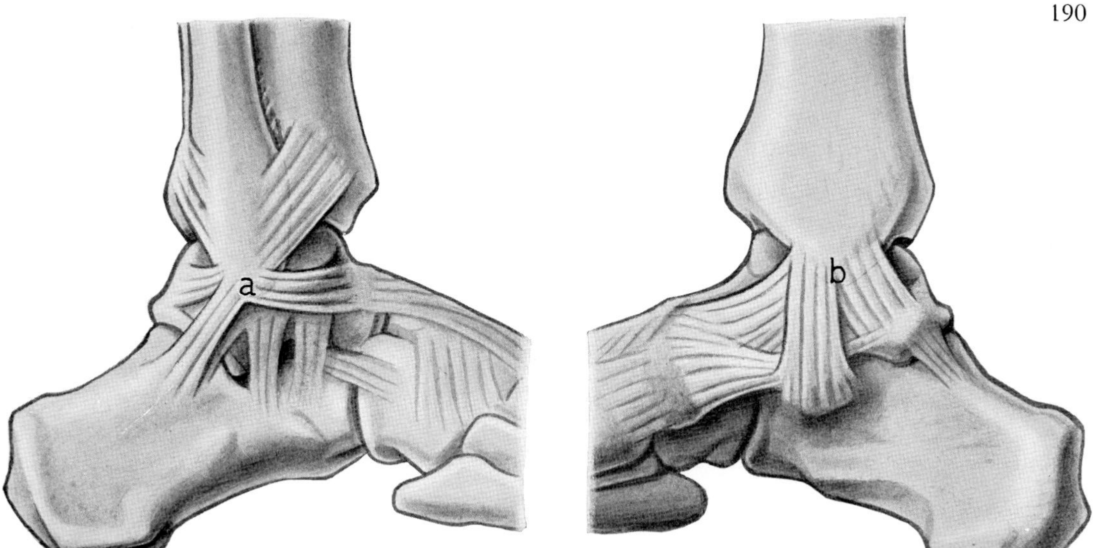

191

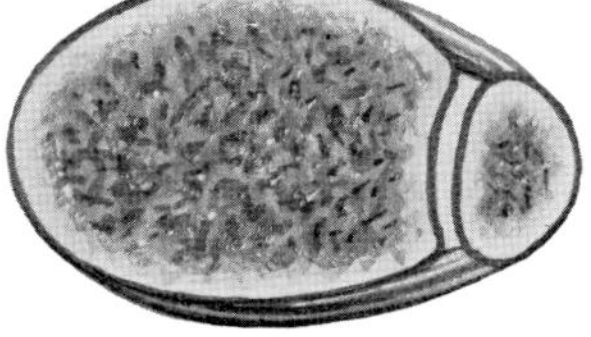

195

Classification of Malleolar Fractures

The higher the fibular fracture, the greater is the damage to the tibio-fibular syndesmosis and the greater the danger of major inefficiency of the ankle mortice. Three basic fracture types are distinguished:

Type A: Fracture of the fibula at the level of the ankle joint or distal (an equivalent injury is rupture of the lateral collateral ligament, which can only be diagnosed on a stress film) with or without a shear fracture of the medial malleolus.

Ligamentous injuries: These are never present in this type. The syndesmosis, interosseous membrane and the deltoid ligament are never involved.

Type B: A spiral fracture of the fibula level with the syndesmosis with or without an avulsion fracture of the medial malleolus or an equivalent rupture of the deltoid ligament.

Ligamentous injuries in this type: Usually associated with disruption of the anterior syndesmosis or its avulsion, and a tear of the deltoid ligament if the medial malleolus remains intact.

Type C: A fracture of the fibula anywhere above the syndesmosis, even as high as the head of the fibula. On the medial side this injury is always associated either with a rupture of the deltoid ligament or avulsion of the medial malleolus.

Ligamentous injuries: Total disruption of the syndesmosis either by tearing of the ligaments or their avulsion, varying degrees of damage to the interosseous membrane, and rupture of the deltoid ligament if the medial malleolus remains intact.

It is important to appreciate that all three types, irrespective of the malleolar element, may be associated with a posterior fragment of the tibia which can be small or large. In type A the posterior fragment is medial, adjoining the medial malleolus. The posterior syndesmosis remains intact. By contrast, in types B, and C, the posterior fragment is lateral, adjoining the lateral malleolus. It always retains its attachment to the lower fibular fragment via the posterior syndesmotic ligament which always remains intact.

Ruptures of the deltoid ligament: This is impossible in type A, but certain in type C, if the medial malleolus is not fractured. In type B, the deltoid ligament may be ruptured if the medial malleolus remains intact. A stress X-ray is necessary to prove it.

The extent of ligamentous damage progresses in severity from types A, to B, to C. The severity of the fracture of the malleoli parallels the severity of the ligamentous injuries.

Fig. 192   *Classification of malleolar fractures.*

Type A: Transverse fracture of the fibula at the level of the ankle joint or below. Possible shear fracture of the medial malleolus.

Type B: Spiral fracture of the fibula level with the syndesmosis, with partial rupture of anterior syndesmosis, with or without rupture of the deltoid ligament, depending on the presence or absence of avulsion fracture of the medial malleolus.

Type C:
a) Oblique fracture of the fibula immediately above the syndesmosis, rupture of the anterior syndesmotic ligament though its substance or at its insertion, and avulsion of the posterior triangle from the tibia (DANIS, group 3).
b) High comminuted fracture of the fibula with tearing of the interosseous membrane and both ligaments of the syndesmosis. If the fracture goes through the head of the fibula, it is called MAISONNEUVE's fracture (DANIS, type 4).

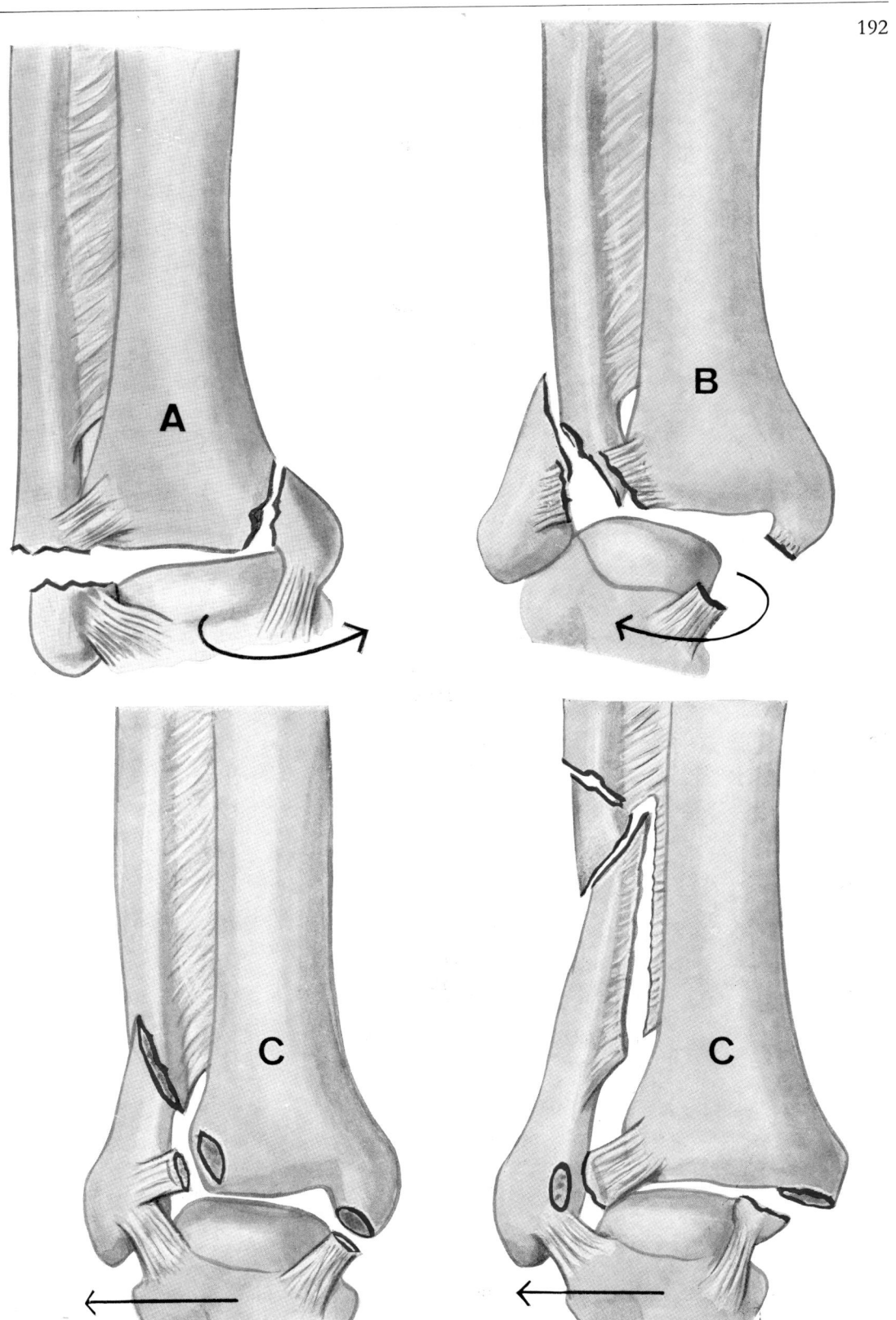

Principles of the Operation

In malleolar fractures, exact anatomical reconstruction of the fibula is mechanically of first importance, and for this reason the fibula must take priority.

The fibula fits into the notch of the tibia only when it is in its full length (Fig. 193). The ligaments of the syndesmosis (anterior and posterior tibio-fibular ligaments) and the interosseous membrane, the two structures responsible for holding together the ankle mortice, will only heal at their proper length and tension if the fibula is restored to its normal length, axial alignment and rotation.

Open reduction and internal fixation therefore must begin with an attack on the lateral malleolus, which must be anatomically reduced and rigidly fixed. The next step is to repair the anterior syndesmosis and if necessary protect it temporarily. The lateral side of the ankle mortice must be reconstructed before beginning on the medial side. A medial reconstruction may involve reduction and fixation of the medial malleolus, or repair of a torn deltoid ligament, and if necessary reduction and internal fixation of the posterior triangular lip fragment from the tibia.

Internal Fixation of Lateral Malleolus

Internal fixation of the lower end of the fibula should be done with a minimum amount of metal. The type of internal fixation depends on the type of fracture that is involved.

Fig. 193   *A cross section through the inferior tibio-fibular joint at the level of the syndesmosis.*

a   The fibula fits into the notch of the tibia only if it is of normal length.

b   If the fibula is shortened, the broader part of the lateral malleolus engages with the fibular notch of the tibia. This notch is too small and the ankle mortice remains permanently widened.

Fig. 194   *Method of internal fixation of the lateral malleolus.*

a   The avulsed tip of the lateral malleolus is fixed with two Kirschner wires and a figure of eight tension band wire. When this fragment is very small it can be fixed with a tension band wire alone.

b   A short oblique fracture of the lateral malleolus can be stabilized with a single malleolar screw inserted from the tip of the malleolus upwards, to lie obliquely in two planes. It must penetrate one cortex of bone proximally.

c   A long spiral fracture just above the syndesmosis can be fixed with two 4.0 mm cancellous screws.

d   A short spiral fracture of the lateral malleolus can be stabilized with a thick Kirschner wire and a single cerclage wire. The Kirschner wire must be bent 2.5 cm from its tip, to correspond to the lateral bend of the malleolus.

e   A short spiral fracture can also be fixed with one 4.0 mm cancellous screw and one cerclage wire.

f   A high transverse fracture is fixed with one thick medullary Kirschner wire.

g   A fracture of the fibular shaft can be stabilized with a small semi-tubular plate.

h   A comminuted lateral malleolus is buttressed with a contoured small semi-tubular plate.

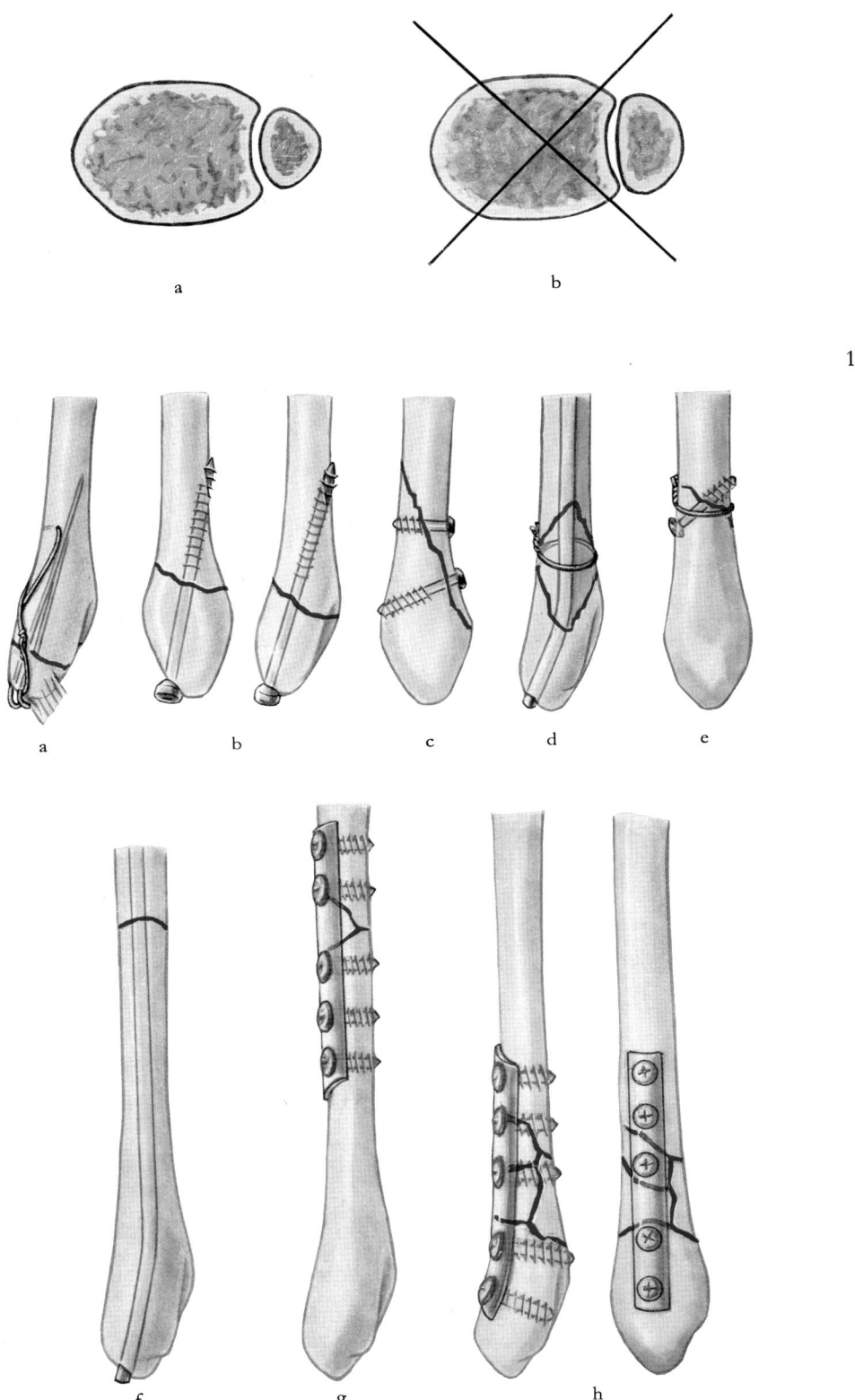

Stabilization of the Syndesmosis

A torn anterior syndesmosis should be repaired by suture or, if it has been avulsed from either tibia or fibula, it may be screwed back with a small cancellous screw. If the interosseous membrane has been torn in addition, the repair of the syndesmosis must be protected temporarily by further stabilization of the fibula.

Fig. 195	The anterior tibio-fibular ligament can be ruptured at three points.
a	At its mid point.
b	It can be avulsed from its insertion into the tibia (avulsion of the tubercle of Tillaux-Chaput) or,
c	it can be avulsed from its insertion into the fibula (Le Fort-Wagstaffe).
Fig. 196	With a high fibular fracture the repaired syndesmosis may be protected in three different ways:
a	Internal fixation of the fibular fracture with a small semi-tubular plate and screws, reduction and fixation with a cancellous screw of the avulsed tubercle of Chaput, and reduction and fixation of the avulsed posterior tibial triangle. No additional protection of the syndesmosis repair is then needed.
b	Intramedullary nailing of the fibula, and suture of the torn anterior syndemosis. A small fragment avulsed from the back of the tibia is not screwed back. Here, however, the syndesmotic repair has to be protected. This is done with a so-called position screw, which is a cortex one for which the thread is tapped in both fibula and tibia, so that it does not act as a lag screw.
c	If the whole interosseous membrane has been disrupted, as for instance in a very high fracture of the fibula, and the posterior syndemosis is not repaired, then one or even two position screws are needed. All the position screws must be removed at the end of six weeks.
Fig. 197	If a ligament of the syndesmosis has been torn it should not be repaired by simply transfixing the inferior tibio-fibular joint with a transverse or oblique screw, as this may so disturb the ligament of the syndesmosis that early post traumatic osteoarthritis may occur. If this method is used, the screw should be removed at the end of a month.

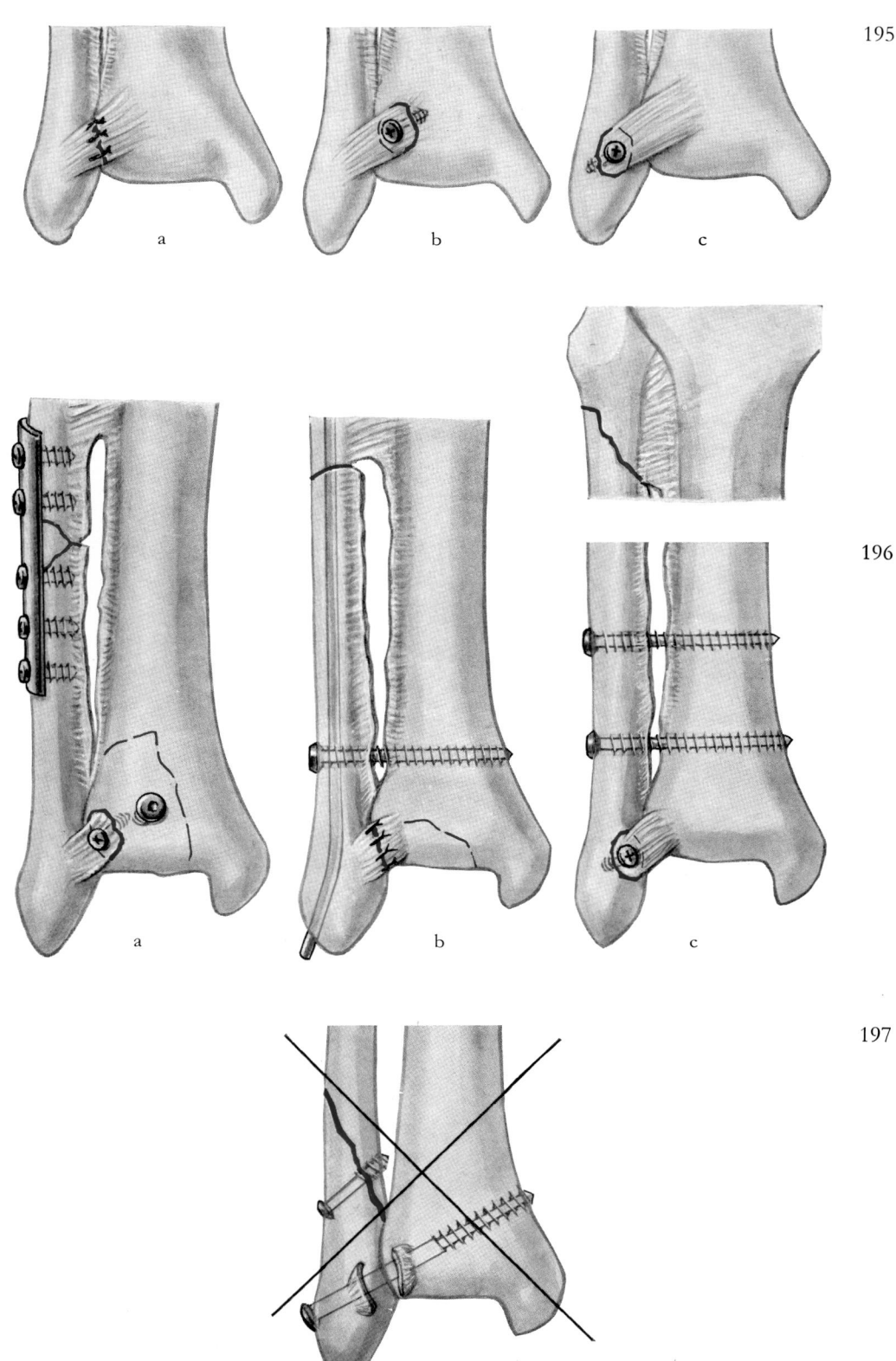

a   b   c

a   b   c

Internal Fixation of the Medial Malleolus and the "Posterior Malleolus" or Posterior Lip Fragment

A single medial incision should be used to expose the fracture of the medial malleolus or a tear of the deltoid ligament and the posterior lip fracture of the tibia. Both may be exposed, reduced and stabilized through this single incision.

Fig. 198

    a   A hemi-cerclage wire is used to fix a small avulsion fragment.

    b   A larger avulsion fragment is fixed with two Kirschner wires and a figure of eight tension band wire.

    c   A larger avulsion fragment fixed with two screws.

    d   A larger fragment, sheared off, is also stabilized with two screws.

Fig. 199   *Internal fixation of the posterior lip fracture of the tibia.*

    a   If this fragment is medial, close to the medial malleolus (type A injury), it is screwed directly from back to front.

    b   If the fragment lies near to the lateral malleolus (type B, and C, injuries) it is screwed from front to back. It is fixed with a cancellous screw, introduced at right angles to the axis of the tibia.

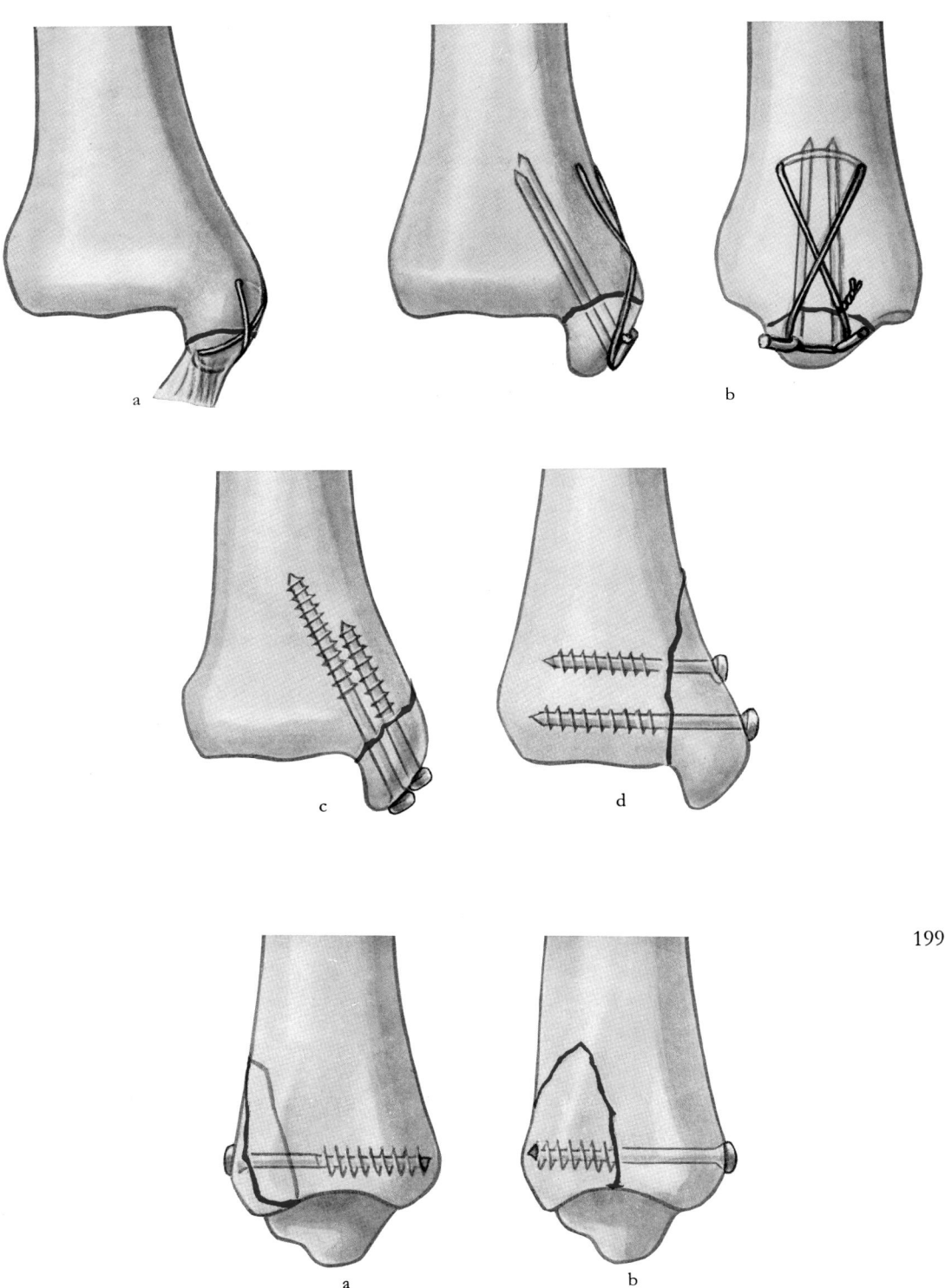

a

b

c

d

a

b

Surgical Exposures

Fig. 200   *Surgical exposure of malleolar fractures.*

1   Exposure of the lateral malleolus and the anterior syndesmosis. The incision runs parallel to the superficial peroneal nerve (musculo-cutaneous nerve) and must not damage this. This incision exposes the anterior border of the fibula and the anterior syndesmosis. Internal fixation of the lateral malleolus is then possible with the least amount of stripping of the malleolus.

2   The standard incision for internal fixation of the medial malleolus. If the anterior capsule of the ankle joint is incised via this incision, the intra-articular aspect of the reduction of the medial malleolus can be seen, as well as the ankle joint.

3   The incision for simultaneous exposure of the medial malleolus and of the posterior tibial triangle.

4   The incision used to expose the posterior syndesmosis and a large triangular fragment from the tibia associated with a fibular fracture. The patient lies in the prone position.

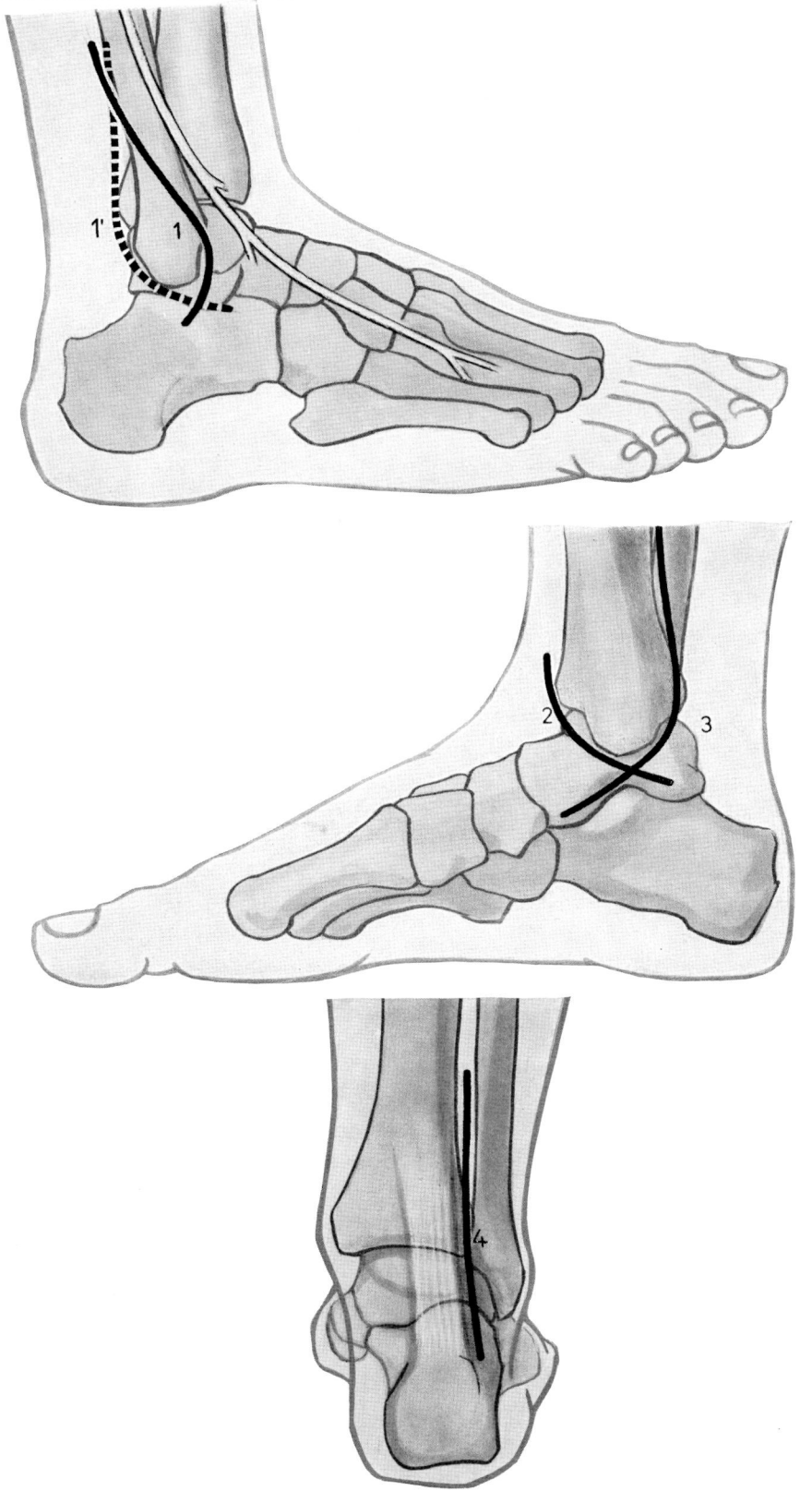

Examples. Simple Malleolar Fractures

Examples of some simple malleolar fractures.

Fig. 201   *Comminuted fracture of the tip of the lateral malleolus (MS 1919).*

The small fragments are transfixed by two Kirschner wires. A supplementary figure of eight tension band wire is used (type A).

Fig. 202   *A bi-malleolar fracture (MS 1933).*

The lateral malleolus is fixed with one malleolar screw running obliquely in two planes. The tip of the screw penetrates the medial cortex of the upper fragment. The medial malleolus is fixed with either a single cancellous screw or two malleolar screws.

Fig. 203   *A spiral fracture of the lateral malleolus at the level of the syndesmosis (MS 446).*

The fixation is done with a 4.0 mm cancellous screw and a cerclage wire. The avulsed tubercle of Chaput has been screwed back with a 4.0 mm cancellous screw (type B).

Fig. 204   *A long fibular fracture above the syndesmosis.*

The fracture is first fixed with two 4.0 mm cancellous or two 3.5 mm cortex screws. In addition, the anterior syndesmosis is sutured (type C).

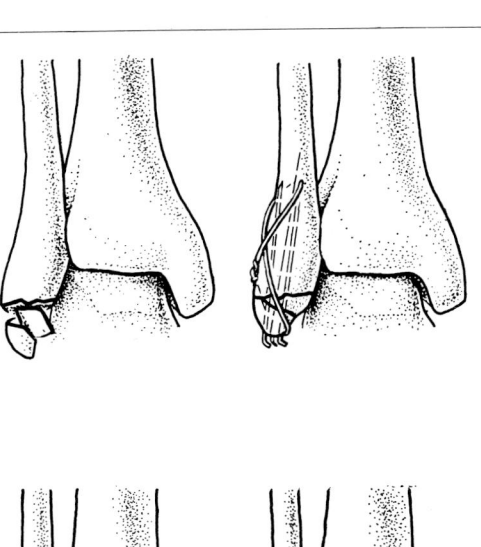

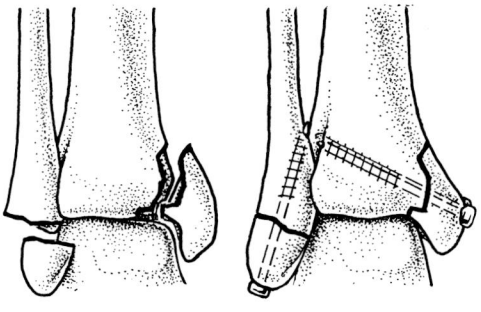

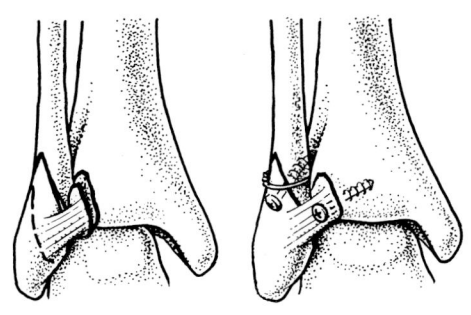

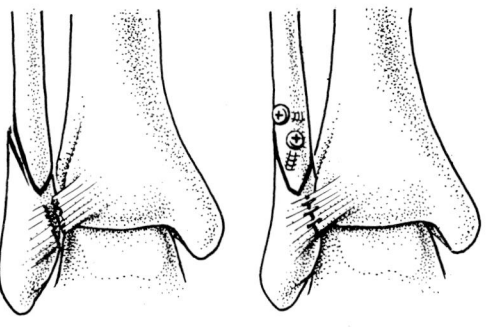

Post-operative Management

After operation all malleolar fractures are drained by suction for 48 hours, and the leg is elevated for four to six days. The leg is immobilized in a plaster splint (Fig. 85a) with the ankle at 90°. After 48 hours, while still in the splint, the patient begins active dorsiflexion exercises of the ankle.

Once the plaster splint is removed, active movement of the ankle is begun and it usually takes about eight days before full range is regained. At about two weeks, partial weight bearing is begun. From now on, post operative management must be made to fit the severity of the initial injury and the rigidity of internal fixation which was achieved at the operation. Thus, a patient is either given a removable splint or a below knee plaster for six to eight weeks.

At the end of this time, if the patient has a position screw, this is removed and only now is full weight bearing allowed.

As a rule, malleolar fractures need ten to twelve weeks to unite and by this time the ankle has regained full function.

Metal may be removed at the end of three months and this can often be done under local anaesthesia, using small stab incisions. Tension band wires are the only things that need a more major re-opening of the wound.

Fracture dislocations of the ankle joint.

Fig. 205   *Fracture dislocation of the ankle joint with comminution of a porotic lateral malleolus (MS 1836).*

The comminuted lateral malleolus is stabilized with a small semi-tubular plate. The avulsed anterior syndesmosis is fixed back to the fibula with a 4.0 mm cancellous screw. The medial malleolus is fixed with two malleolar screws (type B).

Fig. 206   *MS 1899.*

The lateral malleolus is fixed with two 4.0 mm cancellous screws. The anterior syndesmosis is repaired with nylon. The large posterior triangular fragment is fixed with a cancellous screw introduced from front to back, and the medial malleolus is fixed with one malleolar screw (type B).

Fig. 207   A similar case to Fig. 206, but the posterior fragment of the tibia is much larger. In this case because the fragment is large it is fixed with two cancellous screws.

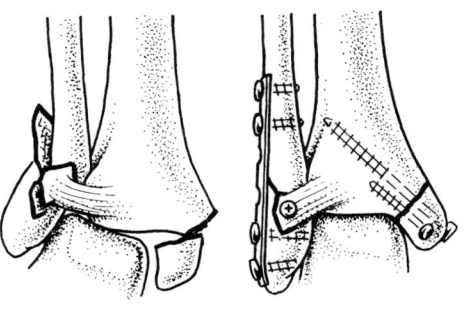

205

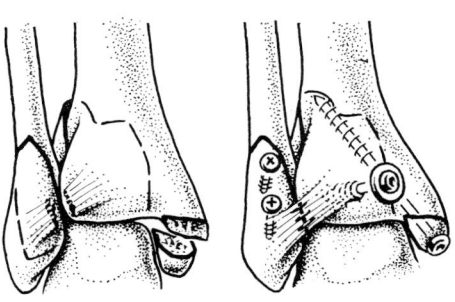

206

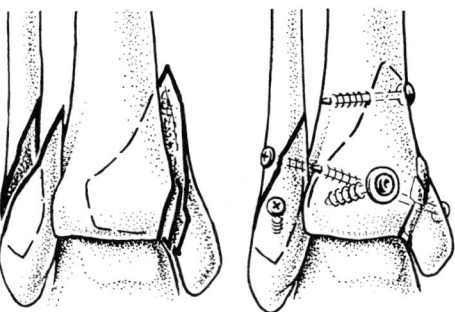

207

II. Compound Fractures in the Adult

Definitive internal fixation of compound fractures in the adult is undertaken either within the first six to eight hours or is deferred for one to three weeks while soft tissue healing takes place. If definitive internal fixation is deferred, temporary fixation of the fracture should be undertaken. If primary internal fixation is decided upon during the first six to eight hours, the surgeon should remember that two-thirds of all compound fractures fail to provide a positive swab culture from the depth of the wound. About one-third of wounds are contaminated. Infections occur when necrotic tissue is left in the wound, as this provides a nidus for bacterial multiplication. Thus, in all compound fractures, secondary hospital infections with resistent bacteria are more of a real problem than primary infection of the wound at the time of the injury.

When treating compound fractures, the surgeon must weigh the pros and cons of trying to prevent a primary wound infection at the time of admission to hospital, and the possibility of secondary hospital infection because of skin necrosis.

The following points are important:

1. The primary wound dressing must be left untouched until it can be removed in a completely aseptic environment. The wound must never be inspected by non-medical personnel or without wearing a mask. If a patient arrives in the emergency department without a dressing on a compound wound, then a sterile dressing should be applied at once.

2. The majority of compound wounds are left open. Even the wounds of fractures compounded from within are left alone. Where there is much skin and muscle contusion, even the surgical wound is left open and simply covered with tulle gauze. Five to eight days later a secondary suture is undertaken or, if this is not possible, a split skin graft applied between ten and twenty days on to the fresh granulations.

3. If primary internal fixation has been undertaken, the minimum amount of metal should be used, as metal should never be inserted under damaged tissue or left exposed to the air.

Classification of compound fractures:

Compound fractures are divided into three grades according to the degree of soft tissue damage.

Grade I: Compounded from within by a bone fragment (about 60%).

Grade II: Compounded from without with skin and muscle contusion (about 30%).

Grade III: Extensive skin and muscle damage with comminuted fractures and often with associated lesions of vessels or nerves, as in a fracture due to a gunshot wound (about 10%).

The following principles of treatment have stood the test of time:

Grade I compound fractures: If the wound does not interfere with a standard surgical approach for the fracture involved, then a clean surgical incision is made at a distance from the wound and the wound left open without débridement. If this is not possible, the wound is extended and the bone is rigidly fixed, as in a simple fracture. In fractures of the tibia we usually secure fixation with lag screws between fragments and a neutralization plate. The skin is closed primarily as above.

Grade II compound fractures: The first step is débridement, which consists of careful excision of all necrotic subcutaneous tissue and muscle. All instruments are discarded. The skin is freshly disinfected, the gown and gloves are changed and a new operation with new instruments is begun. No implant must be left exposed nor should it be covered by devitalized tissue (e.g. contused subcutaneous tissue). No screw should be inserted in such a way that later soft tissue necrosis might expose the screw tip, as might happen in a plate fitted on the posterior surface of the tibia. After internal fixation the skin is almost always left open, and simply covered with tulle gauze. The limb is immobilized in plaster splint, and a delayed primary suture is carried out at five to eight days.

Grade III compound fractures: These wounds are treated like war wounds. The wound is extended in the long axis of the limb, upwards and downwards over some distance. All necrotic tissue is excised, and fascia, especially over closed compartments such as the anterior tibial, is incised. A second operation then follows, as in Grade II fractures. The least amount of metal that can be used is employed and is always left covered by healthy tissue. Cut nerves are approximated with marking sutures and vessels are either tied off or repaired as may be needed. The limb is not placed in plaster as in Grade II injuries, but is suspended on a splint to facilitate wound care. A severe compound fracture of the tibia for instance, is treated by inserting a Steinmann pin through the os calcis and another through the tibial tubercle, and the leg is suspended on a metal frame.

Before beginning the treatment of a compound fracture the surgeon must ask himself the following questions:

1. *The timing of surgery.* We operate on compound fractures usually within the first six to eight hours. After ten hours we speak of "deferred urgency". Such cases are operated upon on the third or fourth day whenever possible, using a separate incision without touching the original wound. A third possibility is to treat the fracture in traction and carry out the internal fixation between one and four weeks later.

2. *Antibiotic prophylaxis.* The more often we leave wounds open, the less we use local antibiotics. We have also given up local irrigation drainage.

Some AO members start an intravenous infusion at the time of admission with 20–40 mega units of Penicillin and 1 gram of Streptomycin and maintain this daily for five to six days. Other AO members, however, are completely opposed to any type of antibiotic prophylaxis, with the exception perhaps of Grade III compound grossly contaminated wounds. During the actual operation, however irrigation of the wound is undertaken with a Neomycin-Bacitracin-Ringer solution.

3. *Internal fixation.* In compound fractures of the tibia of Grade II or Grade III, a plate is never applied to the medial surface of the tibia but always on the lateral or posterior surface. If intramedullary nailing is carried out, it is done without reaming and only a thin nail is used. After three to five weeks re-nailing is carried out. After intramedullary nailing the nail must never shine in the depth of the wound. If there is any bone defect which exposes the nail, it must be filled with cancellous bone grafts to cover the nail completely.

4. *Relaxing incisions.* In Grade I compound fractures the incisions are closed at the end of the procedure. Occasionally edema will prevent a tension-free primary wound closure, and then a posterior relaxing incision should be made (Fig. 211) or, perhaps better, a series of small 4–6 mm long stab incisions, between ten and twenty in number, through the skin on both sides of the suture line. In Grade II and III compound fractures, primary closure of the wound is seldom undertaken and therefore release incisions are not necessary.

5. *Skin closure.* Primary wound closure is carried out only in Grade I compound fractures. A primary split skin graft is never used. There is even less indication for applying a primary cross leg flap.

6. *Functional after-care.* In compound fractures the prevention of infection is paramount, but this does not mean that the objective of early restitution of full function should be lost sight of. The compound fracture is at first immobilized in plaster or suspended in a splint. Three to four days after delayed primary suture or ten days after primary skin closure, the surgeon should assess the whole situation and decide whether mobilization can be begun or whether a longer period of immobilization is still needed.

7. *Repeated internal fixation.* In compound fractures it is often necessary at the end of six weeks to revise the so-called minimal internal fixation where a small amount of metal was used, which may therefore not have provided rigid fixation. Thus, at the end of six weeks a fresh nailing, sometimes combined with medullary reaming, is quite often needed. If revision of the internal fixation is to be avoided, primary cancellous bone grafting must be carried out at the time of the first operation. If this is done, the bone graft should be obtained from the iliac crest at the beginning of the operation.

8. *The management of skin necrosis.* Skin necrosis is uncommon after delayed primary suture. The more often the surgeon attempts primary skin suture, the more often he will encounter the problem of skin necrosis. If skin necrosis occurs, all attempts are made to keep it dry and defer any procedure until healing has taken place under the scab, or until a demarcation line has appeared. We feel that early excision or split skin grafting is never indicated.

9. *Secondary wound closure.* Should be carried out usually after 8 days, and never before 5 days.

Fig. 208   *Compound fracture of the tibia with contusion on the medial side of the leg (MS 1741).*

Internal fixation is carried out using two lag screws supplemented by a neutralization plate on the lateral surface of the tibia.

Fig. 209   *Segmental fracture of the tibia (MS 1597).*

Primary fixation was performed with a thin medullary nail.

Fig. 210   *Segmental fractures of the upper tibia with compounding of the shaft fracture only and extensive skin contusion on the medial side (MS 1735).*

The upper fracture was fixed with a semi-tubular plate and a small tension wire. The shaft fracture was fixed with a very thin medullary nail without medullary reaming.

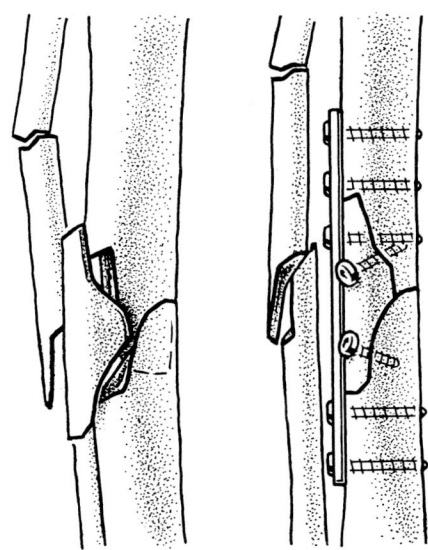

208

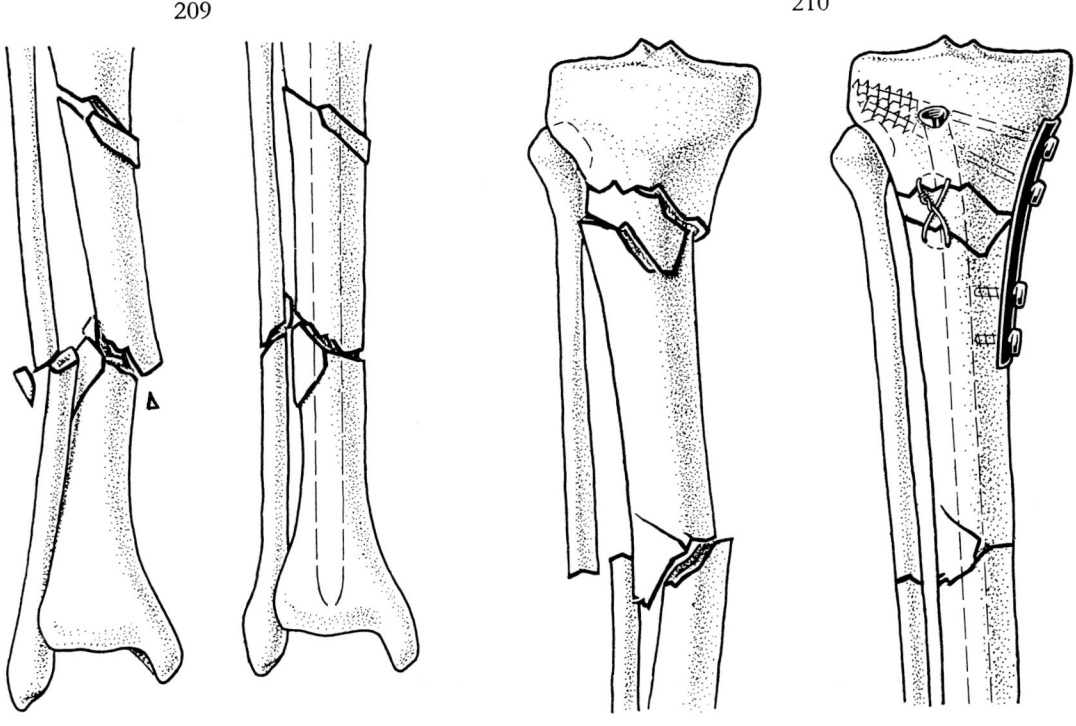

209

210

Fig. 211   *A wide posterior relaxation incision immediately in the mid-line of the calf with simultaneous fasciotomy.*

No split skin graft. The wound is left open and covered with tulle gauze.

Fig. 212   *A compound fracture dislocation of the lower femur (MS 288).*

Primary excision of the patella and of necrotic soft tissues. Minimal internal fixation of the femoral condyles was performed. Full return of function occurred. The patient received a 10% disability pension, because of the patellectomy.

Fig. 213   *A grade III compound fracture of the tibia (AC 29/7a).*

Primary fixation with a posterior plate. To help wound care the lower extremity was suspended on a splint until the wound healed.

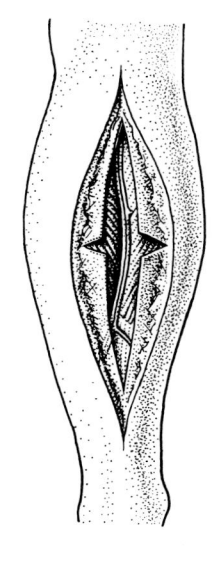

211

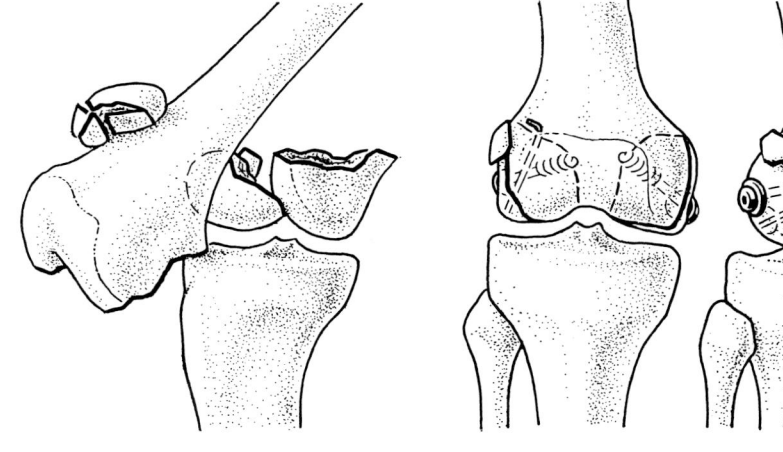

212

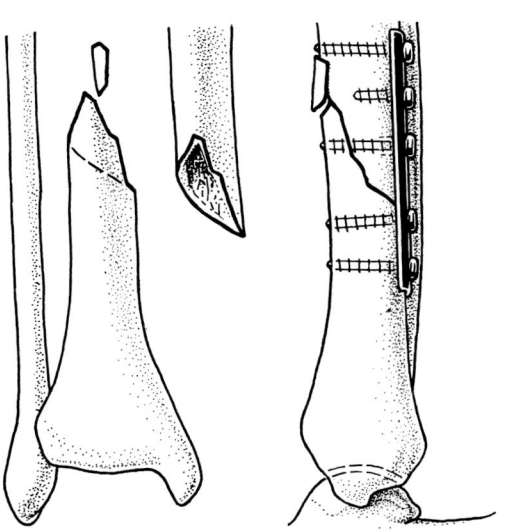

213

Fig. 214   *A compound fracture of the tibia admitted after ten hours with severe skin contusion (MS 27. 12. 66).*

The fracture was fixed with four transverse Steinmann pins, held together with external compression clamps.

Fig. 215   *Compound malleolar fracture dislocation (MS 1592).*

Minimal internal fixation was carried out, Medullary wiring was used to fix the fibular fracture. The large posterior fragment was screwed with an antero-posterior cancellous screw and the medial malleolus was fixed with a single malleolar screw and one Kirschner wire.

Fig. 216   *Fracture dislocation of the lower tibia with severe damage to the talus (MS 1876).*

Primary arthrodesis of the ankle joint was carried out after open reduction and internal fixation of both the fibular and tibial fractures. Two Steinmann pins were used, one on each side of the resected joint surface. They were then placed under compression with the Charnley type of external compression clamps (Fig. 214).

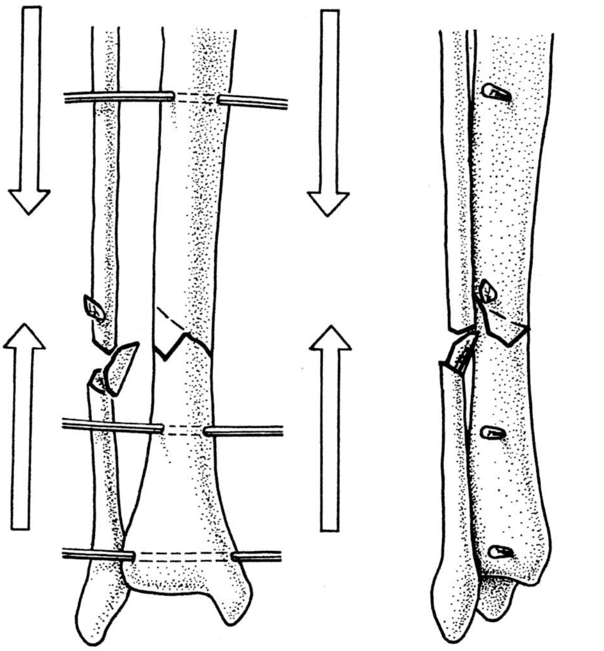

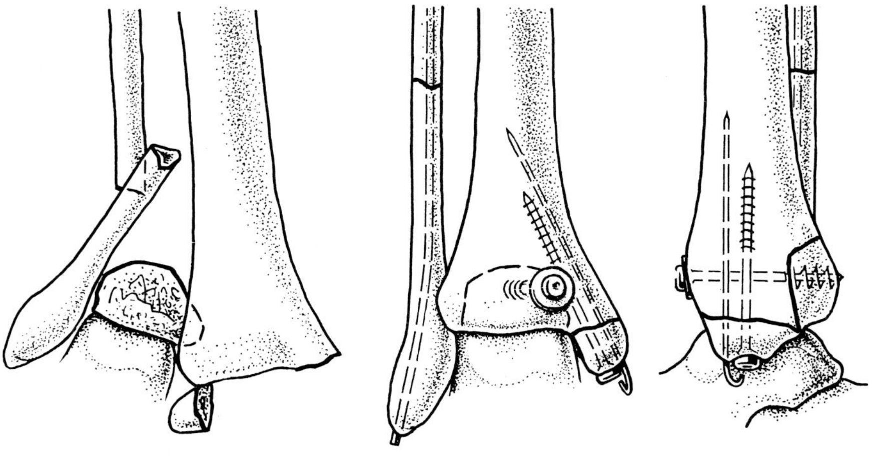

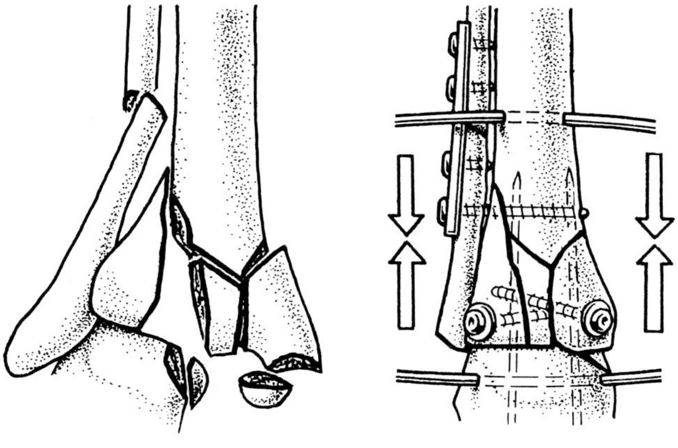

III. Fractures in Children

The treatment of fractures in children is quite different from those in the adult because only 10% require surgery.

Fractures through the shafts of long bones: These fractures are chiefly treated by closed means as they heal up rapidly and axial deformities usually correct themselves during growth at the epiphyseal plates and by remodelling. Shortening corrects itself by accelerated growth of the limb. Rotational deformities are the only ones which do not correct spontaneously. For this reason, in the treatment of femoral shaft fractures in children, WEBER constructed a special traction table which allows full rotational control of the fragments. Exceptions to this rule are fractures of the femoral shaft in children over the age of ten. In these children any sub-trochanteric fracture which cannot be controlled on the traction table should be plated, and any mid-shaft fractures should be nailed with a thin tibial intramedullary nail, without reaming (Fig. 233).

Articular and metaphyseal fractures: These often need open reduction. We feel that open reduction and internal fixation of fractures involving joints are indicated if one cannot obtain a congruent articular surface by conservative means. When we talk about metaphyseal fractures, we mean those involving the epiphyseal plate. Bony bridging of the epiphyseal plate results in its premature closure and subsequent growth disturbance. Where there is fracture separation at an epiphyseal plate which threatens to disturb growth, anatomical reduction and internal fixation is indicated. In fractures of the lower humerus, especially supra-condylar fractures, great attention must be paid to the position of the lower humeral epiphysis after reduction. Any mal-alignment of this epiphysis in relation to the long axis of the humerus is permanent, because the humerus is a non-weight bearing bone, and no spontaneous correction occurs at the epiphyseal plate.

In children, Kirschner wire transfixion is an excellent method of internal fixation. The cancellous bone is very hard and gives good fixation with Kirschner wires. After accurate reduction, the fractures heal quickly and Kirschner wires can be removed at three weeks. Epiphyseal plates can be transfixed with parallel Kirschner wires without any danger of disturbing subsequent growth. The ends of these wires are usually left protruding through the skin, so that they are easy to remove at three weeks. Screw fixation is seldom used (Fig. 236, 241). There are disadvantages to screw fixation in children. The screws have to be removed, which makes a second operation necessary. An epiphyseal plate should only be transfixed with a screw under exceptional circumstances, and then only for a very short period of time (e.g. avulsion fracture of the tibial tubercle, or the repair of a cruciate ligament.) One should never nail fractures of the femoral neck in children as the cancellous bone is very hard and the head may easily be pushed off by the advancing nail. For this reason these fractures should be fixed with cancellous screws.

Fig. 217	*Classification of epiphyseal plate fracture separations.*
	These fractures are divided into two major groups:
A	Simple epiphyseal plate fracture separations, in which the plate remains intact. Growth disturbance in these is rarely encountered and any residual deformity corrects spontaneously by further growth at the plate.
B	Plate separation, where the plate itself is involved. If reduction is not perfect, bone may grow across the epiphyseal plate, interferring with subsequent growth.
a′	Simple epiphyseal plate fracture separations, which are often encountered as birth injuries or just before the cessation of growth. In birth injuries, accurate reduction is not necessary but it is so at the later age.
a″	Growth disturbance is not to be expected. Most imperfect reductions can certainly be accepted. Reduction is maintained in a plaster.
b′	In this case the epiphyseal plate must be accurately reduced. This is usually best done under direct vision. Fixation in these cases is usually secured by a small cancellous screw (Fig. 241).
b″	In these cases accurate reduction of the epiphyseal plate is most necessary. Fixation can be secured with two or three Kirschner wires (Fig. 235).
b‴	In impaction fractures of the epiphyseal plate and of the articular surface, it is more important to obtain accurate reduction of the joint surface. A cancellous graft is usually necessary to fill the defect. These injuries usually result in some growth disturbance, because of the damage to the cells of the plate itself. X-rays during weight-bearing are necessary later. If a deformity begins to appear, it is best corrected through an open wedge lengthening osteotomy, done on the same side as the damage to the plate (Fig. 297 b).

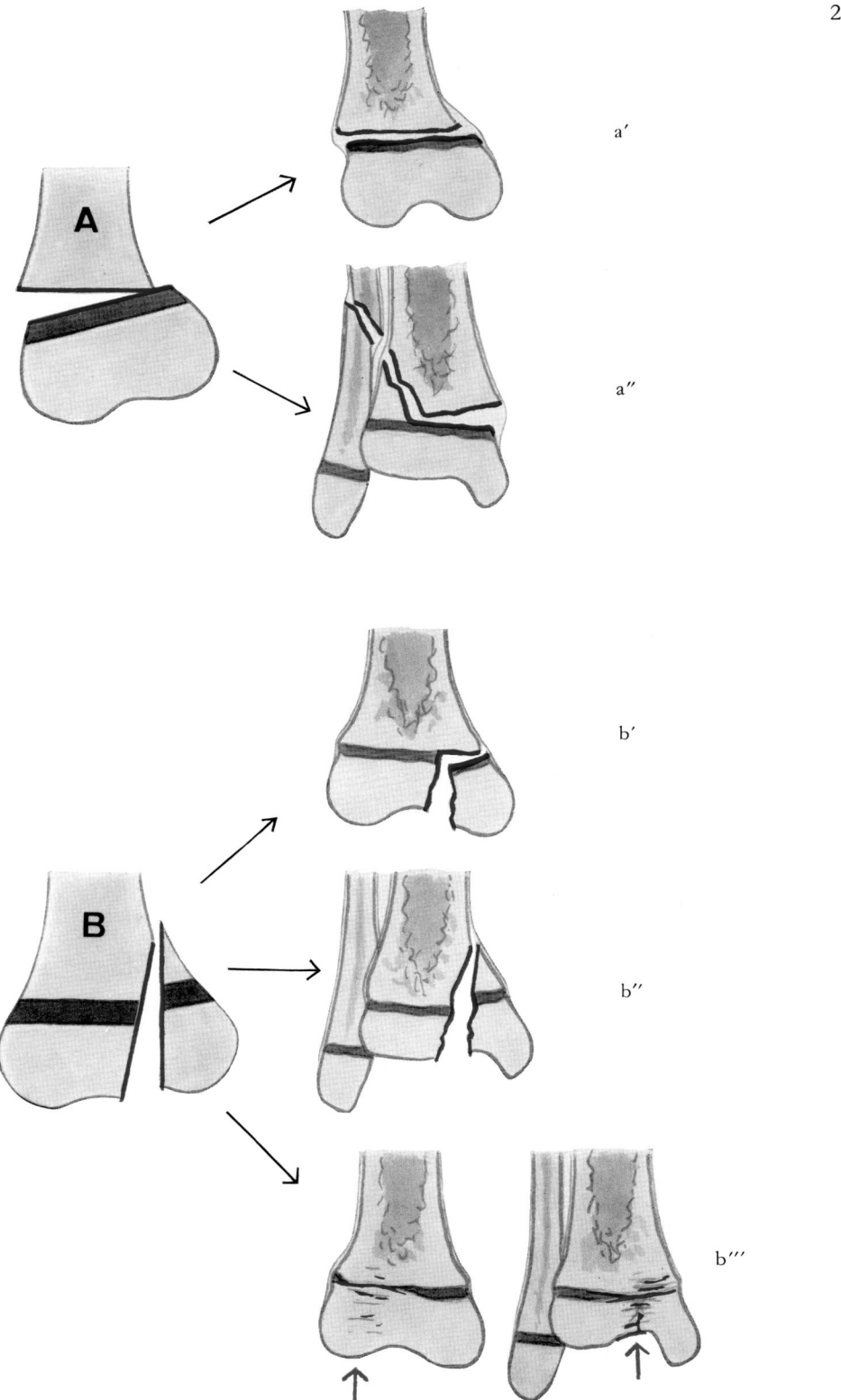

a′

a″

b′

b″

b‴

Fractures of the Humerus in Children

Fractures through the upper humerus: Fractures of the neck and shaft can almost always be managed in vertical traction. We prefer an olecranon cortex screw to the trans-olecranon wire because of the lower incidence of complications (infection, late ulnar palsy). Very occasionally it is necessary to undertake an open reduction of a subcapital fracture or of an epiphyseal plate fracture separation. Fixation of these is usually secured with Kirschner wire transfixion which is left in place for between two and three weeks.

Supra-condylar fractures: Most supra-condylar fractures can be managed conservatively using BLOUNT's method or in traction through the olecranon. Open reduction becomes necessary in irreducible fractures or in those associated with a vascular and/or nerve lesion. Adequate fixation is usually secured with two Kirschner wires. Fractures of the lateral condyle and of the medial epicondyle are also usually treated by open reduction and Kirschner wire fixation for two or three weeks. In fractures of the lateral condyle, it is most important to restore the angle of inclination of the condylar epiphyseal plate to the long axis of the humerus. This plate usually subtends an angle of 70–75° to the axis of the humerus. These fractures usually result in a cubitus valgus and rarely in a cubitus varus. They may also give rise to late ulnar palsy.

Fractures of the forearm: Most fractures of both bones of the forearm can be treated conservatively. The first step in closed reduction is to increase the deformity before securing the actual reduction.

Fractures of the head of the radius: Fractures of the radial head, if displaced, should be treated by means of open reduction and a trans humeral Kirschner wire fixation. This fixation is maintained for three weeks and supplemented with a cast. This is to prevent late deformity and incongruity of this joint.

Monteggia fractures: All Monteggia fractures must be treated surgically (Fig. 124) since the annular ligament can only be repaired or reconstructed surgically.

Fig. 218	*Irreducible subcapital fracture of the humerus (WL 35/8).* Simple Kirschner wire fixation.
Fig. 219	*Irreducible proximal humeral epiphyseal plate fracture-separation (S 1).* Fixation with two Kirschner wires.
Fig. 220	*Fracture of the medial epicondyle (WS 19).* Fixed with two crossed Kirschner wires.
Fig. 221	*Fracture of the lateral condyle (WL 46/11).* This fracture is stabilized with transfixing Kirschner wires.
Fig. 222	*Supra-condylar fracture of the humerus (WL 47/26).* A stable fixation is achieved with two crossed Kirschner wires, which are removed at two to three weeks.
Fig. 223	All supra-condylar fractures must be reduced so that the epiphyseal plate of the lateral condyle subtends an angle of 70–75° to the long axis of the humerus. If reduction does not result in restoration of this normal angle, a varus or valgus deformity will result.
Fig. 224	*Vertical traction through an olecranon cortex screw.* We prefer the screw to a transfixion wire because of the lower incidence of infection and ulnar nerve palsy. This form of traction may need to be assisted by axial skin traction in line with the pronated forearm.

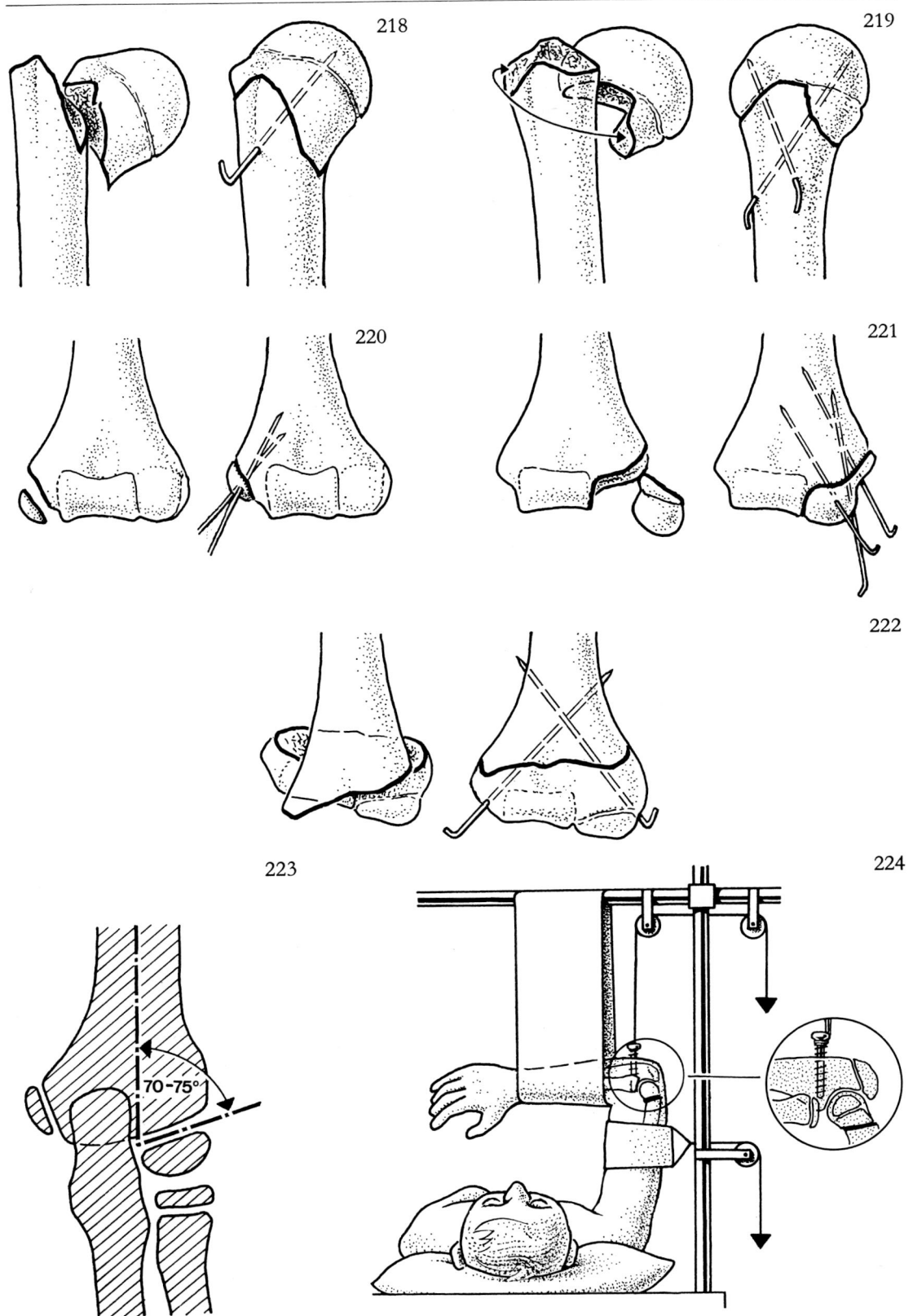

225

Fractures of the forearm.

Fig. 225   *Epiphyseal plate fracture-separation of the radial head (WL 47/33).*
Simple Kirschner wire transfixion.

Fig. 226   *Subcapital fracture of the radial neck (WS 57).*
The fracture is stabilized by a Kirschner wire which is passed through the capitellum with the elbow at 90°. This is supplemented with a full arm plaster.

Fig. 227   *Comminuted fracture of the upper ulna (WS 59).*
This fracture was stabilized with a single Kirschner wire.

Fig. 228   *Distal radial epiphyseal plate fracture-separation (WL 38/10).*
This fracture may be very difficult to reduce and reduction hard to maintain. Fixation of the reduction is secured with two crossed Kirschner wires left protruding through the skin. These wires are removed after two weeks.

Fig. 229   *Unstable lower radial epiphyseal plate fracture-separation (WL 43/26).*
Simple wire transfixion.

226

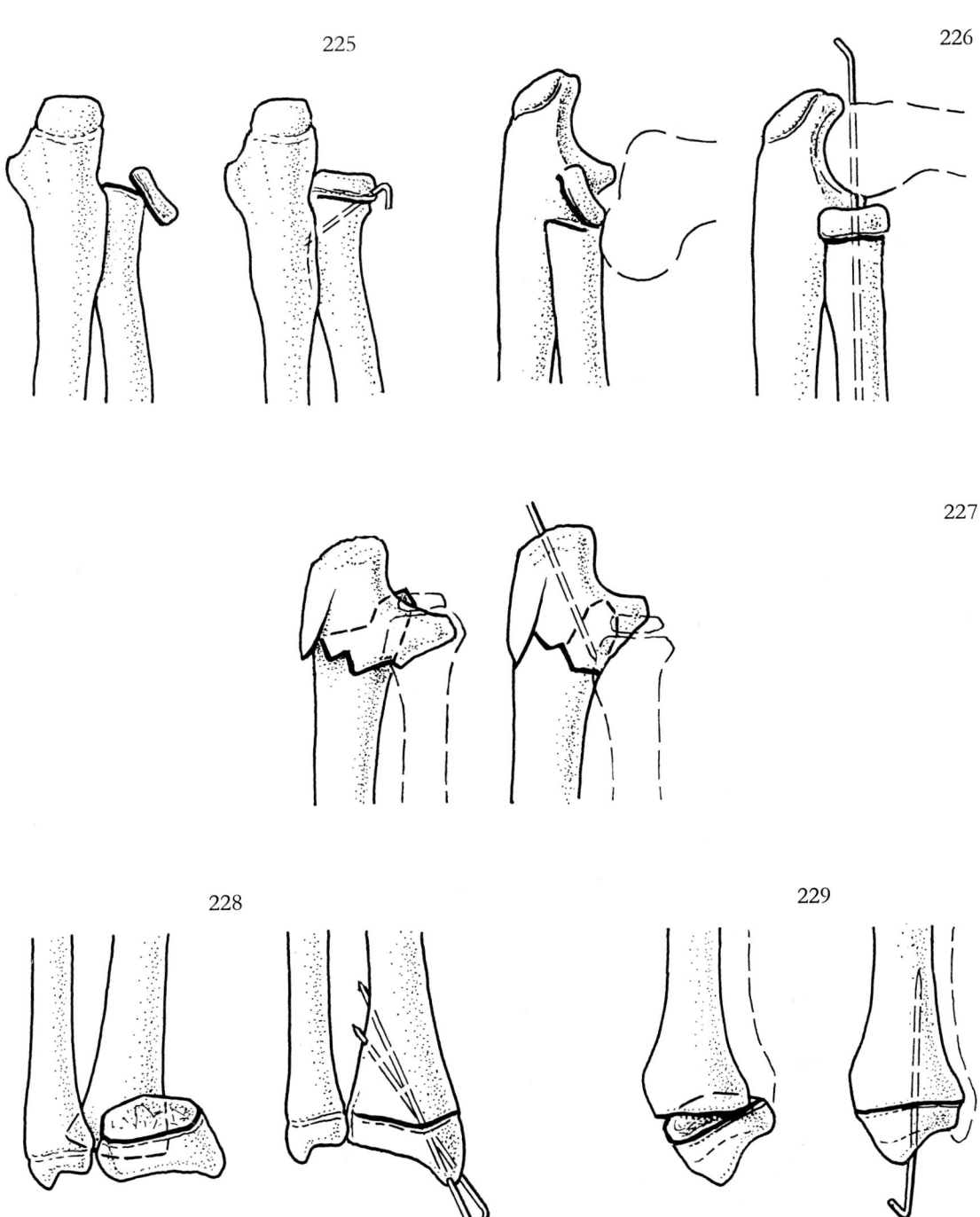

225

226

227

228

229

Fractures of the Femur in Children

Fractures of the femoral neck in children are an absolute indication for open reduction and internal fixation. Stable internal fixation is achieved by means of one or more cancellous screws. The screw must never transfix the epiphyseal plate. These fractures should never be nailed in childhood, as the cancellous bone is very hard and the fracture may easily be opened up further by the nail. This may disturb the blood supply of the femoral head. Open reduction is almost always done, as in the adult, but in children particular care must be taken not to damage the dorsal retinacular vessels while retracting with the Hohmann retractors. The childhood fracture is usually through the base of the neck, and a long threaded cancellous screw is adequate.

Fractures above or below the lesser trochanter in older children which cannot be reduced successfully by closed methods, should be openly reduced and fixed with a small tension band plate.

Fractures of the femoral shaft that need internal fixation, are best fixed with an intramedullary nail. We use a tibial nail and introduce it from the back, just below the epiphyseal plate of the greater trochanter. This avoids any damage to the plate (Fig. 78).

In supra-condylar fractures of the femur, especially in epiphyseal plate fracture-separations, open reduction is carried out and fixation obtained with crossed Kirschner wires.

Fig. 230   *Fracture through the base of the femoral neck (MS 1474).*

This fracture is fixed with cancellous screws and a T-plate. The T-plate acts as a large washer for the three lag screws. The thread of the screws does not transfix the epiphyseal plate.

Fig. 231   *Fracture through the base of the femoral neck (MS 1698).*

This fracture in an eleven year old child was fixed with two long threaded cancellous screws.

Fig. 232   *Subtrochanteric fracture (WL 41/6).*

The fracture was first stabilized with a lag screw and then fixed with a semi-tubular plate used as a tension band plate.

Fig. 233   *Fracture of the femoral shaft (WL 33/9).*

This fracture occurred in a fourteen year old boy. It was fixed with an 8 mm tibial nail, introduced from behind and below the epiphyseal plate of the greater trochanter, so as not to interfere with its growth (Fig. 78).

Fig. 234   *Supra-condylar fracture of the femur (MS 1964).*

Stabilized in a seven year old boy with four Kirschner wires, two on each side.

Fig. 235   *A transverse fracture across the lower epiphyseal plate of the femur (GG 10/12).*

After careful, exact anatomical reduction, fixation was achieved with two Kirschner wires which were left protruding through the skin.

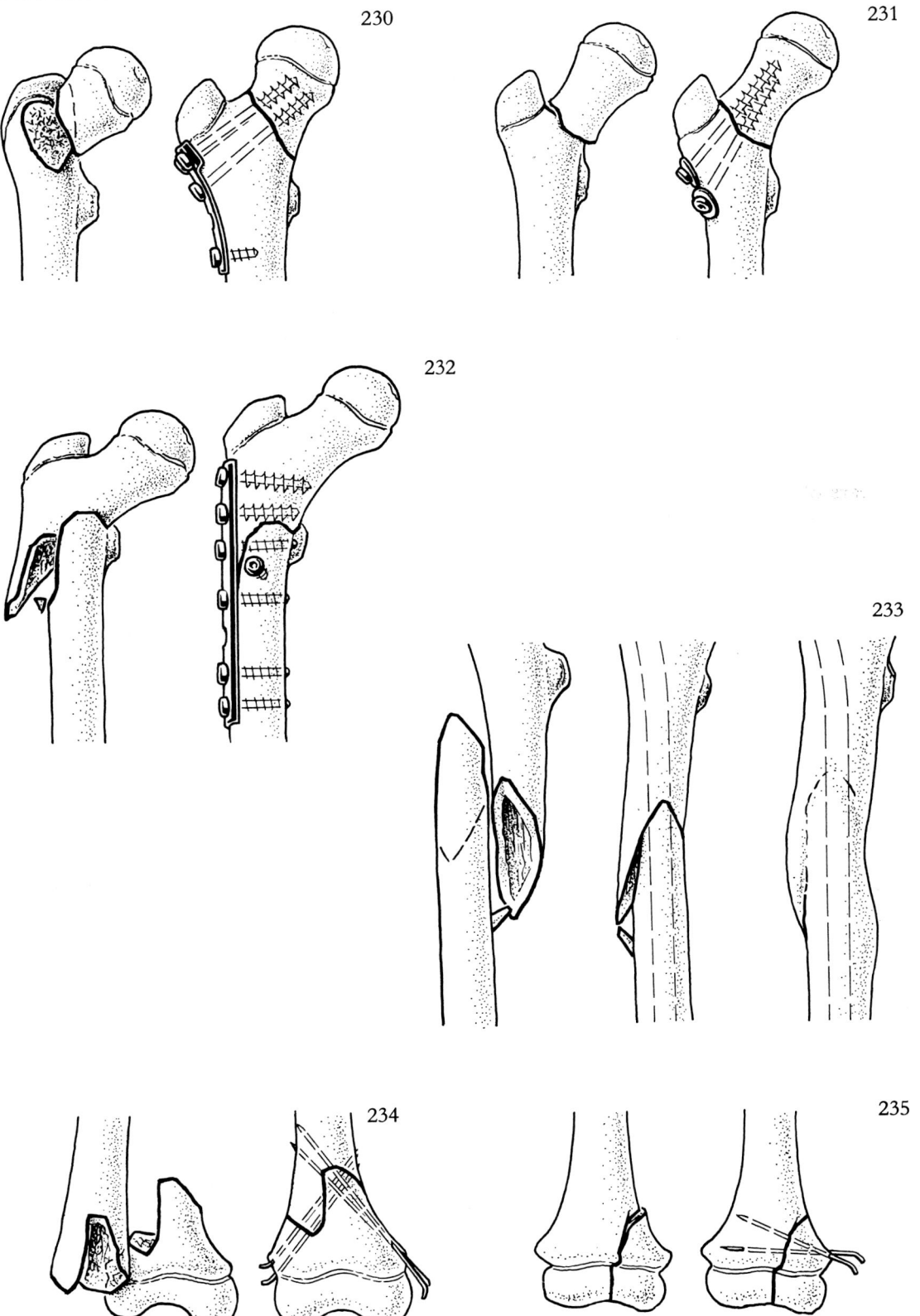

Fractures of the Tibia

Avulsion fracture of the tibial spine should be treated by open reduction and internal fixation. This may be done with a cerclage wire or better with a small cancellous screw passed across the epiphyseal plate.

The operative technique: Before reduction, introduce a 1.5 mm Kirschner wire parallel to the planned position of the cancellous screw. If the wire is properly directed, a hole is made for the screw with a 3.2 mm drill. The reduction is now carried out, and while the fragments are kept reduced, a 2.0 mm drill bit is passed through the 3.2 mm pilot hole and the small fragment is drilled. The small fragment is then secured, either with a small cancellous screw or a malleolar screw, cut to length. This is the only method which makes fixation of this fragment under compression possible. After fixation the wounds are closed and the knee is immobilized in 30° of flexion for five weeks. The screw is removed between six and nine weeks later.

Fractures of the tibial shaft are on the whole treated conservatively. The only time open reduction and internal fixation is indicated, is when growth is almost complete i. e. after 12 years of age, and axial malalignment cannot be corrected conservatively. In such cases, one can use one screw for the fixation of oblique fractures of the tibia in the presence of an intact fibula. The fracture is drifting into varus.

Fig. 236   *Avulsion of the tibial spine (MS 1912).*

     This fracture was stabilized with a small cancellous screw. The screw was removed after six weeks so that it would not result in premature closure of the epiphysis.

Fig. 237   *Fracture of the shaft of the tibia (GG 11/27).*

     A fracture of the tibial shaft, just before growth ceased. It was stabilized with a single lag screw.

Fig. 238   *Fracture of the lower tibia (FW 10/25).*

     A sixteen year old boy. The lower fracture could not be reduced conservatively, so fixation was achieved with a single screw, resulting in only moderate fixation. The leg was then immobilized in plaster.

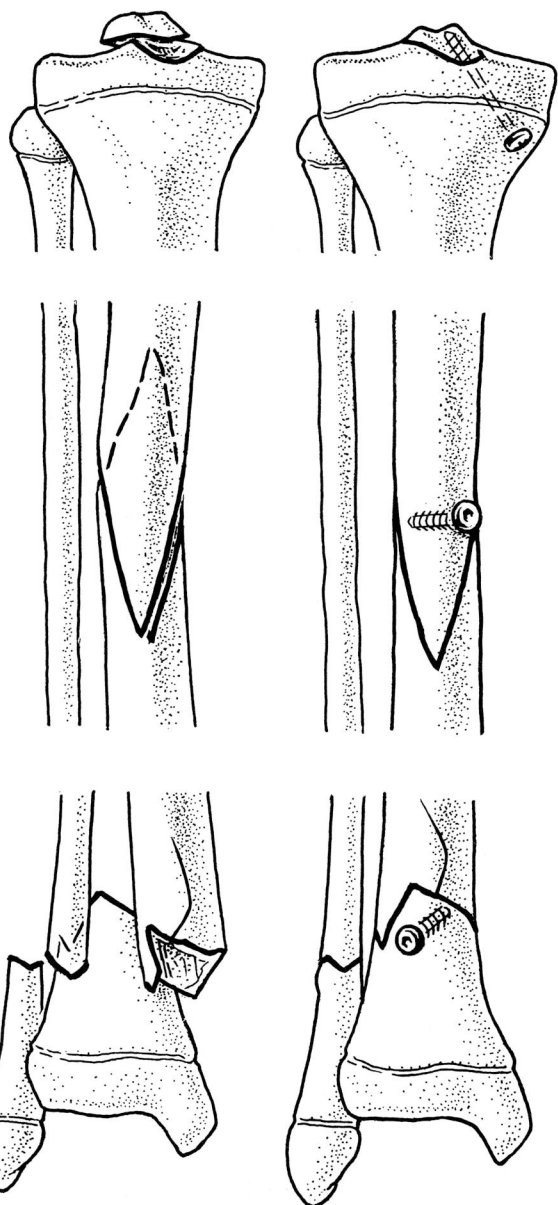

236

237

238

Malleolar Fractures

Surgery is only needed if the epiphyseal plate has separated with widening of the ankle mortice, or where the fracture crosses the epiphyseal plate. Fixation is carried out with one or two small cancellous screws. Kirschner wires are seldom used as the only method of fixation here. If 4.0 mm cancellous screws are used as the method of fixation, no callus forms.

Fig. 239   *A malleolar fracture with a huge posterior tibial fragment, the so-called Volkmann triangle (fracture always crosses the epiphyseal plate) (BI 26/26).*

Fourteen year old boy. The fixation should be obtained with two cortex screws used as lag screws or better with two malleolar screws, inserted from front to back.

Fig. 240   *A supra-malleolar fracture involving the epiphyseal plate (MS 1645).*

These fractures are usually treated conservatively. Occasionally, if the fracture cannot be reduced, open reduction and Kirschner wire fixation is indicated.

Fig. 241   *A fracture transversely crossing the epiphyseal plate (MS 1879).*

After exact reduction, fixation with two 4.0 mm cancellous screws. This was a fourteen year old boy.

Fig. 242   *Avulsion fracture of the tubercle of Chaput (MS 1422).*

Fixation with Kirschner wires or finally with a 4.0 mm cancellous screw. A fourteen year old girl.

Fig. 243   *A fracture of the medial malleolus traversing the epiphyseal plate (BI 30/18).*

After exact open reduction, transfixion with two Kirschner wires.

Fig. 244   *Bi-malleolar fracture dislocation (MS 20/18).*

Open reduction and fixation with Kirschner wires. A perfect reduction with correspondingly good result.

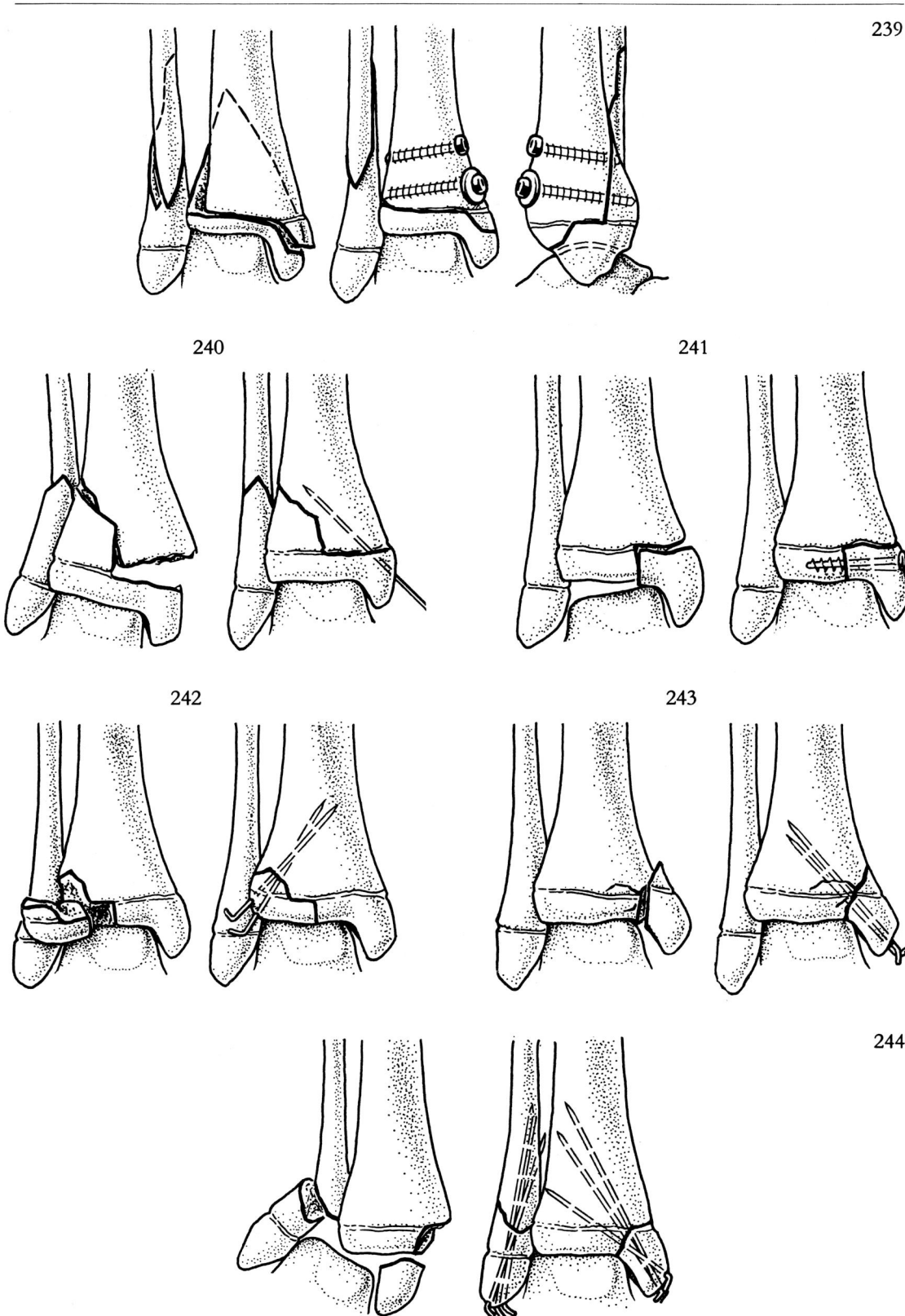

240

241

242

243

244

Supplement

Reconstructive Bone Surgery

M. E. MÜLLER

Introduction

Internal fixation with compression has led both to a profound change in the treatment of fractures and to a change in the techniques of reconstructive bone surgery. It is for this reason that we now present as an appendix to the manual a comprehensive treatise on reconstructive bone surgery.

In this appendix we shall not discuss the normal functional anatomy, the indications, the complications nor the postoperative treatment. We shall discuss only those procedures which have been developed over the years with the help of the AO instrumentarium and which have stood the test of time.

Our reconstructive bone surgery is characterized not only by *rigid internal fixation,* achieved with the help of compression, but also by *exact pre-operative planning* of all corrections and by a method of carrying out these corrections precisely so that *radiological control* during the operative procedure is hardly ever necessary. We shall also discuss in detail the technique of *decortication,* so often necessary in reconstructive bone surgery, as well as the indications for *autogenous cancellous bone grafting* in bridging areas of bone loss or regions of devitalized bone.

I. Pseudarthroses

Under *pseudarthroses,* we include not only the rare cases of true false joint formation in which the medullary canal is sealed off, with the development of new cartilaginous surfaces as well as a joint capsule and synovial lining, but *all fractures which have not united within eight months from the time of injury.*

We define as *delayed union* a fracture which has not united within four to five months from the time of injury.

Delayed union of a fracture after anatomical reduction of the fragments, rigid internal fixation, and early post-operative mobilization, presents no great therapeutic problems. In the *lower extremity* we remove all previously introduced implants. In the femur we ream the medullary canal to a diameter of 14 to 15 mm and in the tibia to a diameter of 12 to 14 mm and introduce the corresponding intramedullary nails. In most cases the patients require only a few days in hospital and are soon able to resume full weight bearing. In the *upper limb* the problem is somewhat more complicated, particularly if the fracture has been originally plated. Here bone necrosis is the usual cause of delayed union or non-union. Therefore the plate which has loosened has usually to be removed. A decortication or "shingling" (Fig. 247) must be carried out together with an autogenous cancellous bone graft. A longer tension band plate than the one previously used must be employed. The holes for the new screws are frequently drilled at 90° to the old holes. In the arm, loss of rigidity of fixation is the only indication for intervention. As long as the screws are not loose and as long as the patient has no symptoms, one must wait. In most cases, despite partial necrosis of the fragments, as long as fixation is rigid, slow remodelling will take place and union will ensue.

Classification of Pseudarthroses
A. Non-infected
B. Previously infected
C. Infected

A. Non-infected Pseudarthroses

The non-infected pseudarthroses are subdivided according to their position into: 1. *diaphysial* and 2. *metaphysial*.

1. *Diaphysial Pseudarthroses* are subdivided into two types:

   a) *The classical "elephant foot" type pseudarthrosis.* The classical elephant foot type pseudarthrosis represents 85 to 90% of pseudarthroses which develop in conservatively treated fractures. Radiologically they show a proliferative bone reaction, the so-called sclerosis. This sclerosis does not represent dead bone as one might surmise, but is due to an over-production of well vascularized bone. When such a pseudarthrosis is rigidly immobilized, the interposed cartilage or fibrous tissue rapidly ossifies. In dealing with these pseudarthroses therefore, it is not necessary to freshen up the bone ends or to apply a bone graft. These pseudarthroses *will heal as soon as they are completely immobilized with a straight tension band plate or with an intra-medullary nail after medullary reaming.*

b) *The non-reactive atrophic pseudarthroses.* The atrophic pseudarthroses radiologically show no bone reaction and are either poorly vascularized or avascular. To induce such a pseudarthrosis to heal, it is necessary to secure *rigid internal fixation* with a medullary nail or tension band plate, to perform extensive decortication or shingling, and to apply an *autogenous cancellous bone graft.* These non-reactive pseudarthroses are becoming more and more common as open reduction and rigid internal fixation gain wider acceptance. *

2. *In metaphysial pseudarthroses,* in addition to securing the broadest and closest contact between the fracture fragments, the most important factor in securing union is absolute rigid immobilization. At these sites, however, one cannot obtain rigid immobilization with straight tension band plates or with intramedullary nails. A pseudarthrosis of the proximal humerus is immobilized with the T-plate. In the distal humerus and proximal tibia we employ double plates, and in the proximal and distal third of the femur, condylar plates. In pseudarthroses of the femoral neck, healing depends on the angle of the pseudarthrosis relative to the resultant of forces acting on the femoral head. It is for this reason that in pseudarthroses of the femoral neck with a viable head, we prefer the repositioning osteotomy of PAUWELS.

B. Previously Infected Pseudarthroses

In dealing with previously infected pseudarthroses, we must distinguish between those in which there is some contact between the fragments and those with bone loss. If there is *wide contact between the fragments,* to obtain healing of such a pseudarthrosis, it is sufficient to place the fragments *under high compression,* either by means of a tension band plate, omitting the middle four or five screws, or with double compression clamps using four to six Steinmann pins. (Example: pseudarthrosis of the tibia.) In *pseudarthroses with bone loss,* we bridge the defect in the upper extremity with one semi-tubular plate and in the lower extremity two semi-tubular plates (Fig. 270). The viable bone is decorticated over an appreciable distance and the defect filled with pure autologous cancellous bone (Fig. 88). At the same time an antibiotic irrigation system is set up for a few days to prevent a flare up of the infection.

C. Open Infected Draining Pseudarthroses

In the open infected pseudarthroses we have two problems to deal with: namely, the *healing of the pseudarthrosis and the eradication of the infection.* The healing of the pseudarthrosis depends on the distance between well vascularized bone surfaces and on the stability of the internal

---

* A pseudarthrosis should never occur after an AO rigid internal fixation. If a diagnosis of delayed union is made at the 4 months follow-up a reoperation is mandatory (see page 237).

fixation. Infection is most often propagated by the presence of dead bone which acts as a foreign body. This dead bone is present either in the form of sequestrum or is still firmly united to the healthy viable bone. Inadequate skin cover is also a contributing factor in the maintenance of infection.

We are of the opinion that in such a situation, *the first step is to obtain bone union*. After bone union is obtained it is frequently possible to clear up the infection in a relatively short period of time by carrying out a sequestrectomy and autologous cancellous bone grafting. Skin grafting is rarely indicated.

Before any bone procedure is undertaken, we attempt first, for a period of two to three weeks, to reduce both the drainage and the bacterial virulence by immobilization and elevation of the affected limb, and by local instillation of Neomycin/Bacitracin solutions.

In infected pseudarthroses, metal implants should be left undisturbed as long as they afford rigid immobilization of the fragments. In those cases in which internal fixation is providing rigid immobilization, extensive dorsal autogenous bone grafting or a decortication is first carried out. As soon as a sufficiently strong bony bridge is obtained both implants and sequestra are removed. In those cases in which internal fixation is not providing rigid immobilization we remove all implants and radically resect all dead tissues (both soft tissue and bone) until fresh healthy tissues are exposed. Irrigation drainage with antibiotics (mostly Neomycin and Bacitracin) is always used in addition. In the tibia, if a tibio-fibular graft cannot be performed, other methods have to be used. If after resection there is still adequate contact between the fragments, it suffices to carry out a decortication and stabilize the pseudarthrosis under compression with external compression clamps. If, however, resection leaves a gap, then the external compression clamps can only maintain stability and the defect must be filled in with a cancellous autograft.

The Fundamental Principles in the Treatment of Pseudarthroses

A. Non-Infected Pseudarthroses

Introduction and the Principles of Treatment:

a) *The elephant foot type of reactive pseudarthrosis heals after stable internal fixation (intramedullary nail, tension band plate) without resection of the soft tissue between the bone ends, or bone grafting, or post-operative immobilization in plaster.*

In the elephant foot type of pseudarthrosis, if in addition significant axial mal-alignment must also be corrected by an osteotomy or by opening up the pseudarthrosis, decortication ("shingling") must be carried out to ensure quick healing of the pseudarthrosis. If, in addition to the pseudarthrosis, shortening has occurred, this too can be corrected at the same time. For the technique of lengthening osteotomy see Fig. 289/295.

b) *In treating the atrophic non-reactive type of pseudarthrosis, extensive decortication of the viable fragments must be combined with cancellous bone grafting and stable internal fixation.*

The same principles apply in the treatment of pseudarthrosis with bone loss (page 254). In dealing with an atrophic pseudarthrosis one must first obtain rigid internal fixation. In the upper extremity this is achieved by means of a tension band plate and in the lower extremity by intramedullary reaming and nailing. Once rigid internal fixation is secure, decortication of one half to two thirds of the bone circumference is carried out and is extended to include healthy bone. Cancellous autologous bone grafting is then carried out.

Note: If a bone graft is necessary only autologous cancellous bone is to be used.

Fig. 245   *The two types of diaphysial pseudarthroses.*

     a   The elephant foot type, the hypertrophic well vascularized, reactive pseudarthrosis.

     b   The atrophic, non reactive, avascular pseudarthrosis.

Fig. 246   *Removing of bone grafts from the ilium.*

     For some pseudarthroses we recommend the small cortico-cancellous bone grafts (see also Fig. 87).

Fig. 247   JUDET's *technique of decortication (pedicled bone grafts).*

     The bone is exposed by chiselling away the outer layer of the cortex and leaving the small pieces of bone attached to the periosteum and soft tissues. In this way the small bone fragments retain their blood supply and remain viable. The decortication should be carried out over a half to three quarters of the bone circumference and over a length of to 8–10 cm.

     These mobile and viable small bone grafts ossify rapidly and result in a strong bony bridge. This holds true for both the non-infected and infected pseudarthroses. In treating a pseudarthrosis with a defect, the ends of both fragments should be decorticated. Into the pockets left between the main cortex and the small fragments with their soft tissue pedicles, insert enough cancellous bone to provide a graft, bridging the defect (Fig. 177). Decortication is also indicated when a corrective osteotomy is performed through fracture callus (Fig. 295).

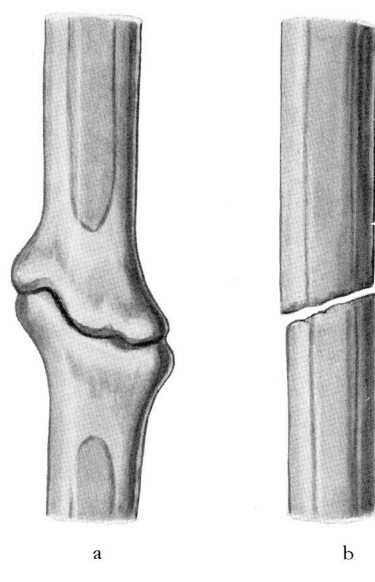

a

b

 245

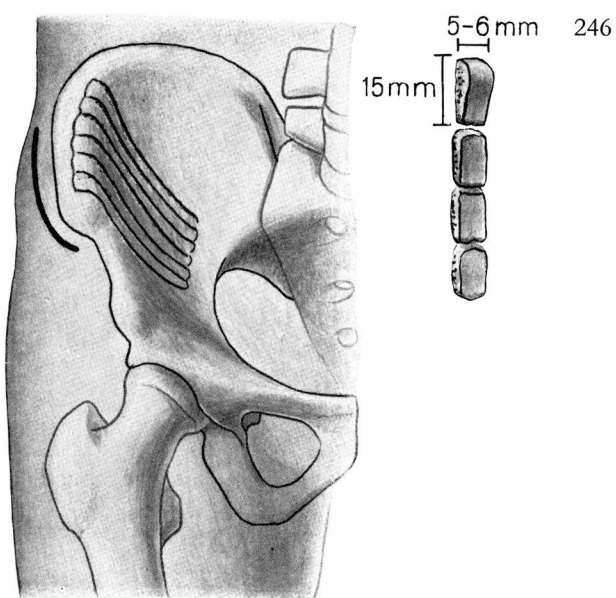

5–6 mm 246

15 mm

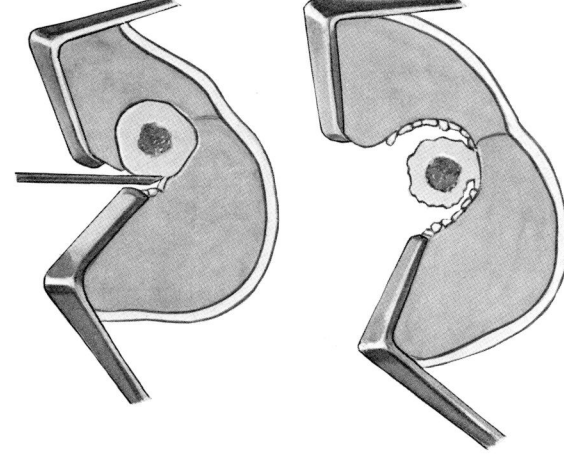

247

The Different Techniques Employed in the Treatment of Non-Infected Pseudarthroses

Medullary Nailing: Medullary nailing is indicated in pseudarthroses of the tibial and femoral diaphyses when no significant axial mal-alignment is present. The sclerotic bone is opened at the pseudarthrosis and the medullary canal entered either with a hand or motor-driven drill prior to reaming.

Only rarely is it necessary to break or to osteotomize through a pseudarthrosis. If this is anticipated, an extensive decortication must first be carried out. The medullary canal of both fragments is then first opened into with a standard 4.5 mm drill and is then reamed with the hand reamer to 9 mm. If this technique is needed in the tibia, a fibular osteotomy is almost always necessary to allow sufficient bending of the tibia to allow access to the medullary canal of each fragment.

Re-Nailing: Most often reaming is carried out to a diameter 2 to 3 mm greater than the previous nail. In the femur 14 mm and in the tibia 12 mm are the minimum nail dimensions. In addition one must get an excellent purchase with the nail in both fragments. In order to accomplish this, the proximal femur has to be reamed on occasion to 18 mm and more. A new nail must always be longer and must be advanced for at least 1 cm distal to the sclerotic plug in the medullary cavity.

Tension Band Plates: In the upper limb, tension band plates are the method of choice. In the tibia, tension band plating is contraindicated if previous medullary nailing has been carried out. In the tibia, the tension band plate is always placed on the convex surface. This means that in a varus deformity it comes to lie on the lateral surface, in a valgus deformity on the medial surface, and in the case of recurvatum on the dorsal aspect. If excessive callus is present, a bed must be cut in it for the plate.

Fibular Osteotomy: Fibular osteotomy is necessary if there is much deformity of the fibula or if it becomes necessary to disrupt the pseudarthrosis by bending the tibia in order to expose the medullary canal (see above). The correction of mal-alignment of the tibia results in lengthening of the tibia despite the use of a tension band plate. This frequently results in gaping of the fibular osteotomy and in its delayed union.

Fig. 248   *Perforation of the closed medullary canal* with the 6 mm hand reamer.

Fig. 249   *The technique of correcting significant varus deformity with the tension band plate.*

The plate is first fixed with four screws, most commonly to the distal fragment. The tension device is then fixed to the other fragment with a long screw and then, as correction proceeds, the tension device is brought closer and closer to the cortex by tightening of the long screw.

Fig. 250   *Fibular osteotomy.*

We see here how the correction of a varus deformity results in lengthening of the tibia.

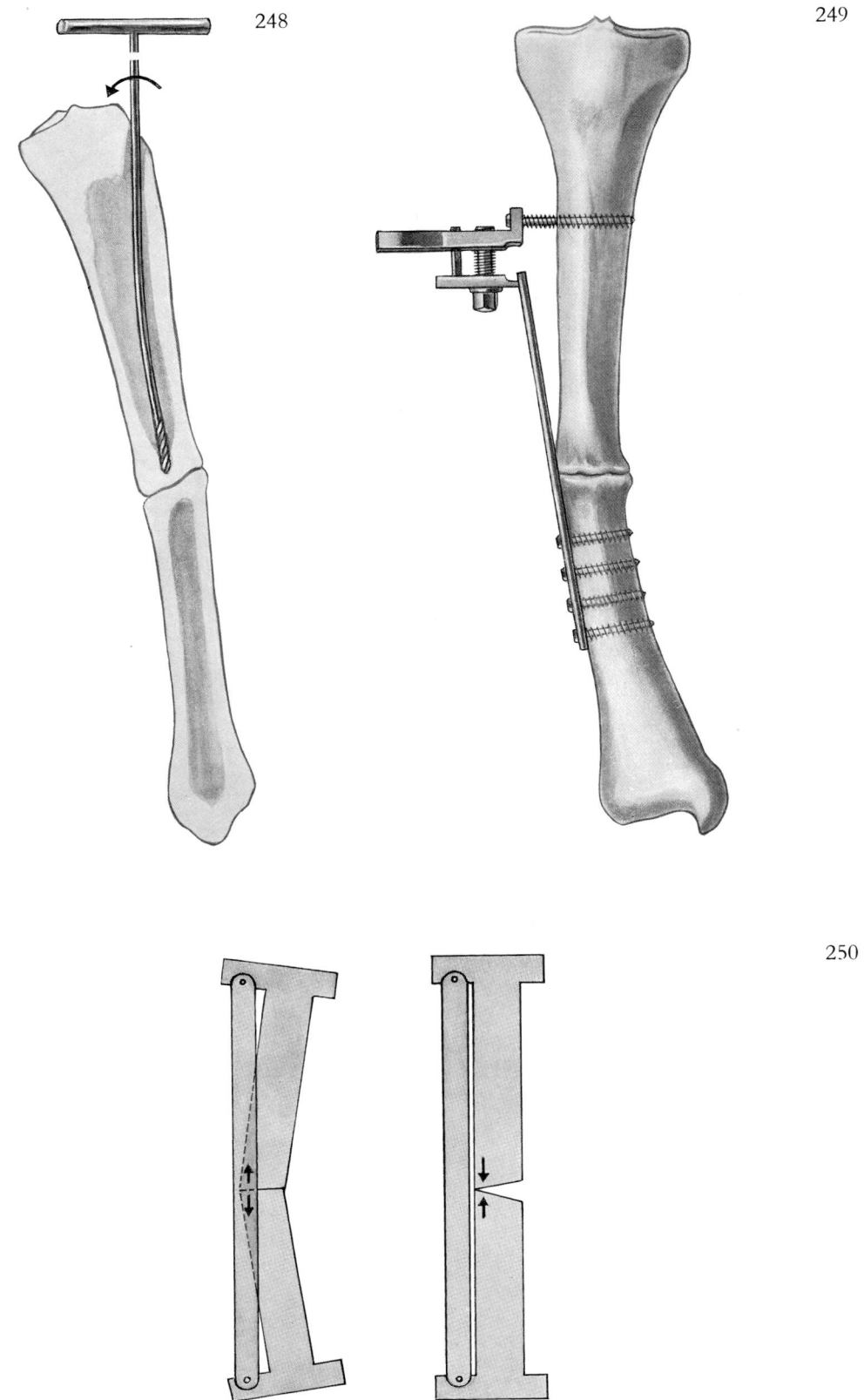

Fig. 251   *Pseudoarthroses of the clavicle.*

In a pseudarthrosis of the clavicle, stable internal fixation is usually achieved with the aid of a five or six hole semi-tubular plate. The anatomical length of the clavicle must always be restored. The procedure is begun by carrying out a decortication, then by freshening up of the bone ends, securing stable internal fixation, and finally supplementing the procedure with a cancellous bone graft.

Fig. 252   *Pseudarthroses of the humerus.*

In a pseudarthrosis of the humerus one should use a broad six to eight hole plate because the screws must have a good purchase in at least six cortices on each side of the fracture line. The wide plate is chosen not because of its greater strength but because of its offset screw holes. The humerus, more often than any other bone, produces the atrophic type of pseudarthrosis. Even if the pseudarthrosis is of the hypertrophic type, the proximal fragment is frequently very osteoporotic. We feel that decortication and bone grafting is most necessary in dealing with these pseudarthroses to ensure rapid bone healing.
N.B.: If the elbow is stiff or if absolutely rigid fixation is not obtained (e.g. in severe osteoporosis), we recommend a double U plaster splint as a supplement for four to six weeks, in order to decrease the stresses on the screws.

Fig. 253   *The forearm.*

In the forearm, we advocate a six hole tension band plate. On the ulna we use mostly a straight plate and on the radius a semi-tubular or a narrow straight plate.

Fig. 254   *The femur.*

Whenever possible, it is best to treat a pseudarthrosis of the femur with a medullary nail. Tension band plates may be used in hypertrophic pseudarthroses without running the risk of subsequent refracture (see Fig. 44b).

Fig. 255   *Tibia.*

Whenever possible the tibia should be re-nailed or nailed with a medullary nail as shown in the illustration. Whenever a tension band plate is used, the plate must always be put on the convex side of the bone (Fig. 34).

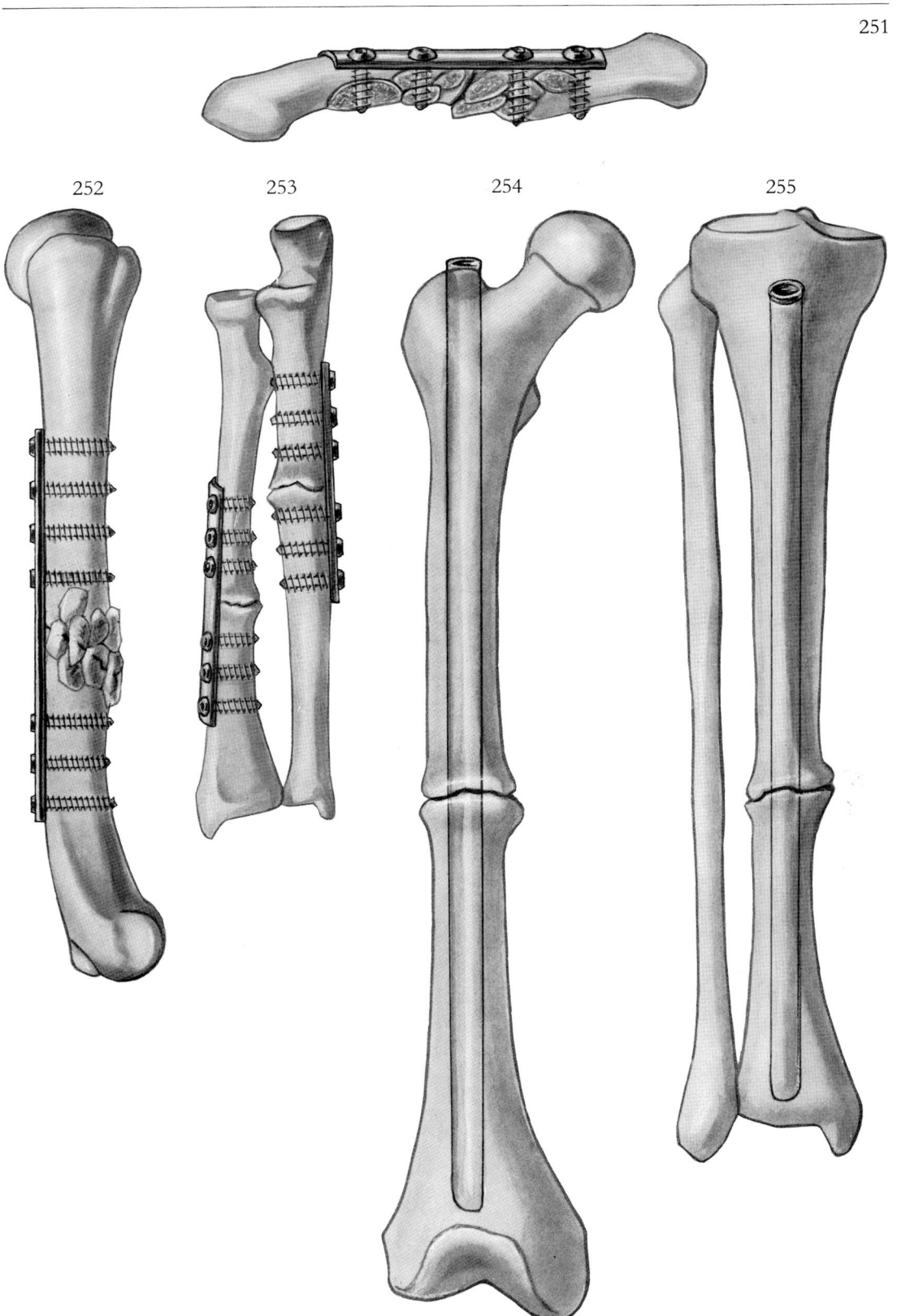

252   253   254   255

Metaphysial Pseudarthroses (Excluding Pseudarthroses of the Femoral Neck

In metaphysial pseudarthroses rigid internal fixation is also absolutely necessary to obtain rapid ossification of the pseudarthrosis. It is for this reason that we use different plates or combination of plates.

Pseudarthroses of the femoral neck present different problems (see page 248).

Fig. 256   In the region of the head of the humerus, we employ the T-plate.

Fig. 257   In the region of the elbow joint, two plates are necessary.

a   A supracondylar pseudarthrosis usually does not require bone grafting.

b   Pseudarthrosis after a Y-fracture is dealt with by means of two small semi-tubular plates and an autogenous cancellous bone graft. The ulnar nerve must be transposed anteriorly.

Fig. 258   In the intertrochanteric region, the right angle plate is used. The blade of the plate must be hammered into the proximal fragment as far cephalad as possible to preserve a wide bridge of bone between the blade of the plate and the fracture line.

Fig. 259   In treating supracondylar pseudarthrosis of the femur, the condylar plate is used for rigid internal fixation.

Fig. 260   In a double pseudarthrosis, that is one on each side of the knee joint, with extensive damage to the knee, two compression plates at 90° to another are indicated. In this way the knee joint is stiffened in its physiological position (see page 284).

Fig. 261   In pseudoarthrosis of the medial malleolus, compression fixation with a lag screw is impossible because of extensive osteoporosis. For this reason we cut a small trough across the pseudarthrosis and fill it with an autograft, as a supplement to the internal fixation.

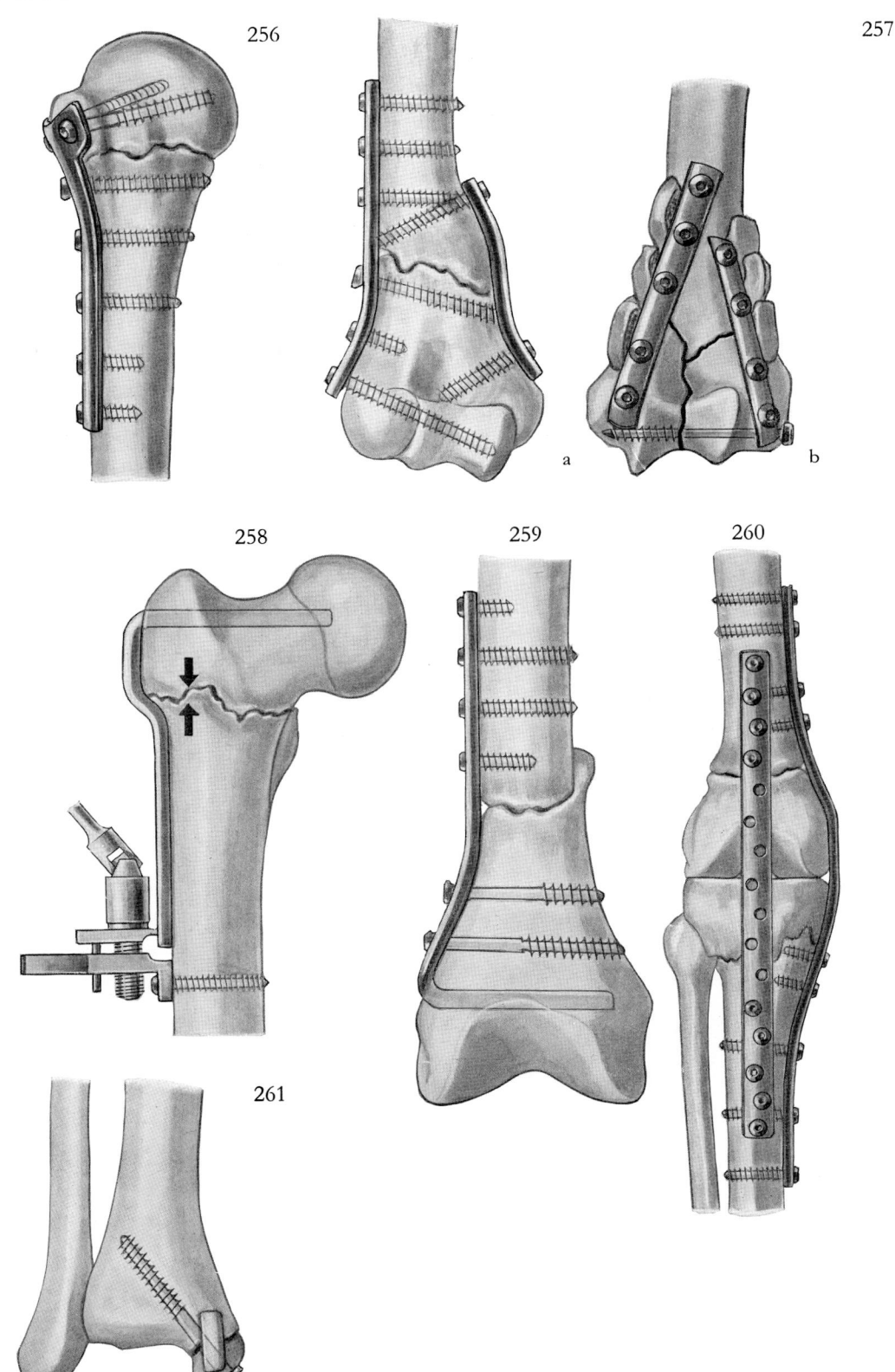

256

257

a   b

258   259   260

261

247

Pseudarthroses of the Femoral Neck

The best solution for a pseudarthrosis of the femoral neck in patients over 70, or for patients who are in poor health, is a total prosthetic replacement. In young patients in whom consolidation of the pseudarthrosis is desirable, we recommend most strongly the corrective osteotomy of PAUWELS.

Before this is undertaken, however, the *viability of the femoral head* must be established, for in patients over 30 repair of the pseudarthrosis should be undertaken only when the femoral head is viable. In children and in patients under 30 a repositioning osteotomy should be undertaken even in the presence of necrosis of the femoral head.

Avascular necrosis is unlikely in those cases in which radiology shows hypertrophic new bone formation in the head fragment at the pseudarthrosis or where no flattening of the head has occurred eight months after fracture.

In order to stabilize the pseudarthrosis, the repositioning osteotomy is carried out in such a way that the fracture line is made to lie at 90° to the resultant of forces (PAUWELS). Following a successful operation the pseudarthrosis usually ossifies with surprising rapidity.

The relationship of the two fragments to one another is best determined from two orthograde X-rays. The antero-posterior projection is taken with the lower limb in 20° of internal rotation. For the technique of the axial projection see Fig. 263.

Fig. 262   In order to determine the angle of correction for the repositioning osteotomy, it is necessary to know the direction of the resultant (R) of forces acting on the hip joint. The direction of the resultant (R) in the presence of a negative Trendelenburg-Duchenne sign is largely dependent on the line of action of the abductors. According to PAUWELS, the resultant (R) subtends an angle of 16° with the vertical axis of the body (V) and an angle of 25° with the femoral shaft axis (A). The femoral shaft axis subtends an angle of 9° with the vertical (V). The pseudarthrosis is then under compression when it subtends an angle of 30° or less with the vertical (S) to the femoral shaft axis. If for example, a fracture line subtended an angle of 75° with the vertical (S) then the angle of correction, the *repositioning angle*, would amount to 50°. The *repositioning angle is the angle between* the fracture line and the vertical to the resultant R.

Fig. 263   *The technique of the axial projection:* The patient lies supine, or slightly turned to the side, with the hip and knee joints bent to 90° and the thighs in 25° of abduction (when the femoral neck/shaft angle is 115°).

a   As seen from in front.

b   As seen from the side.

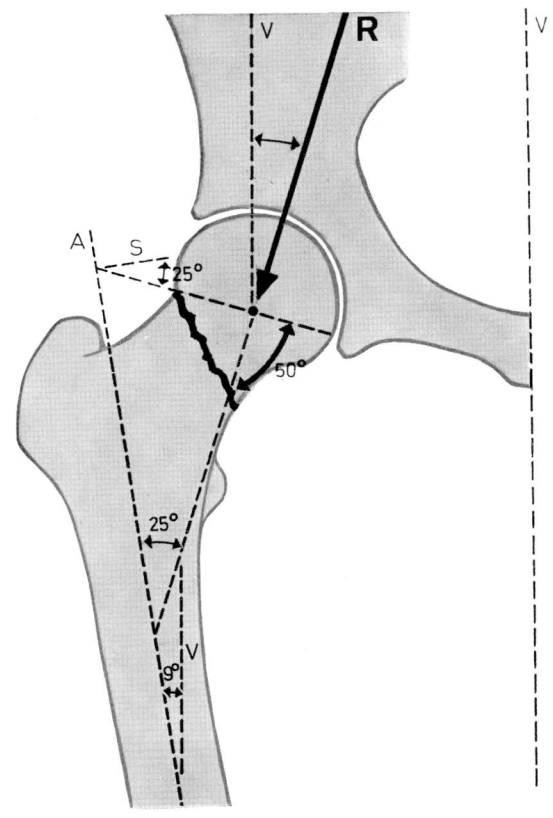

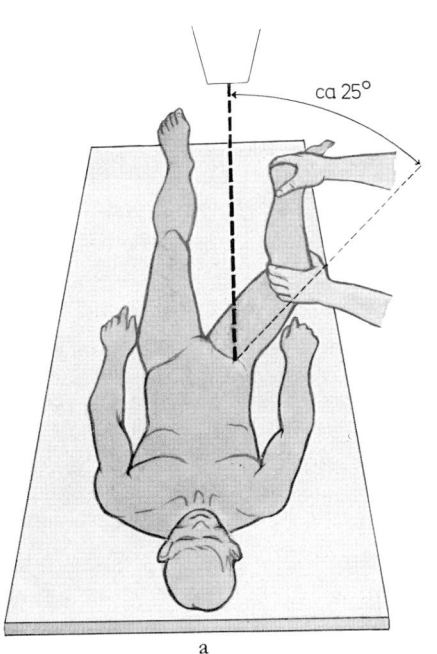

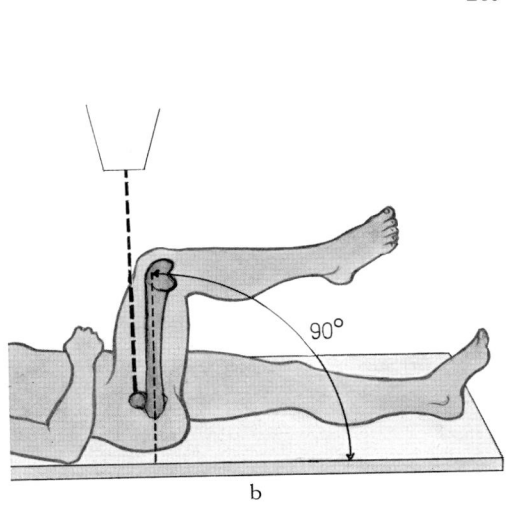

Fig. 264   *Pre-operative drawing.*
Draw an exact copy of the antero-posterior roentgenogram and draw, in the following order:

a   The femoral shaft axis and a perpendicular to it.

b   Draw a line through the fracture line to determine the angle between this line and the perpendicular to the femoral shaft axis. In this case it amounts to 75°. The corrective angle is next determined. In this particular case it amounts to 50°.

c   Draw another perpendicular to the femoral shaft axis, in such a way that it meets the edge of the calcar.

d   Draw in the downward slip of the femoral head. This distance can be measured along the femoral neck, either at the proximal or distal end of the fracture line. Mark off this distance on line c beginning at the medial femoral cortex (d').

e   From this point (d'), draw an angle of 30° with line c in a caudal direction giving line e. (You are using a 120° blade plate, less 90° equals 30°.)

f   Beginning at d' on the proximal side of c, draw a line making an angle of 50° with line e. This is line f, and the angle f–d'–e is then equal to the repositioning angle.

g   Draw in the line for the Kirschner wire as far proximal as possible and parallel to f.

h   Next, draw in the special seating chisel parallel to f and g (the tip of the chisel should extend as far as possible into the lower quadrant of the femoral head. At the same time, great care must be taken that the bone bridge between the chisel and line f is not less than 15 mm).

i   Calculate the angle between the seating chisel and the femoral shaft axis (60° plus the corrective angle = 110°). (This identifies the wedge of 50°, based laterally, which is to be excised.)

k   Check your drawing with a 120° blade plate, positioning it in such a way that the blade of the plate lies parallel to the seating chisel. The angle between the femoral shaft axis and the side portion of the plate must correspond to the repositioning angle, that is 50°.

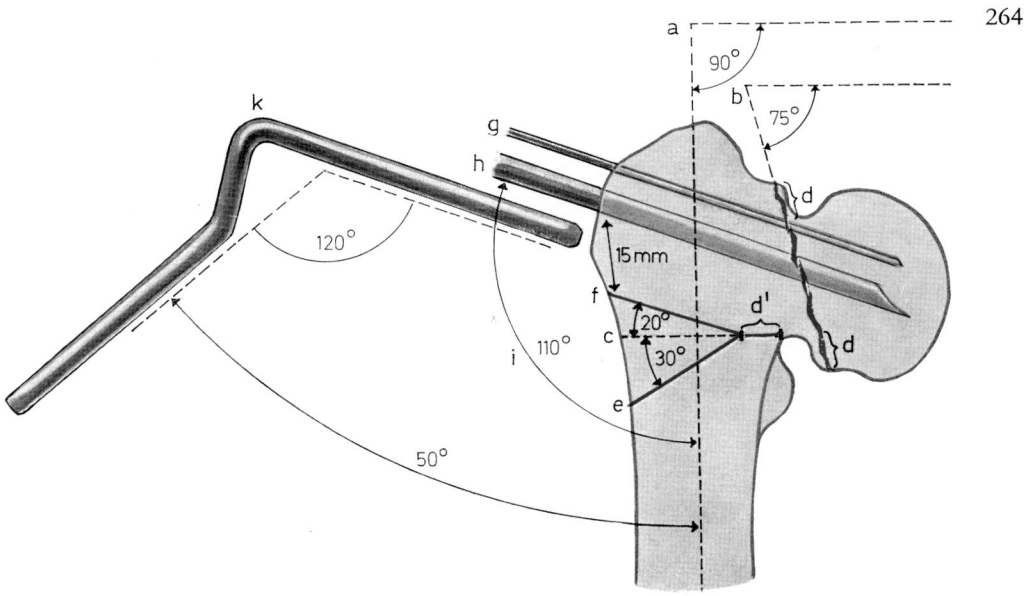

Repositioning osteotomy for pseudarthroses of the femoral neck.

Fig. 265   *Operative technique.*
(same notation as in illustration 264).

1   Introduce the Kirschner wire (g) and the seating chisel (h) with its chisel guide set at 110°. Next, take an X-ray and check the blade length and its inclination to the femoral shaft axis. After it has been established that no correction is necessary, excise the wedge. In this case a 50° wedge with its base laterally.

2   Remove the seating chisel and hammer in the 120° blade plate. If necessary, take another X-ray and check whether the blade of the plate is of the right length and whether it subtends the correct angle with the femoral shaft axis. Only if no corrections are necessary, is the next step undertaken. The next step consists of a cut at a right angle to the femoral shaft axis (d′) which divides the distal from the proximal fragment.

3   Abduct the leg until the osteotomy surfaces come to lie together. Increase the abduction slightly, so that the femoral shaft makes contact only with the distal end of the plate, and so that a gap is created between the shaft and the plate. This gap should not exceed 5 mm. Insert now the short diatal screw. With the insertion of the proximal screws, the femoral shaft is pulled in towards the plate. This impacts the osteotomy surfaces and brings them under compression.

4   Small grafts are placed medially between the fracture and the distal fragment. The fracture line is now at a right angle to the resultant of forces (R).

5   *N.B.:* If there is less than 15 mm of bone left laterally between the blade of the plate and the osteotomy, an additional tension band wire fixation is necessary. This tension band wire is passed around the insertion of the abductors and through a drill hole in the distal fragment.

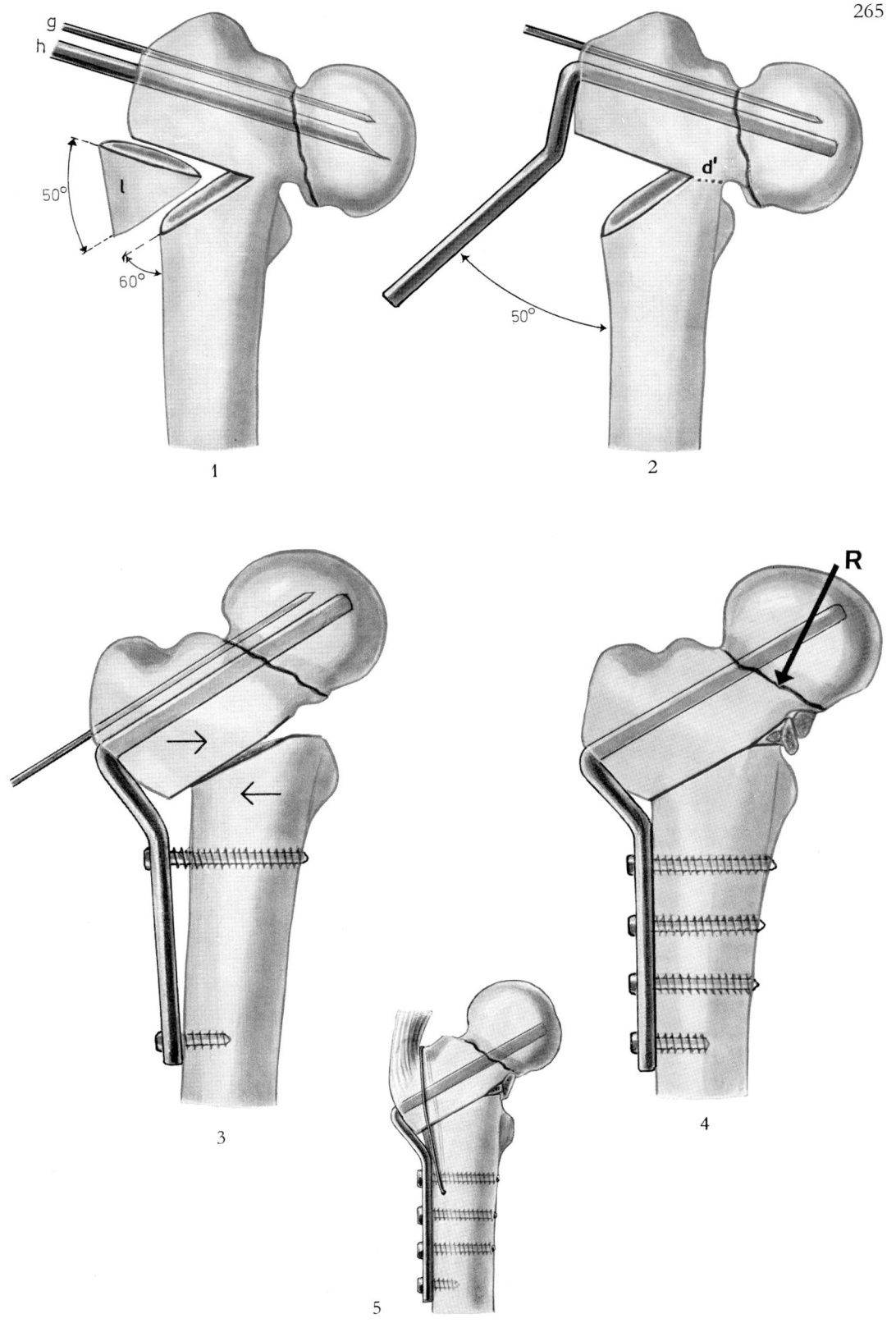

B. Previously Infected but now Dry Pseudarthroses and Pseudarthroses with Bone Loss

In dealing with previously infected pseudarthroses, one must always remember that even after many years of quiescence the infection may flare up. It is also important to know whether there is contact between the fragments or whether there is bone loss with a gap.

The treatment of these pseudarthroses consists of providing a stable rigid fixation in combination with decortication of the bone. Whenever a defect is present autogenous cancellous bone must be used to fill it.

Fig. 266		
	a	Whenever wide contact exists between the hypertrophic bone ends and a deformity is present, the pseudarthrosis is fixed with a very long eleven to sixteen hole "tension band" plate, applied on the convex side of the deformity. In the middle of the plate, that is in the region of the pseudarthrosis and of the previously infected bone, no screws are inserted. Thus the pseudarthrosis and its immediate vicinity is left completely untouched by the procedure.
	b	Whenever a fibular osteotomy becomes necessary, as for example when a small defect is present, the osteotomy must always be carried out distally and never at the level of the pseudarthrosis. External compression clamps should be used to provide rigid fixation. A decortication should also be carried out.
Fig. 267		Whenever a small defect is present and a small cancellous graft is required to bridge the defect, the bone may be obtained from the greater trochanter and placed in between the freshened bone surfaces. Afterwards a tension. band plate is applied, as for an example, in pseudarthrosis of the clavicle.
Fig. 268		A pseudarthrosis with bone loss of the humerus is adequately treated by extensive decortication and cancellous grafting. Additional metal fixation is not necessary. If bony union does not occur subsequently, fixation with a tension band plate is indicated.
Fig. 269		In dealing with a pseudarthrosis with bone loss of either the radius or the ulna, a long semi-tubular plate is employed and is fixed proximally and distally with screws with the forearm maintained in full supination while the fixation is carried out. In the trough of the plate, cancellous bone autografts are laid. Additional plaster fixation is almost always necessary because of the rotational stress even if one of the two bones is intact.
Fig. 270		In pseudarthroses of the femur, we prefer to use two (specially made) semi-tubular plates applied at 90° to one another. These are left *in situ* even if the infection flares up. The cancellous bone autograft which is placed in the defect between the two semi-tubular plates often leads to consolidation. Here we have an example of such a pseudarthrosis in the femur. The same applies also for the tibia, particularly if the fibula is intact.

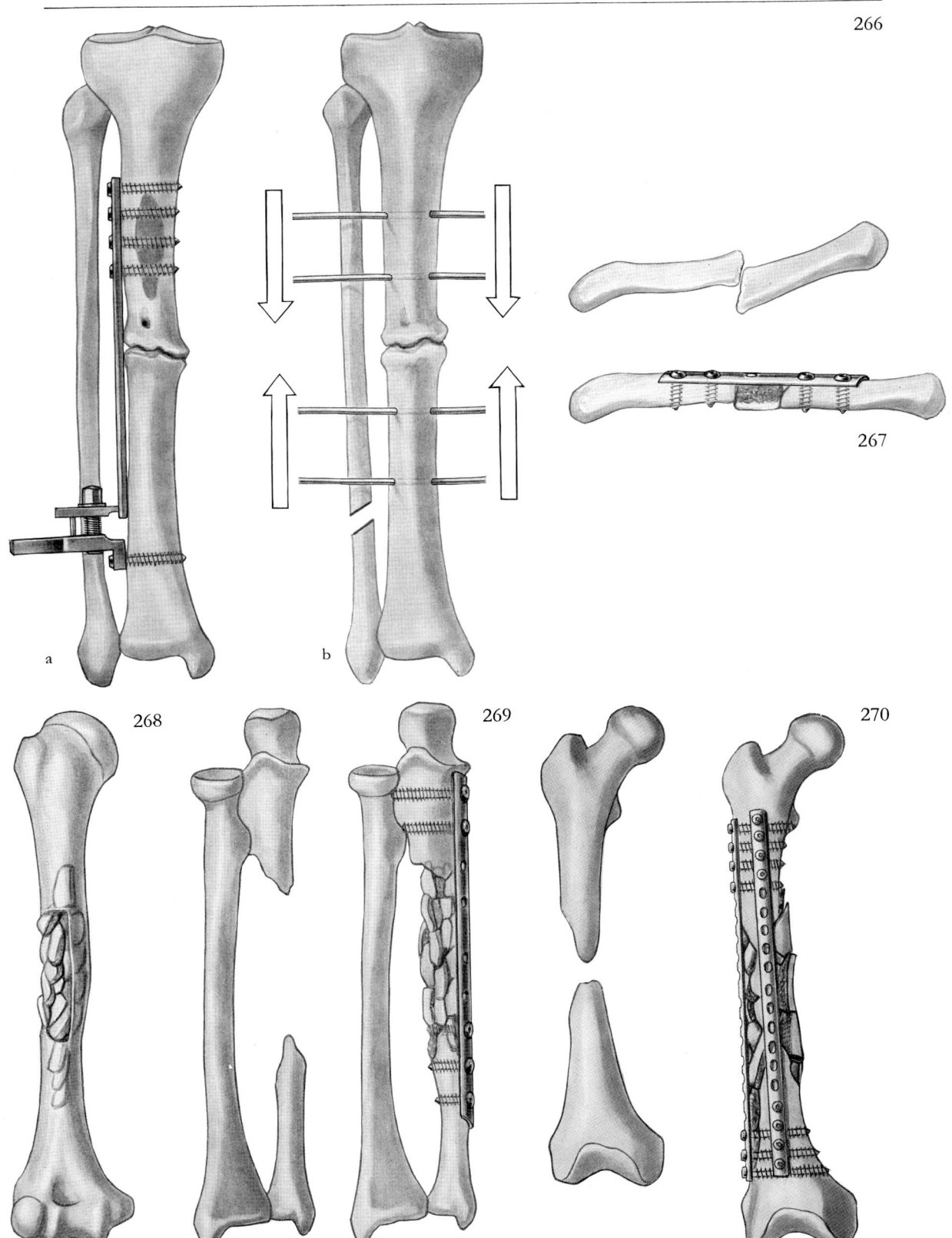

267

269

270

a

b

C. Open Infected Draining Pseudarthroses

Infected Pseudarthroses of the Femur

These pseudarthroses present the greatest problems because of their tendency to shortening and because it is impossible to employ a second bone as in the tibia, for immobilization. It is for this reason that whatever method of fixation had originally been used, so long as it still provides fixation, must be left alone. If no internal fixation was used, this must now be provided in addition to wide decortication and autogenous bone grafting. Infection will persist as long as the implant is *in situ,* but as long as the implant provides rigid fixation, the pseudarthrosis will usually heal. Once the pseudarthrosis has healed, the implant can be removed and the infection will usually subside. Whenever good contact between the bone fragments is present, external compression clamps can be used as a means of rigid immobilization.

Possible methods for stabilizing infected femoral pseudarthroses.

Fig. 271	If an intramedullary nail is rigidly fixed in the proximal fragment but is moving distally in a large medullary canal, fixation can be obtained by simply advancing the nail 2–3 cm through the distal sclerotic bone plug in the medullary canal. If there is good contact between the fragments, this must be supplemented by decortication. If there is a small local defect at the fracture site, cancellous bone grafting must also be carried out in addition to the decortication.
Fig. 272	*Sub-trochanteric pseudarthroses.* We recommend that such pseudarthroses be stabilized under compression by means of a condylar plate and that cancellous bone grafting be carried out on the dorsal surface of the pseudarthrosis. A discharging sinus may persist as long as the plate is in place, but within a few months the pseudarthrosis will usually unite. The implant can then be removed and the infection usually subsides.
Fig. 273	*Mid-shaft pseudarthroses.* In an infected pseudarthrosis in the middle third of the femur, stabilization can be obtained by means of four Schanz screws and two external compression clamps, placed side by side to apply compression. The stability, however, is not as great as by the application of compression clamps on opposite sides. This method is not recommended because one can easily damage blood vessels.
Fig. 274	*Infected pseudarthroses of the distal femur.* An infected pseudarthrosis of the distal femur can be stabilized and brought under compression by introducing two Steinmann pins into each fragment and then applying two external compression clamps, which bring the pseudarthrosis under compression and afford stabilization.
Fig. 275	In dealing with a badly infected pseudarthrosis of the lower femur, one can, if the lateral cortices are viable, secure bone union between these cortices by abducting the distal fragment to 60°, and immobilizing the leg in this position in plaster for six weeks. After six or seven weeks, as the distal fragment is straightened out and brought into alignment with the proximal fragment, strong interfragmentary compression is achieved and the pseudarthrosis goes on to rapid union. This is an example of using a primary bony bridge as a tension band.
Fig. 276	Saucerization should be sufficiently thorough to lay widely open the medullary canal in each fragment, leaving bleeding bone only. It should be possible to line the resulting cavity with healthy vascular muscle.

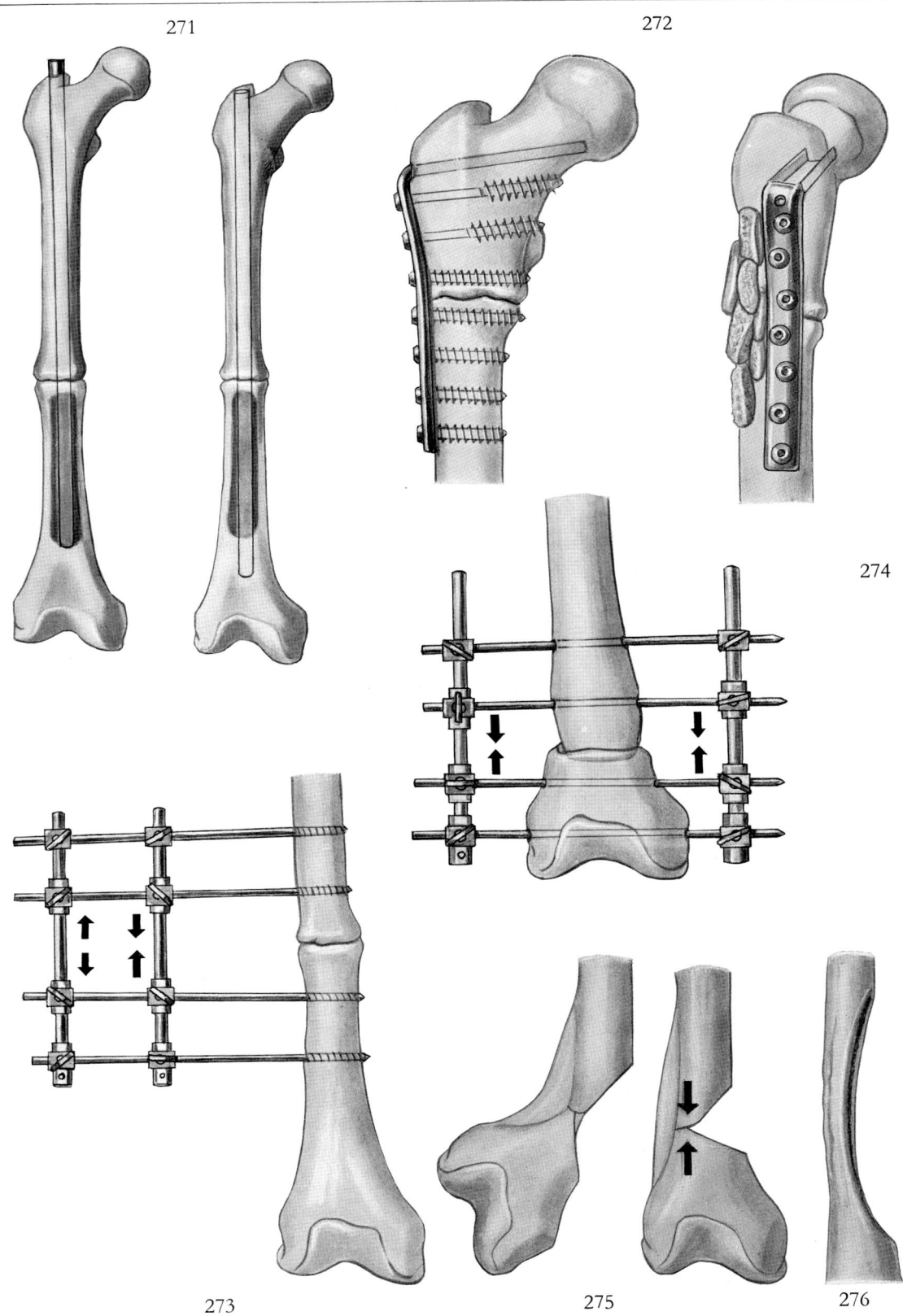

271

272

274

273

275

276

Infected Pseudarthroses of the Tibia

Healing of such a pseudarthrosis is usually achieved after sequestrectomy, rigid internal fixation and decortication. Whenever a defect is present, it must be filled in with cancellous bone. Usually one can achieve a stable fixation only by means of a tibio-fibular synostosis. Such a synostosis is a very dependable method of treatment but it should be remembered that it may compromise the ankle joint.

Fig. 277   As long as the metallic implant, as for example, an intramedullary nail, provides some stability to an infected pseudarthrosis, it should be left in place. In such a case, a dorsal decortication is carried out through a posterior approach and whenever a defect is present, a cancellous bone graft is used to fill the defect.

Fig. 278   If good contact is present between the fragments, sequestrectomy, dorso-lateral decortication and immobilization are indicated, bringing the pseudarthrosis under compression by means of four Steinmann pins and two external compression clamps. Occasionally, a distal fibular osteotomy may be necessary.

Fig. 279   Whenever one is dealing with a pseudarthrosis of both the fibula and the tibia at the same level, one must first obtain fixation by means of six Steinmann pins and external compression clamps. As soon as the infection has become quiescent, a dorso-lateral decortication is carried out and if a defect is present it is filled in with cancellous bone.

Fig. 280   *Tibio-fibular synostosis* with cancellous bone removed from the ilium.

   a   In a case such as this, where the fibula is intact, where there is a medial sinus and good bone contact, the pseudarthrosis should be approached from its lateral aspect, the tibia and fibula freshened up and extensive cancellous bone grafting carried out.

   b   In an infected pseudarthrosis with much bone loss, the cancellous bone grafting must extend as far as possible above and below the pseudarthrosis. Proximally, one must take great care not to injure the anterior tibial artery.

   c   In a distal infected pseudarthrosis with extensive bone loss, the only way to obtain rigid immobilization of the small distal fragment is by securing bony union between the small distal fragment and the fibula.

Fig. 281   Residual osteomyelitis and skin loss after healing of an infected pseudarthrosis.

   a   After a radical sequestrectomy, pull together the skin edges as much as possible with adhesive strips and change these daily.

   b   Subsequently a second sequestrectomy and bone grafting is frequently necessary. The skin is closed primarily with the aid of a few retention sutures (Dermalon 0) which must be removed, at the latest, after 48 hours, when the skin tension is considerably lessened.

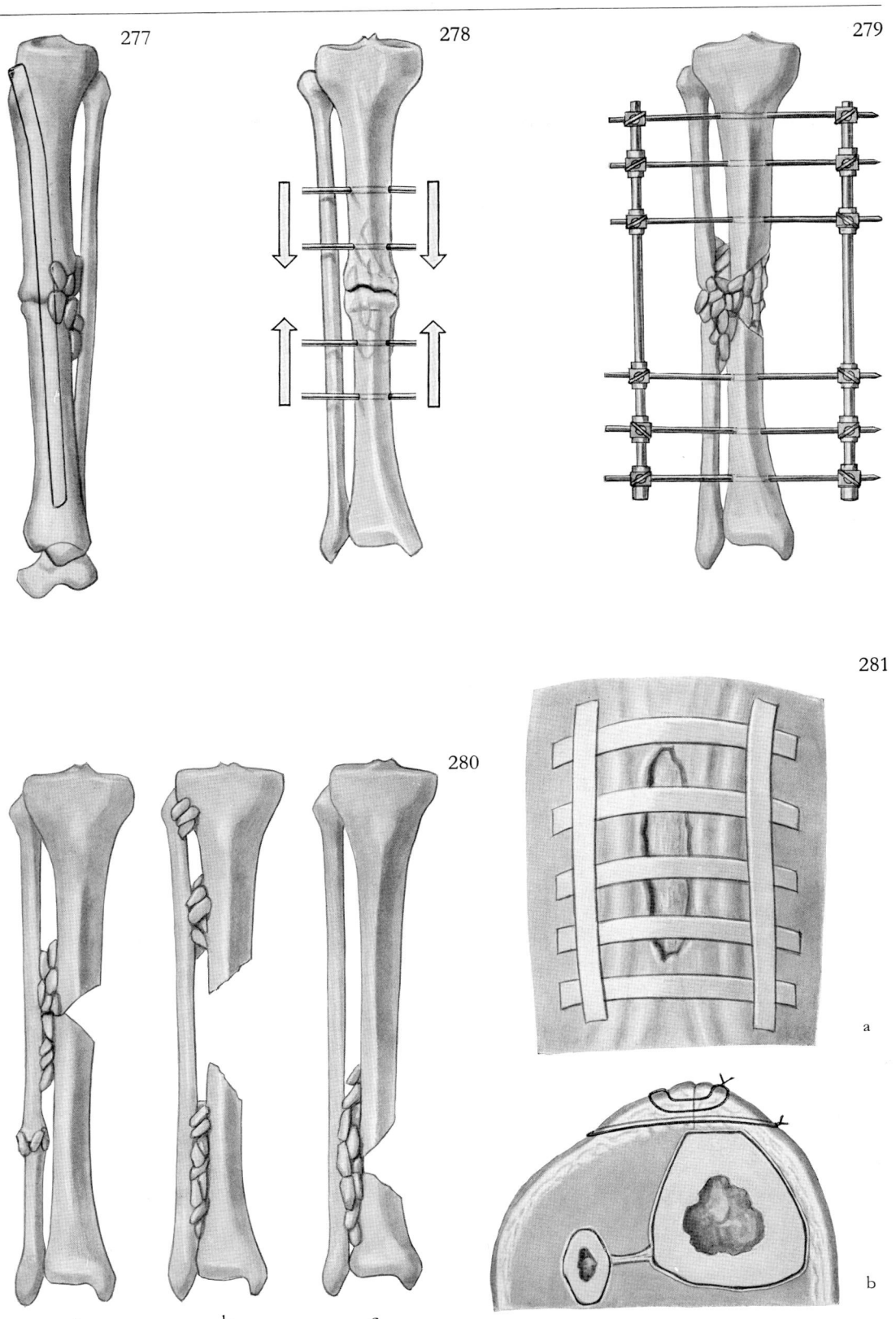

277

278

279

280

a   b   c

281

a

b

Remark to page 261:

Shortening should be corrected whenever possible. This is of particular importance in juvenile patients who have premature incomplete epiphysial plate closure leading to genu valgum or genu varum. In these cases correction is frequently carried out by open osteotomy and bone grafting, rather than closed osteotomy with wedge resection. It should be appreciated that in the former, compression can only be exerted on one cortex.

It should be appreciated that in the adult *lengthening procedures* for healed fractures with shortening, can present great difficulties. In the femur, one can obtain a lengthening of 3 cm without any appreciable problems. In the tibia, however, a lengthening of even 1 or 2 cm can lead to skin necrosis and damage to nerves and vessels.

II. Osteotomies

An osteotomy is the division of bone which is carried out for the purpose of axial correction, for shortening, or for lengthening of the bone. We use *rigid internal fixation* to make absolutely certain that no displacement of the osteotomy fragments takes place, and that no loss of the desired new relationship between the two fragments occurs. *Intramedullary nails* are used very rarely. *Axial compression* with the aid of tension band plates, double plates or external compression clamps is used very frequently. The real advantage of rigid internal fixation is two fold. Post-operative plaster fixation is no longer necessary and early mobilization of all joints can be begun. After a few days, most patients can usually begin partial weight bearing.

An osteotomy is usually carried out through the *metaphysis* because in the diaphysis there is danger of delayed union. Rapid bony consolidation of large cancellous surfaces, immobilized rigidly under compression, is no great biological problem. Whenever an osteotomy is carried out through a large area of callus surrounding the diaphysis, before the osteotomy is done, extensive decortication must be carried out. Whenever, in addition to axial correction, lengthening is also carried out, the resulting defect in the bone must always be filled in with cancellous bone.

An osteotomy allows for six *simultaneous corrections;* namely, valgus/varus, flexion/extension, internal/external rotation, lengthening/shortening, medial or lateral displacement, and dorsal or ventral displacement.

Before operation, one must determine with great precision, *the existing deformity, what corrections are to be undertaken,* and one must draw up a very *detailed plan of the surgical approach* and the procedure contemplated.

Beginners have the greatest difficulty in diagnosing *rotational deformities.* In order to diagnose these in the femur, one makes use of the Dunn-Rippstein-Müller X-ray projection. In the tibia, one uses the patellar position in the upright posture and the position of the foot when the person is sitting. A deformity most commonly ignored is lateral displacement. It should be appreciated that a 5 mm lateral displacement of the tibia can result in a 50% reduction of the pressure exerted on the talus. It is for these reasons that we recommend, before any osteotomy that *full length X-ray films* be taken in at least two but preferably four planes.

In considering technical points, we recommend that after the skin incision, two Kirschner wires be inserted on each side of the osteotomy to allow for a check to be made at any time on the correction that is being carried out. Two of the Kirschner wires are introduced parallel to each other and are left in place, while the other two Kirschner wires form the desired angle of correction in the plane in which the main correction is being carried out. In the case of the tibia, whether in the proximal or distal metaphysis, the ventral Kirschner wires usually remain parallel to each other because anti-curvatum or retrocurvatum rarely require correction. The remaining two Kirschner wires which are introduced at 90° to the ventral ones, represent the angle of desired correction in the frontal plane.

A. Osteotomies in the Upper Extremity

In osteotomy of metaphysial bone we use an oscillating saw. The oscillating blade is cooled with physiological saline. Whenever cortices have to be osteotomized, we employ an osteotome to prevent bone necrosis from the heat generated by the oscillating saw. In osteotomy through diaphysial bone, we recommend thorough decortication to provide an additional osteogenic stimulus to union. In lengthening procedures we feel that the defect created must always be filled with autogenous cancellous bone.

Fig. 282	*Osteotomy through the surgical neck of the humerus.*
	Such an osteotomy is indicated for fractures through the surgical neck of the humerus, treated on an abduction frame, which have healed with painful limitation of adduction. The fixation of such an osteotomy is carried out with a T-plate as in fractures in this region.
Fig. 283	A deformity in the supracondylar region of the humerus is usually the result of a poorly reduced supracondylar fracture in either children or teenagers. A valgus deformity should be corrected long before ulnar palsy becomes manifest.
	The procedure is carried out through a dorsal approach (see Fig. 103c) with anterior transposition of the ulnar nerve and fixation of the osteotomy with a suitably bent narrow plate. Great care should be taken that no screw is inserted into the olecranon fossa, for it would lead to limitation of extension.
Fig. 284	*Shortening of the radius for Kienböck's Disease.*
	We have found two procedures useful in treating osteochondritis of the lunate: namely, shortening of the radius or lengthening of the ulna. It appears that whenever the head of the ulna is made to protrude distal to the articular surface of the radius, it results in decompression of the lunate. At any rate, whatever the explanation may be, the subjective improvement and the objective radiological evidence is so convincing that we strongly recommend these procedures. A lengthening osteotomy of the ulna heals rather slowly, and it is for this reason that we prefer to shorten the radius. A 4–6 mm wide wedge is excised from the radius. For fixation we employ a narrow 4 hole plate placed under tension with a tension device.

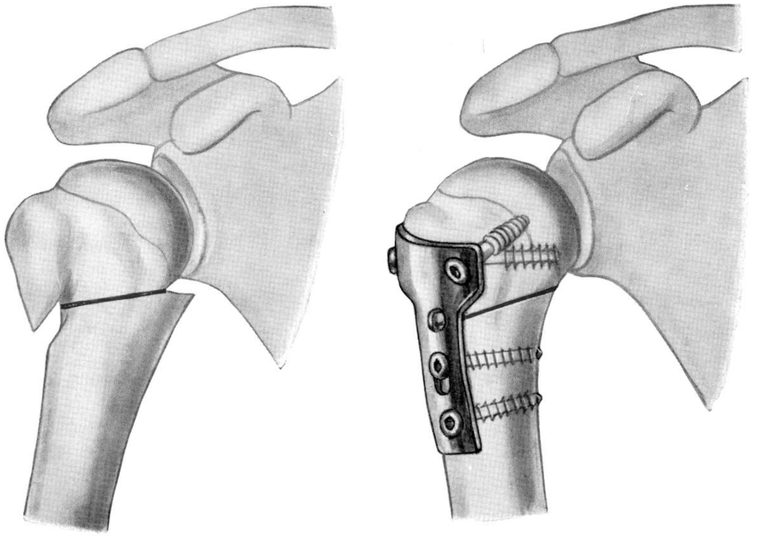

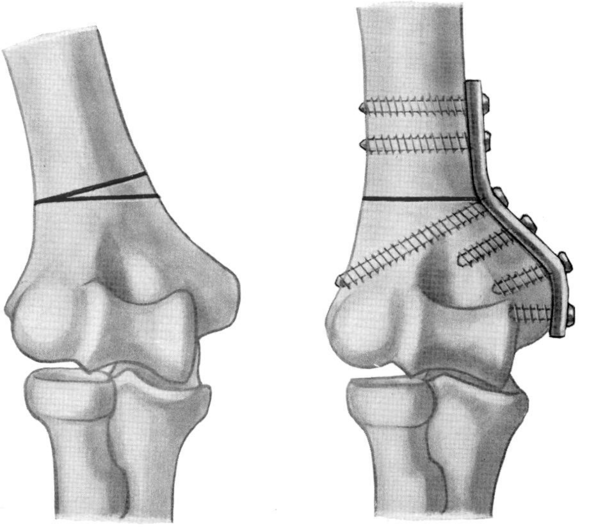

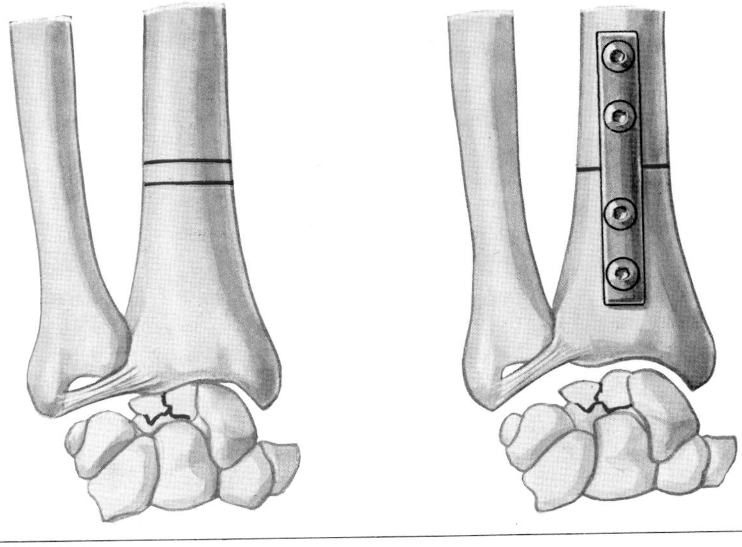

B. Intertrochanteric Osteotomies

A number of post-traumatic deformities in the region of the femoral neck can be corrected by means of intertrochanteric osteotomy. The different intertrochanteric osteotomies using the right angled plate have already been discussed (Fig. 63). The technique of the intertrochanteric varus osteotomy, however, will now be described in detail. It may be indicated for example in an abduction deformity resulting from an abduction femoral neck fracture.

Fig. 285   *Intertrochanteric varus osteotomy.*

1   Make a lateral incision through skin and fascia lata, extending it from the tip of the greater trochanter 20 cm distally. Reflect forwards the vastus lateralis and then insert one Hohmann retractor below the calcar and one above the neck just medial to the greater trochanter. Next, do a wide anterior capsulotomy in line with the femoral neck and examine the joint. Introduce one Kirschner wire (a) along the front of the femoral neck and advance it into bone at the head neck junction. This Kirschner wire (a) corresponds to the *femoral neck axis.* A second Kirschner wire (b) is introduced into the greater trochanter parallel with the first Kirschner wire and parallel with the quadrangular positioning plate (c) (Fig. 63d). This gives us both the *horizontal and frontal planes.*

2   Approximately 2 cm proximal to the point where the osteotomy is to be carried out, with an osteotome cut a hole in the cortex wide enough to receive the seating chisel (d). This hole should be as anterior as possible. The chisel is fitted with a removable chisel guide (e). The chisel is hammered into the middle of the femoral neck to a depth of 4.5 cm and parallel to the second Kirschner wire. The small flap on the chisel guide (e) serves here to indicate the sagittal plane.

3   Introduce a wide Hohmann retractor behind, to protect the soft tissues. The osteotomy is now carried out with the oscillating saw (f). A cut is made parallel to the seating chisel. The blade of the oscillating saw is irrigated with cold physiological saline to prevent bone necrosis from over heating.

4   Using the seating chisel as a lever, open up the osteotomy by tilting the proximal fragment into varus. It is now possible to excise a small wedge (g), based medially, by beginning in the middle of the osteotomy surface of the distal fragment, and making the cut at right angles to the long axis of the femoral shaft.

5   Remove the small medial wedge (h).
This small wedge should subsequently be inserted laterally between the osteotomy fragments.

6   Hammer out the seating chisel. Now insert the right angle blade plate, making certain that it is inserted exactly into the channel cut for it by the chisel.

7   Reduce the osteotomy and maintain the reduction by fixing the plate to the femoral shaft with a Verbrugge clamp. Check now for rotational position of the lower extremity in extension. If the osteotomy has been correctly reduced and if no rotational deformity is present, a 3.2 mm hole is drilled and tapped 2 cm distal to the plate. Now insert the tension device, and fix it to the femoral shaft and begin tightening the screw on the tension device, first with the socket wrench with cardan joint and subsequently with the open-end wrench. Once the osteotomy surfaces have been placed under maximal compression, flex the hip as much as possible and again check for rotation. If everything appears perfect, screw the plate to the femoral shaft and remove the tension device.

8   Now insert a short screw into the last hole of the plate. This screw is short in order to smooth out the gradation between normal elastic bone and the rigid plated segment.

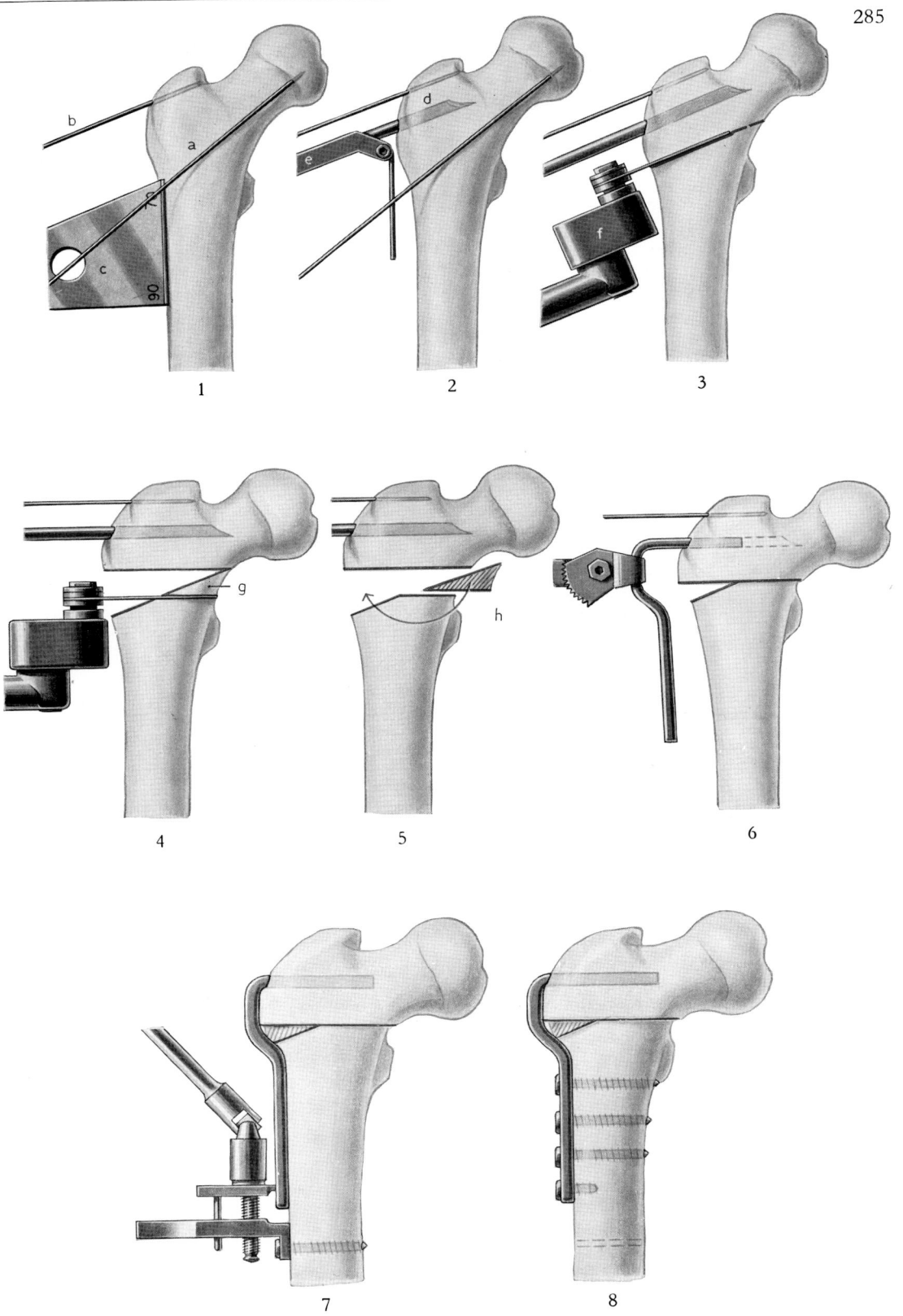

1

2

3

4

5

6

7

8

Shortening of the Leg by Means of an Intertrochanteric Osteotomy

This procedure allows a shortening of 2 to 4 cm and allows ambulation of the patient within a few days.

Fig. 286   *The operative technique.*

1   Expose the intertrochanteric region and insert three Kirschner wires at right angles to the long axis of the femoral shaft. The first Kirschner wire (a) is inserted into the greater trochanter parallel to the axis of the femoral neck and, as previously stated, at a right angle to the femoral shaft axis. The other two Kirschner wires (b) and (c) are inserted into the femoral shaft at an angle of 45° to the frontal plane and somewhat more ventrally than (a). These serve as distance markers and as checks of rotational alignment. Measure the distance between b and c. This means of course that b is inserted into the proximal fragment and c is inserted into the distal fragment, and that the shortening wedge will be removed between these two Kirschner wires. Note the special protractor which allows us to insert the most proximal Kirschner wire (a) at a right angle to the long axis of the femoral shaft (d).

2   Insert the seating chisel at right angles to the femoral shaft in line with the axis of the femoral neck and in the center of the femoral neck. The Kirschner wire is the directional guide. With the oscillating saw, now shorten the femur to the desired length (maximum 4.5 cm). Carry out the osteotomy so that the lesser trochanter remains fixed to the proximal fragment. With a flat chisel, shape the distal fragment into a cone.

3   Remove the seating chisel and replace it by the right angle blade plate. As soon as the fragments are reduced and the Kirschner wires b and c are parallel to one another, maintain the reduction with a Verbrugge clamp and apply the tension device.

4   As compression is applied, the two fragments are impacted, the distal one into the proximal. As soon as the desired shortening and stable fixation are achieved, screw the plate to the shaft.

Fig. 287   *Intertrochanteric derotation varus osteotomy in children.*

For children we have a special right angle blade plate which is fitted with a T-section blade. We also have a corresponding T-blade seating chisel. The technique for this osteotomy in children is almost the same as for intertrochanteric varus osteotomy in the adult. The difference, however, is that the rotational component is very carefully calculated with the help of Kirschner wires inserted on both sides of the osteotomy. In small children the intertrochanteric osteotomy is placed under compression by means of Schanz screws and external compression clamps (see Fig. 43).

1

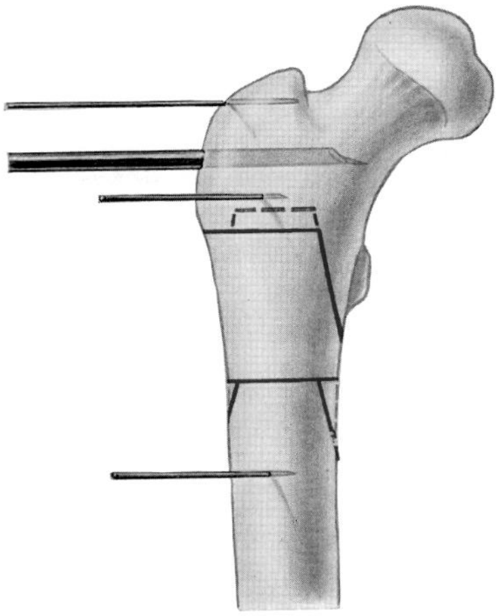

2

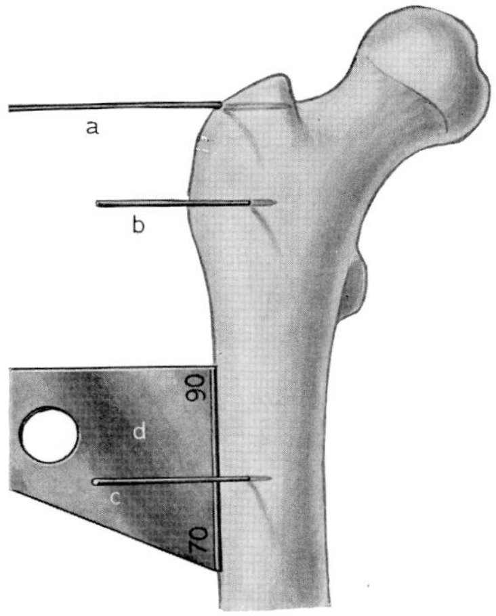

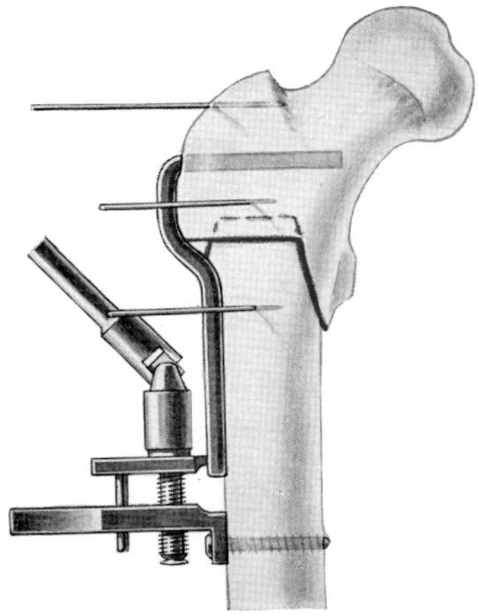

3

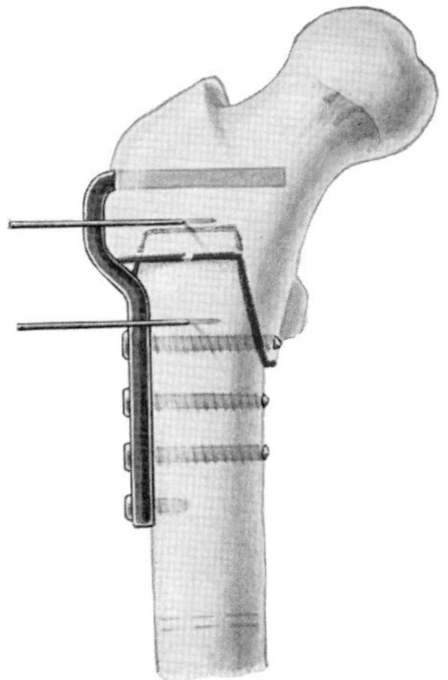

4

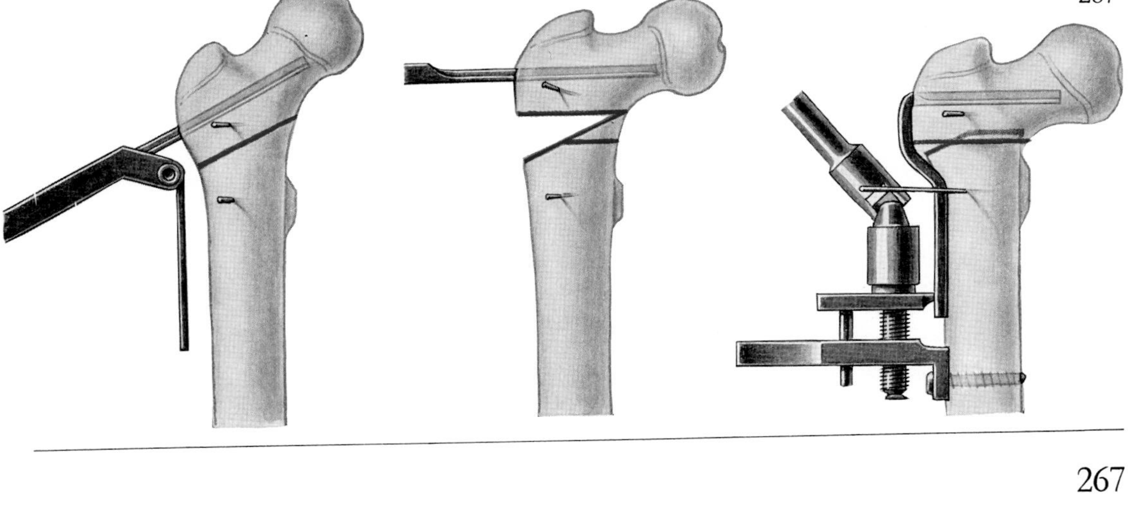

C. Femoral Shaft Osteotomy through old Fracture Callus

Fig. 288   *Simple abduction osteotomy of the femur through callus.*

First of all a wide decortication is carried out. A transverse osteotomy is then done and autogenous cancellous bone grafting is carried out to fill the defect, if such is created. In the proximal and distal femur we employ the condylar plate for fixation. For osteotomy of the middle third we prefer intramedullary nailing.

Fig. 289   *Lengthening osteotomy of the femur for a fracture healed with significant shortening.*

a   The transverse osteotomy through the callus (dotted line) as recommended by CHARNLEY, would of course be the simplest and safest procedure. In general we employ a step osteotomy in order to obtain as much length as possible. Prior to the osteotomy, decortication is carried out over a distance of 10 to 14 cm.

b   Reduction is achieved with the help of a strong osteotome which is used as a lever. A tension band plate is used for fixation, even though osteotomy surfaces appear to be under high compression due to the soft tissue tension. A cancellous bone graft is always used whenever a defect results.

c   Fixation can also be obtained by means of intramedullary nailing with reaming. At times when rotational stability seems to be in doubt, medullary fixation has to be supplemented with a semi-tubular plate applied to the lateral side of the bone and fixed with 14 mm screws (the smallest AO cortex screws) which are short enough to miss the nail. The plate must be removed after 4 to 6 weeks.

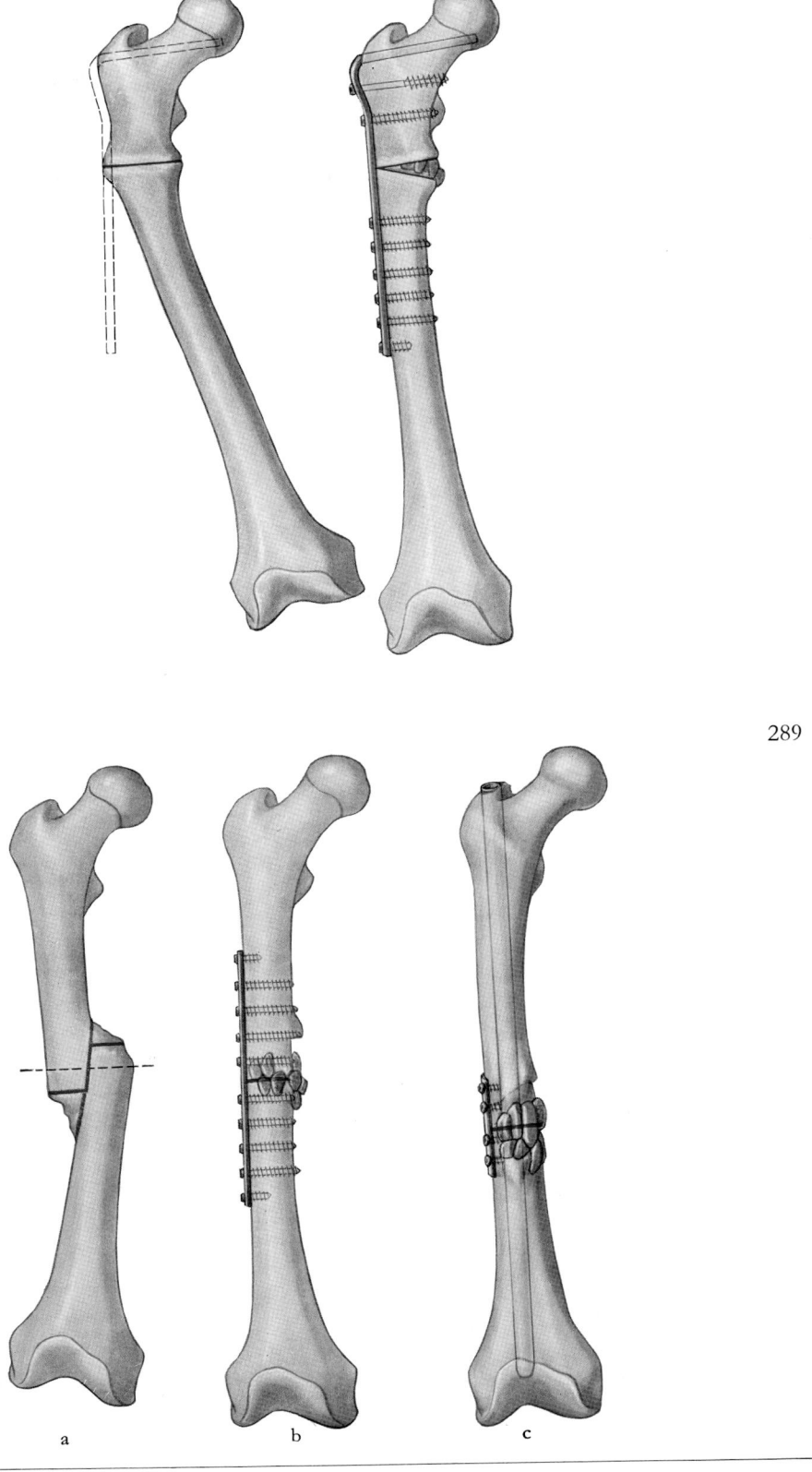

a   b   c

D. Supracondylar Osteotomies

We have found that it is possible to correct through a lateral approach both a varus and valgus deformity. To correct a valgus deformity, however, by a varus supracondylar osteotomy through the lateral approach is not only technically difficult, but the axial compression achieved with a laterally inserted condylar plate following a medial wedge resection, occasionally leaves a great deal to be desired. It is for this reason that we prefer to employ the right angle blade plate and to approach the femur medially.

Fig. 290   The profile of the distal femur makes it obvious that in a valgus osteotomy the condylar plate, and in a varus osteotomy the right angle plate, should be employed to obtain rigid internal fixation.

Fig. 291   *The technique of valgus supracondylar osteotomy.*

Expose the femur through a lateral approach. With the aid of the condylar plate guide and a triangular positioning plate, calculate the desired angle of correction and insert a Kirschner wire into the femoral condyles anticipating the direction of the blade of the condylar plate. Usually this Kirschner wire comes to lie parallel to the plane of the knee joint. The seating chisel is now inserted parallel to the Kirschner wire and the osteotomy is carried out. After the osteotomy is completed, the seating chisel is removed, the condylar plate inserted and fixed to the distal fragment with the first cancellous screw. The osteotomy is now reduced, the reduction maintained with a Verbrugge clamp and the tension device inserted. Once the osteotomy has been compressed the plate is screwed to the shaft and the tension device removed. Knee movement is begun on the first post-operative day and the patient is allowed out of bed on his fourth or fifth day. In between, the knee is held at 90° on a special splint.

Fig. 292   *Varus supracondylar osteotomy for marked genu valgum.*

Here we make use of the quadrangular positioning plate for varus osteotomies. With this and with a triangular positioning plate, the angle of correction is calculated and the position of the blade marked in the femoral condyle by the introduction of a Kirschner wire. From this point on, the procedure is the same as in Fig. 291, but a standard right angle plate with a 60 to 70 mm cortex screw, instead of the condylar plate and a cancellous screw are used to obtain fixation in the distal fragment.

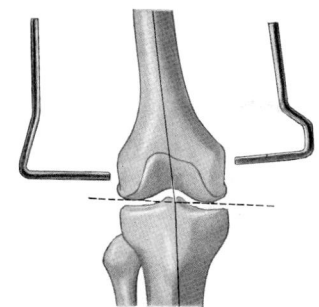

290

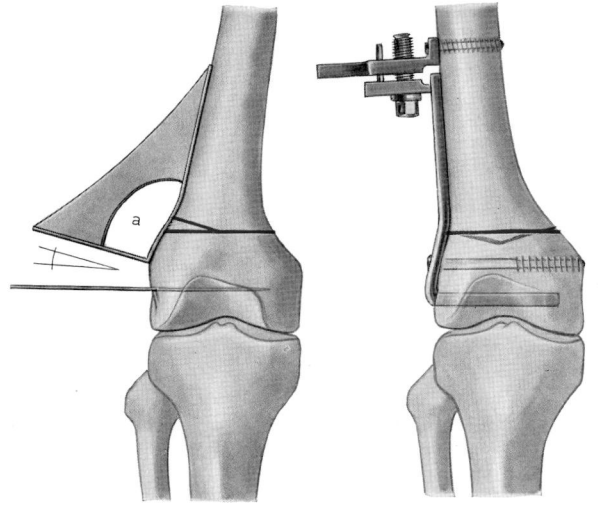

291

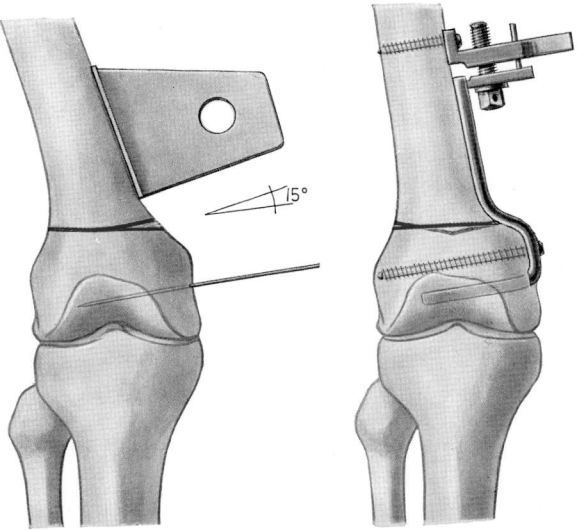

292

E. Osteotomy of the Proximal Tibia

This osteotomy is stabilized either with two Steinmann pins and external compression clamps, or with two plates. As long as we are dealing with non-osteoporotic bone, a two hole plate is sufficient on the lateral side for a varus osteotomy or on the medial side for a valgus osteotomy. In patients in whom the bone is osteoporotic, as in advanced age, one or even two T-plates with corresponding cancellous screws must be employed to obtain the required rigid fixation.

Fig. 293	*The operative technique for proximal tibial osteotomy.*
	Fixation with Steinmann pins and external compression clamps.
1	After the fibular osteotomy and the anterior skin incision is carried out, a Steinmann pin is inserted 1 cm distal to the knee joint. The Kirschner wire (b) subtends with the Steinmann pin (a) an angle which corresponds to the angle of correction. The Kirschner wires (c) and (d), one on each side of the osteotomy, are inserted at right angles to the Steinmann pin and parallel to each other.
2	The osteotomy with the removal of a laterally based wedge for a valgus osteotomy.
3	Close the osteotomy and check that the Steinmann pin is parallel to the Kirschner wire. If this is found to be the case the Kirschner wire is now replaced by a 4.5 mm Steinmann pin.
4	Apply compression and impact the fragments by means of external compression clamps.
Fig. 294	
a	The fixation with plates of non-osteoporotic bone: valgus osteotomy: short plate medially, long plate laterally with the corresponding tension devices and application of tension. A fibular osteotomy is also carried out.
b	Fixation of osteoporotic bone. The shoulder T-plate is employed, as for example here in a varus osteotomy. (The fibula is left intact.) In carrying out a valgus osteotomy through very osteoporotic bone, employ the T-plate on the lateral side and a four hole plate on the medial side. Whenever a rotational element needs correction, one must carry out a fibular osteotomy (see Fig. 44a).

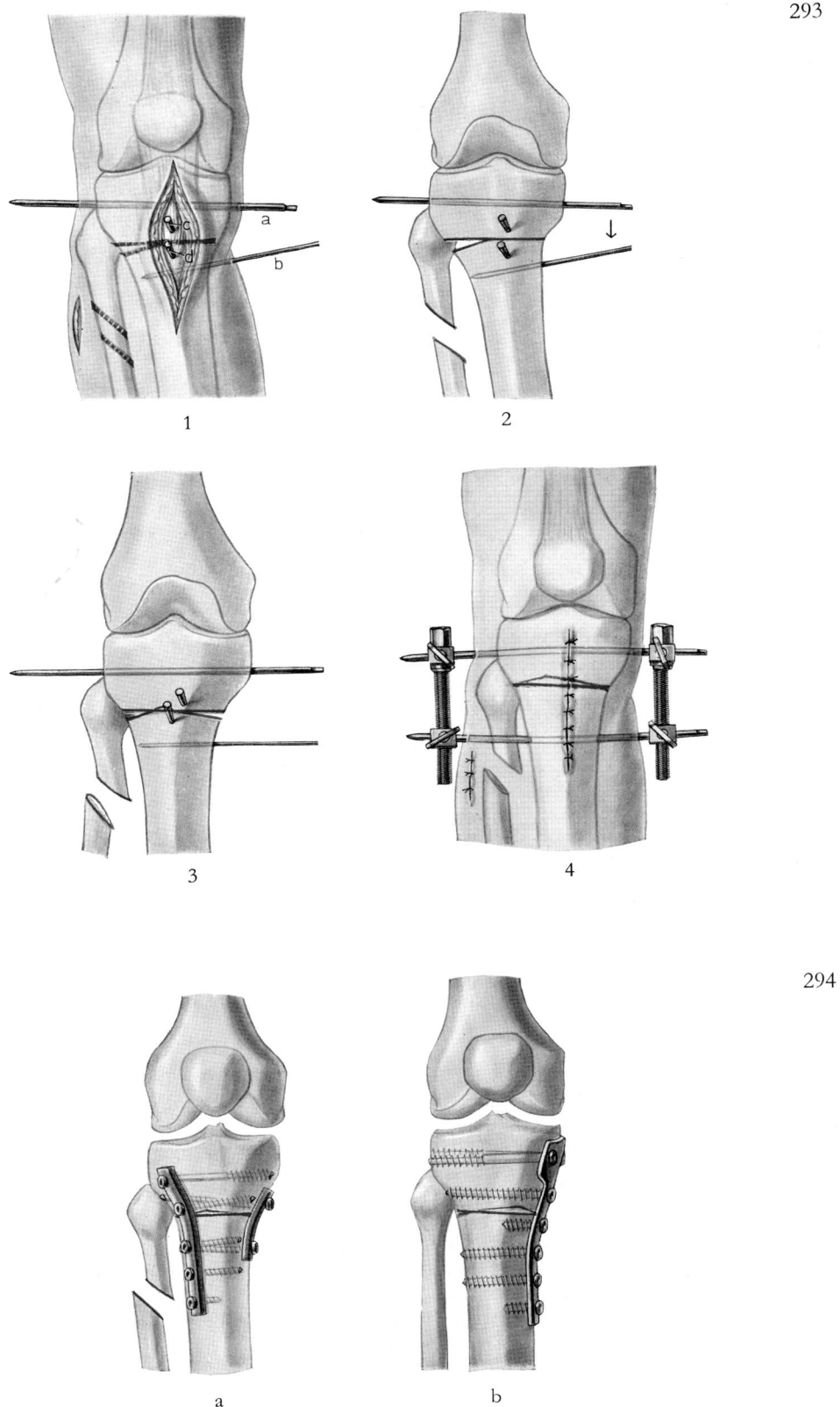

1   2

3   4

a   b

F. Osteotomy of the Tibial Shaft

Osteotomies of the tibial shaft should be done only when there is no problem with the skin, least necrosis of the wound margins occurs. The incision should be straight and very long. Extensive decortication is necessary.

Whenever a lengthening osteotomy is carried out, the resultant bone defect must be filled with autologous cancellous bone.

Fig. 295   *The operative technique.*
A corrective lengthening osteotomy of the tibial shaft through fracture callus.

a   Two Kirschner wires are inserted into the metaphyses, one on each side of the proposed osteotomy. These serve as direction guides. An extensive decortication is carried out followed by an oblique osteotomy.

b   A lateral tension band plate is applied for a valgus osteotomy. The defect is filled with cancellous bone.

c   When the osteotomy is carried out through the mid-shaft of the tibia, after correction of the deformity, it is occasionally possible to ream out the medullary canal and use a medullary nail for fixation. Rotational fixation, if necessary, can be achieved with a 4 hole semi-tubular plate which is applied either on the anterior or medial crest of the tibia.
The plate should be removed after one month or as soon as the danger of rotational instability has passed.

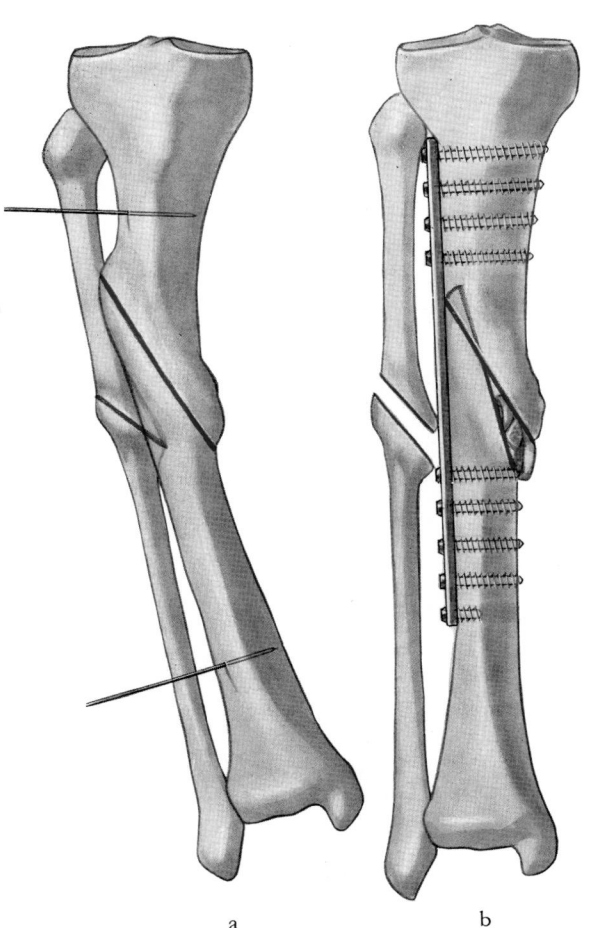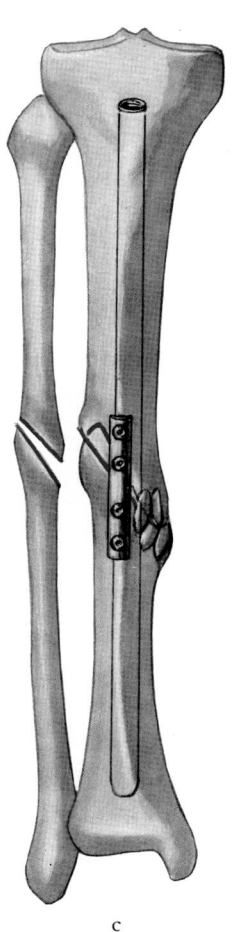

a   b   c

G. Osteotomy of the Lower End of the Tibia

a   Osteotomize the fibula and then insert a Steinmann pin parallel to the plane of the ankle joint through the distal fragment. Proximal to the site of the planned osteotomy, insert from the medial side a 3.2 mm drill. This drill should subtend with the Steinmann pin the desired angle of correction. In addition, insert into the anterior crest of the tibia two Kirschner wires parallel to each other, one above and one below the planned osteotomy site. These will serve subsequently as guides to maintain rotational alignment.

b   An osteotomy is carried out between the two Kirschner wires.

c   Malalignment is now corrected.

d   The drill is now replaced with a Steinmann pin and the osteotomy surfaces are brought under compression by means of two external compression clamps.

Fig. 297

a   A tibial osteotomy can be fixed with two plates in adults, if they need to be discharged from hospital very quickly.

b   In children in whom a deformity is the result of premature incomplete epiphyseal plate closure, the osteotomy surfaces are not impacted but an open wedge osteotomy is carried out and the defect is filled with cancellous bone. The osteotomy is fixed usually with a small semi-tubular plate.

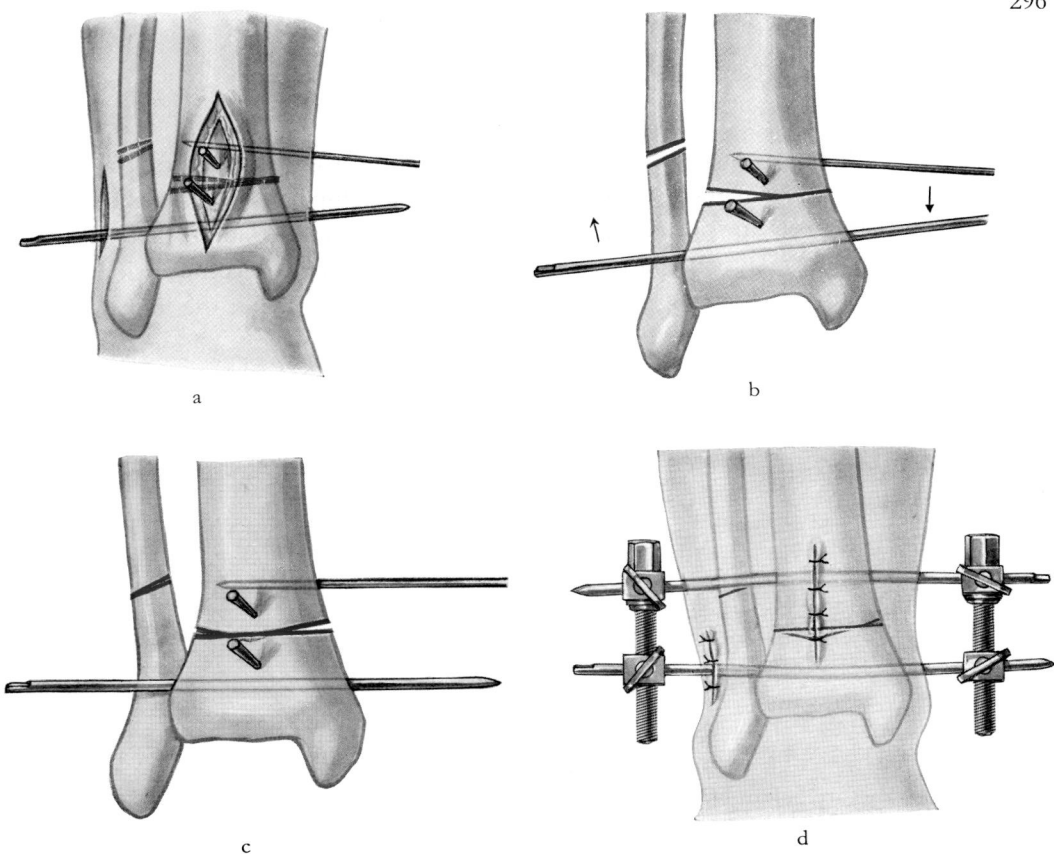

a

b

c

d

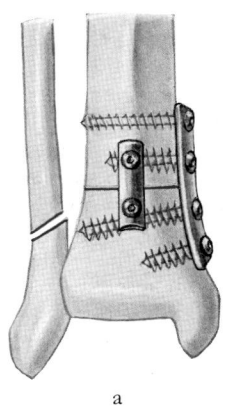

a

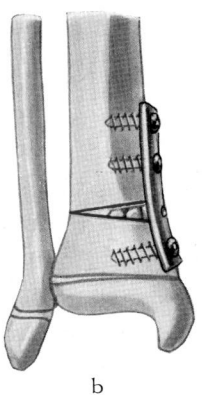

b

III. Arthrodeses

A. Shoulder Arthrodesis

The technique of compression arthrodesis has opened up for the skillful orthopedic surgeon procedures which a few years ago could not even be imagined. Plaster fixation is no longer necessary and after compression arthrodesis of the hip or the knee joint, the patient can be mobilized within a few days and partial weight bearing begun. After compression arthrodesis of the shoulder or the wrist, the patient usually regains active use of the limb within a few days.

Fig. 298   Before beginning the procedure, the desired angle between the medial border of the scapula (vertebral border) and the humerus is determined. Generally abduction of 50°, external rotation of 10° and forward flexion of 25° are taken to be the ideal position for a shoulder arthrodesis. On abduction of the upper extremity to 50° the lateral border of the scapula forms with the humerus an angle of approximately 80°.

The operation is carried out with the patient lying on his side. A straight incision is made from the spine of the scapula to the insertion of the deltoid. The crest of the scapula is exposed to within 1 cm of the lateral edge of the acromion. The acromion is osteotomized at this point and reflected distally together with the deltoid. The capsule is widely opened and all articular cartilage resected and the undersurface of the acromion freshened. In the glenoid, one must not only resect the articular cartilage, but also the labrum. Finally, the upper limb is placed in the desired position and the bone surfaces are trimmed to fit.

The first drill hole is made so that it goes through the acromion and through the neck of the scapula. This hole is particularly important because it is the medial fixation for the plate which is fixed with a 50 to 60 mm cortex screw (a). This hole should be made approximately 1 cm medial to the glenoid.

A 7 to 8 hole plate is contoured to fit using both the bending press and the bending irons. Fixation begins with the insertion of the two medial screws into the crest of the scapula and the acromion. The shoulder is now put in the desired position. It should be noted that in doing this it is frequently necessary to displace the humeral head upwards so that it gains good contact with the freshened acromion. Once the desired position is obtained, the two cancellous screws are inserted through the plate into the glenoid. Care should be taken, if possible, that these two cancellous screws do not come into contact with the previously inserted cortex screws which must be left undisturbed.

A straight 6 hole plate should be used posteriorly to supplement the fixation, particularly if the bone is at all porotic.

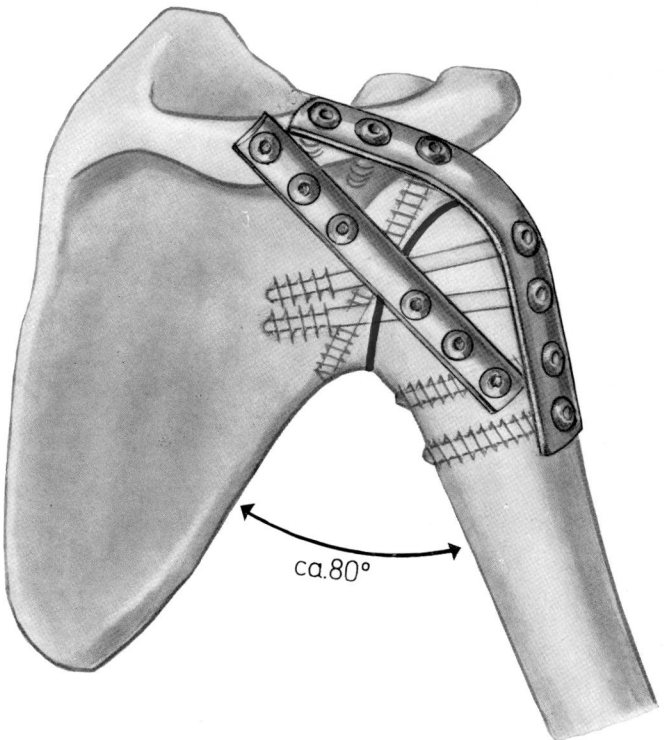

ca.80°

B. Technique of Arthrodesis of the Elbow and Wrist Joint

Arthrodesis of the elbow joint.

Fig. 299   An elbow arthrodesis is the most difficult to perform because the nerves and vessels make it impossible to carry out a tension band fixation. In general, we combine compression systems of external clamps together with an axial cancellous screw. The arthrodesis is most commonly carried out with the elbow at 90°. After resection of the articular cartilage and fitting the fragments, temporary stabilization is achieved by means of a thick Kirschner wire which is introduced through the olecranon into the medullary canal of the humerus. The radial head is then resected as far as the insertion of the biceps tendon. Next a Steinmann pin is inserted into the olecranon in line with the anterior border of the humerus. The Kirschner wire is removed and replaced by a long cancellous screw with a washer. The second Steinmann pin is now introduced into the humerus, the external compression clamps applied, and the cancellous screw finally tightened.

Wrist arthrodesis.

Fig. 300   First resect all articular cartilage and prepare a bed for the cortico-cancellous graft. Next, take a wide cortico-cancellous graft from the iliac fossa and lay it so that it spans from the radius to the base of the second metacarpal, bridging the carpal bones. On top of the graft, extending from the radius to the shaft of the metacarpal lay on a contoured 7 to 9 hole plate, bent so that the wrist is arthrodesed at an angle of 160 to 140°. Fixation is achieved by screwing the plate with three screws to the radius and three screws into the shaft of the second metatarsal. The system can be placed under compression by means of the tension device, but only when the distal ulna has been resected.

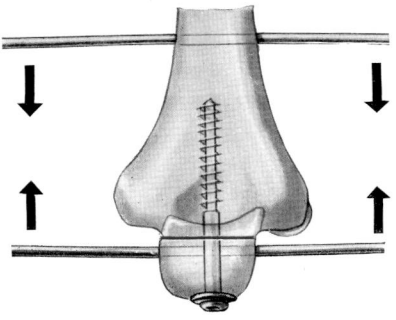

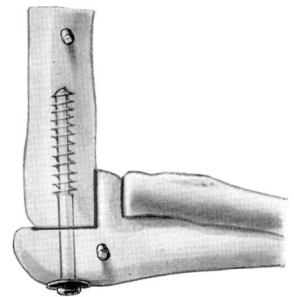

299

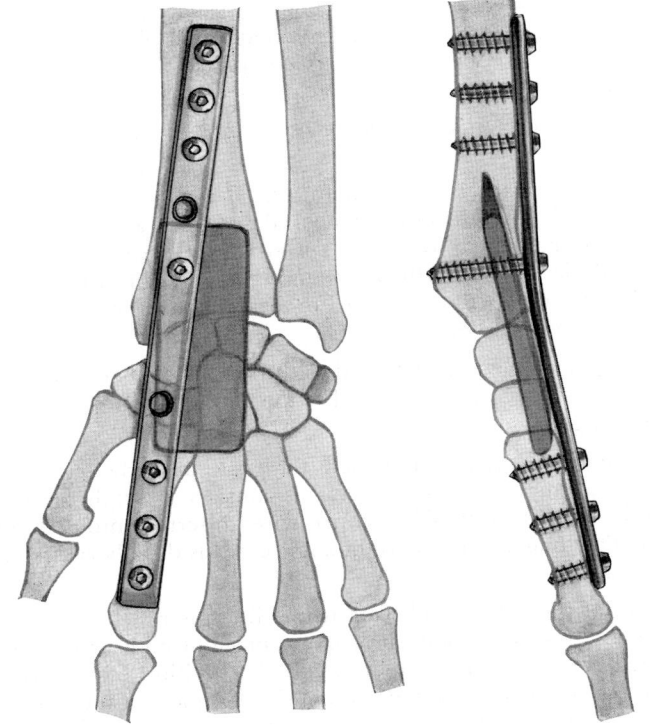

300

C. Hip Arthrodesis with the Cobra Head Plate

Fig. 301

a   Make a 25 cm long incision.

b   Osteotomize a small piece of the greater trochanter together with the insertion of the gluteus medius and minimus and retract the muscles with the fragment of the greater trochanter upwards, exposing the lateral surface of the ilium. Next do an osteotomy through the ilium immediately above the acetabulum, employing wide Hohmann retractors and the AO bone spreader. The osteotomy is carried out with a broad osteotome. The Hohmann retractors displace the sciatic nerve dorsally and protect it. After the osteotomy is completed, both surfaces of the hip joint are exposed, and the articular cartilage is resected.

> *The pelvic osteotomy must be horizontal or even directed slightly upwards. Otherwise an abduction deformity will result.*

c   The vastus lateralis is reflected forwards, exposing the femoral shaft. The leg is placed in 10° of adduction, in neutral rotation, and according to the age of the patient and his lumbar lordosis, in 10 to 25° of flexion. The cobra head plate is now taken and placed against the ilium and the lateral surface of the femur, and checked for fit. Occasionally more bone from the greater trochanter must be osteotomized or the cobra head plate bent.

d   The cobra head plate is next fixed to the ilium with one screw placed 1 cm above the osteotomy surface. It is then fixed to the femoral shaft with the tension device which is gently tightened.

e   As the tension device is tightened, the position of the leg is constantly checked by means of a simple aiming device. This consists of a right angle which is fixed to the pelvis by means of two Kirschner wires inserted into the anterior superior iliac spines. The long arm of the right angle extends distally and is made to lie just lateral to the patella.

f, g   Fixation of the cobra head plate to the ilium is now completed with six additional screws and the osteotomy surfaces are brought under compression. As soon as the maximal compression is achieved and the position of the extremity is perfect, the plate is screwed distally to the femoral shaft. A piece of the resected greater trochanter is used as a bone graft and is placed between the plate and the femoral head. Another piece is placed anterior to the hip joint in a specially cut trough. Before the final tightening of all screws, the position of the extremity should be checked once more.

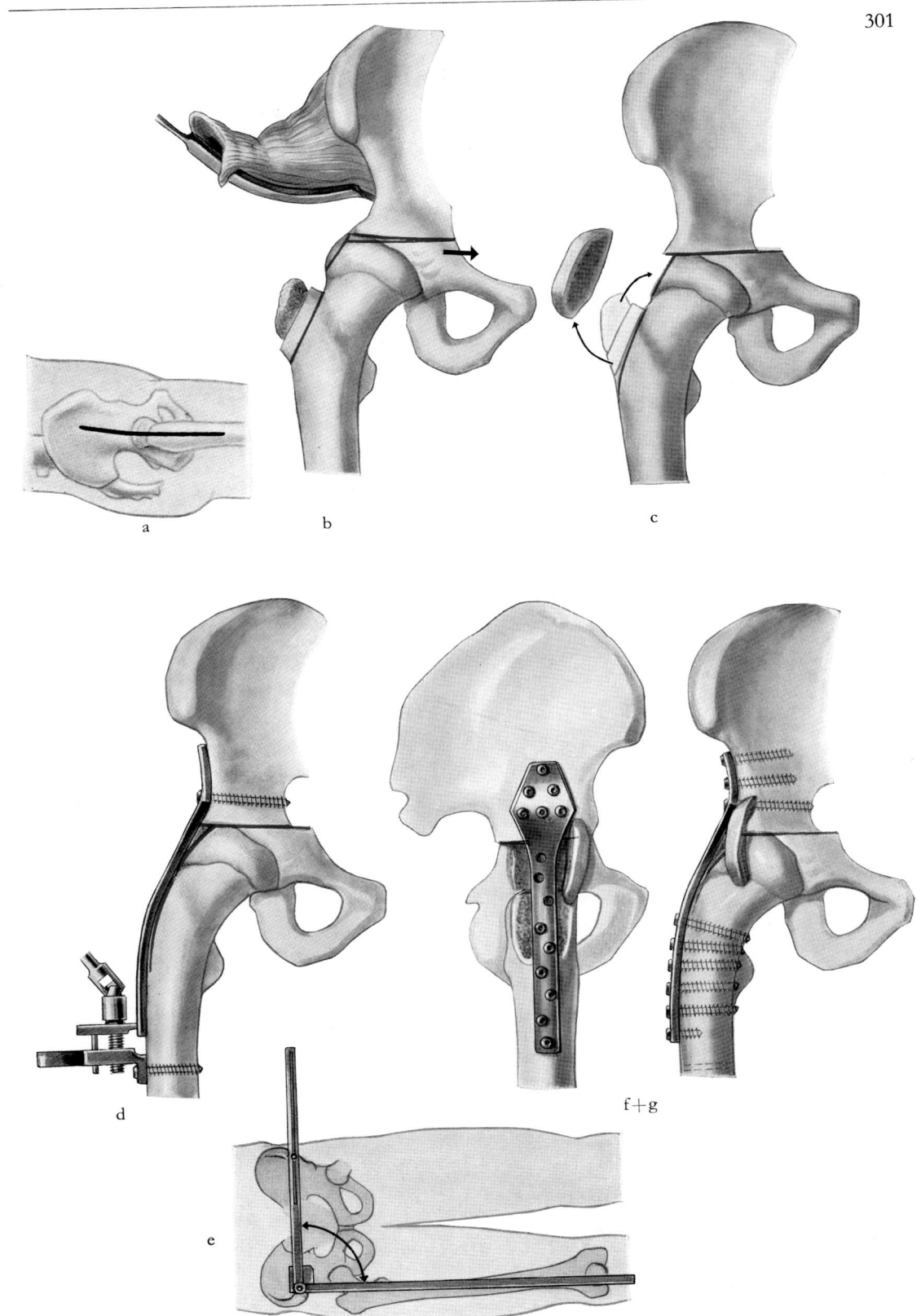

a

b

c

d

e

f+g

D. The Technique in Arthrodesis of the Knee

Fig. 302

a   Make a longitudinal incision. Expose and excise the patella. With a broad osteotome shape it into a cube to be used as a bone graft.

b   Incise the joint capsule widely and flex the knee to 90°. Next, using the oscillating saw, resect the femoral condyles in a plane parallel to tibial axis. The tibial plateau is resected obliquely so that when the fragments are reduced mild flexion of the knee joint will result.

c   Check that the anterior iliac spine, the middle of the knee joint and the space between the first and second metatarsal are all in a straight line.

d   The angle between the axes of tibia and femur should be 170° in both antero-posterior and lateral views.

e   When a correct position of the knee joint has been achieved, four Steinmann pins are driven in. The two posterior ones are driven in as close to the resected surfaces as possible, while the two anterior ones are inserted approximately 4 cm from the resection line. The external compression clamps are applied and the position is checked one again. Finally, use the patellar bone graft to bridge the joint anteriorly.

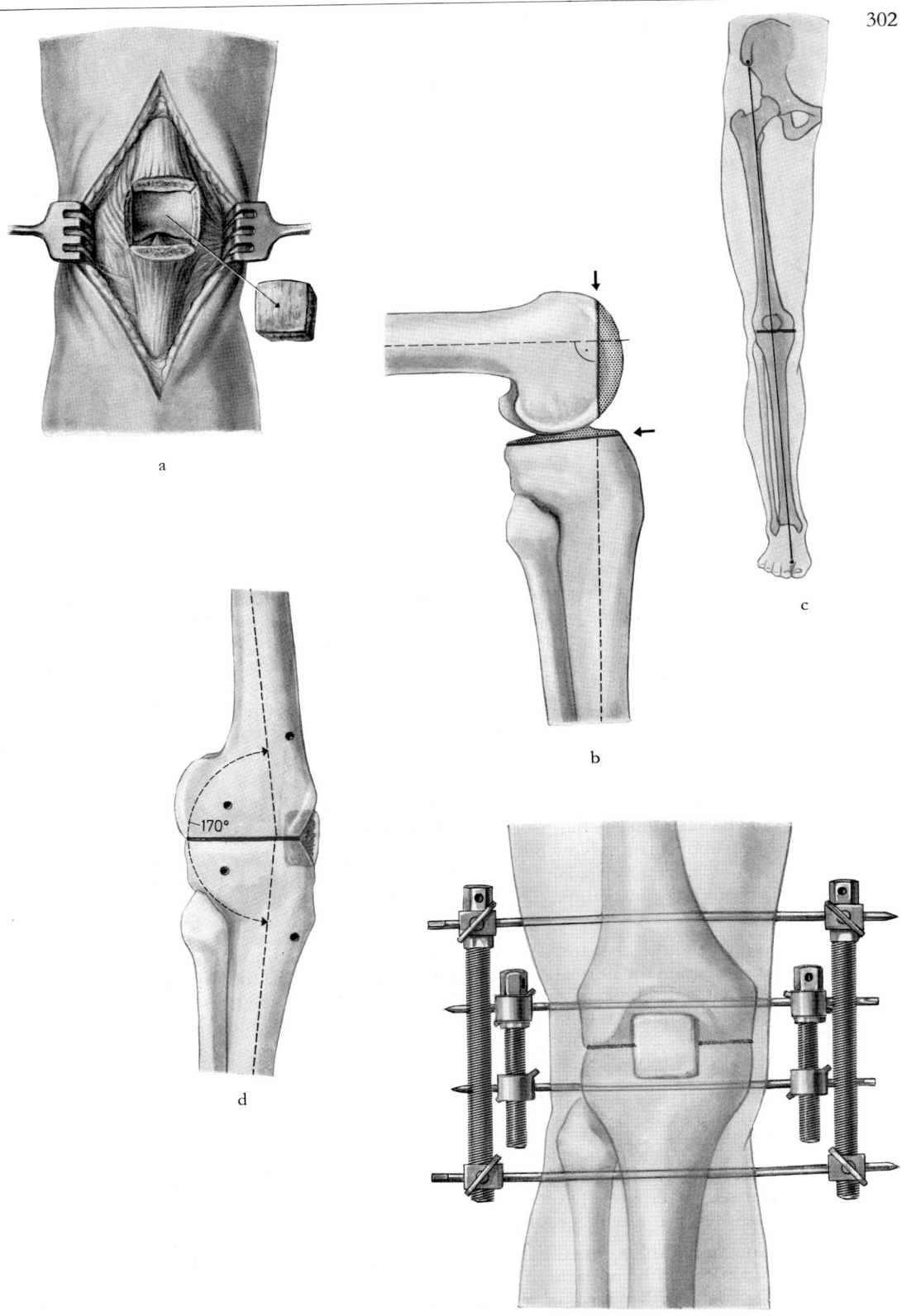

a

b

c

d

e

170°

302

285

E. Technique of Compression Arthrodesis of the Ankle

Fig. 303

a   Apply a pneumatic tourniquet. Drape the leg so as to expose both the knee and ankle joints. Insert the first Steinmann pin from the medial side, 6 to 7 cm proximal to the ankle joint, making certain that it is in 20° of external rotation relative to the axis of the knee joint. This pin should emerge from the leg just in front of the fibula. The pin is more easily inserted if a hole is first drilled in the correct direction, using a 3.2 mm bit. Make an incision of 8 cm over the lateral malleolus and one of 5 cm over the medial malleolus. If there is no deformity of the foot, and particularly if it is in the correct rotational position, insert a 2.5 mm Kirschner wire where the second pin is to be; namely into the talus just at the level of the anterior tibial border and parallel to the first pin.

b   The Steinmann pin and the Kirschner wire are now removed so that they will not be in the way during the procedure. Make an oblique osteotomy through the fibula 3 cm above its tip. Now resect the tibial articular surface, either with a chisel or with an oscillating saw, making absolutely certain that the dorsal lip of the tibia is resected. Through the medial incision resect the medial malleolus and smooth off the medial surface.

c   Now bend the knee to 90° and give the foot the same amount of external rotation as is present on the normal side. Control the position of the foot by placing two Kirschner wires through the previously drilled holes, one in the tibia and one in the talus. These two wires should be parallel to each other. In women the ankle joint should be arthrodesed at 90°. In men who have a good range of movement in the midtarsal joint, we recommend 80° as the best position for arthrodesis.

d   Now resect the dome of the talus to give a flat surface parallel to that of the lower end of the tibia.

e   Now insert the proximal Steinmann pin. Check the position of the foot again and insert the second Steinmann pin into the hole in the talus which previously housed the Kirschner wire. Displace the talus posteriorly to preserve the tendo-Achillis-os calcis lever arm which results in better gait.

f   Now apply the external compression clamps to compress the arthrodesis strongly. Again check the position of the foot and the stability of the fixation. We usually use the lateral malleolus after resecting its articular surface as a bone graft between the talus and the tibia and hold it in place with a small malleolar screw.

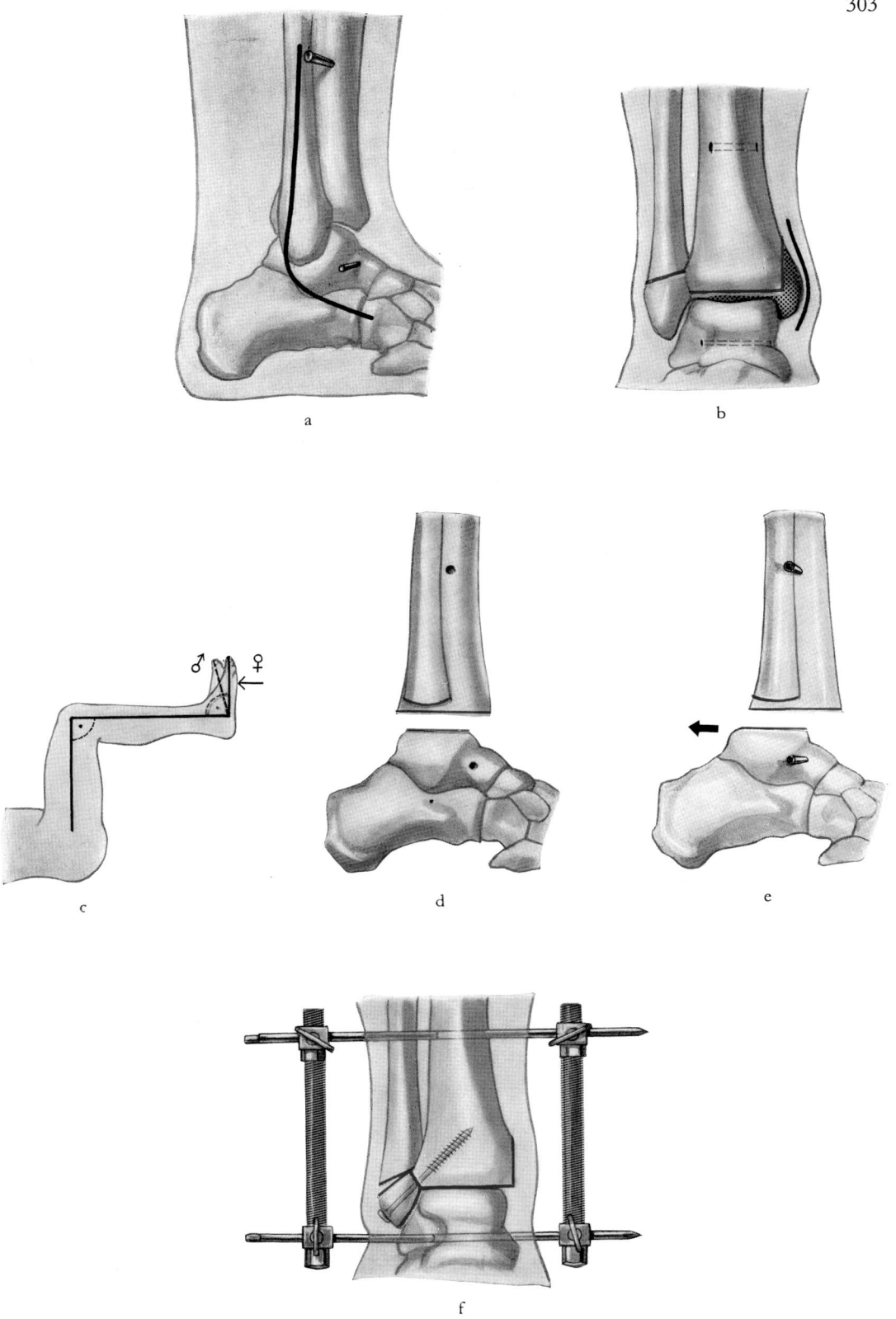

a

b

c

d

e

f

Fig. 304   *Primary arthrodesis of the ankle.*

In those injuries in which the articular surface of the talus and that of the distal tibia are severely damaged, secondary osteoarthritis of the ankle joint is a certainty and subsequent ankle arthrodesis must almost always be carried out to alleviate the pain and disability. It is for these cases that we recommend primary ankle arthrodesis. The articular cartilage is resected before internal fixation is begun. The comminuted fracture of the distal tibia is carefully reduced and fixed as rigidly as possible with screws. Finally Steinmann pins are inserted into the tibia and talus and the two cancellous surfaces are brought under compression by means of the external compression clamps (see also Fig. 216).

Fig. 305   *Pan-arthrodesis.*

Excise the whole talus, resect the articular cartilage from the mid-tarsal joint as well as from the distal articular surface of the tibia and the os calcis. Reduce the fragments and remodel the talus so that it fits exactly as a wedge between the tibia, os calcis and the navicular. Finally introduce Steinmann pins into the tibia, the os calcis as well as into the cuboid and navicular and obtain rigid fixation with four to six external compression clamps.

Arthrodesis of the interphalangeal joint of the great toe.

Fig. 306   An arthrodesis of this joint is indicated in trauma to the joint, in osteoarthritis and in paralysis of the extensor hallucis longus. The ideal position for arthrodesis is 180°.

a   Two incisions are made. The first is 10 to 15 mm in length and is made along the tip of the toe; the second is a transverse one and is made in the skin crease directly over the joint.

b   Resect the articular surfaces with a small saw and then drill through the distal phalanx with a 2 mm drill.

c   The drill is now reversed and the bit is pushed backwards through the distal phalanx without drilling it. The fragments are now reduced into the optimum position and the osteotomy surfaces are further trimmed if necessary. The drill is now advanced into the proximal phalanx and a 2 mm hole drilled in line with that in the distal phalanx. The drill is removed, and while the osteotomy surfaces are held together, fixation with a long, small cancellous screw is carried out.

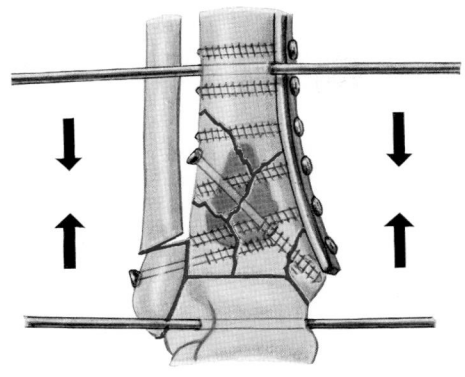

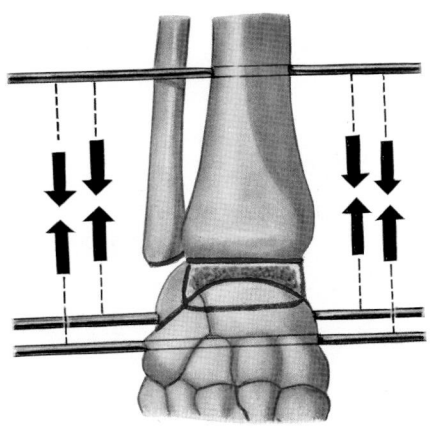
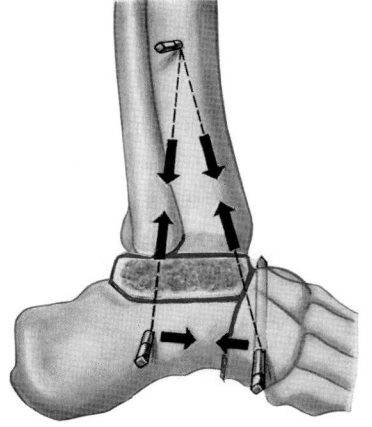

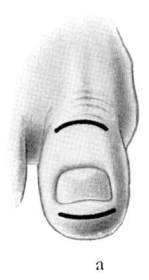
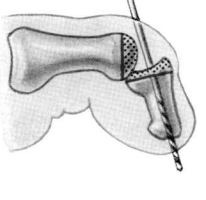

a b

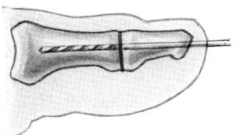
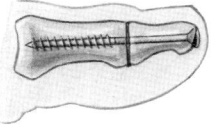

c

References

ALLGÖWER, M.: Funktionelle Anpassung des Knochens auf physiologische und unphysiologische Beanspruchung. Langenbecks Arch. klin. Chir. **319**, 384–391 (1967).
— Healing of clinical fractures of the tibia. C. Rigid internal fixation. Reprint from "The healing of osseous tissue". Nat. Acad. Sciences–Nat. Res. Council p. 81–89 (1967).
— Die intraartikulären Frakturen des distalen Unterschenkelendes. Helv. chir. Acta **35**, 556–582 (1968).
BANDI, W.: Zur Problematik der Korrektur posttraumatischer Achsenfehlstellungen der kindlichen Tibia. Z. Unfallmed. Berufskr. **4**, 289–294 (1966).
— ALLGÖWER, M.: Zur Therapie der Osteochondritis dissecans. Helv. chir. Acta **26**, 552 (1959).
BLOCH, H. R.: Die Druckplatten-Osteosynthese der Vorderarmschaftfrakturen. Helv. chir. Acta **30**, 98 (1963).
BLOUNT, W. P.: Knochenbrüche bei Kindern. Stuttgart: Thieme 1957.
— Fractures in children. Baltimore: Williams & Wilkins 1955.
BÖHLER, L.: Gelenknahe Frakturen des Unterarmes. Chirurg **40**, 198–203 (1969).
BÖHLER, J.: Die Technik der Knochenbruchbehandlung. Wien: Maudrich 1953 und 1957.
— Neues zur Behandlung der Fersenbeinbrüche. Langenbecks Arch. klin. Chir. **287**, 698 (1957).

BOYD, H. B., see CRENSHAW, A. H.: Campbell's Operative Orthopaedics. Saint Louis: Mosby 1963.
CHARNLEY, J.: Compression arthrodesis, Including central dislocation as a principle in hip surgery. Edinburgh: Livingston 1953.
— The closed treatment of common fractures, third edit. Edinburgh and London: Livingston 1961.
DANIS, R.: Théorie et pratique de l'ostéosynthèse. Paris: Masson 1947.
— Le vrai but et les dangers de l'ostéosynthèse. Lyon chir. **51**, 740 (1956).
HACKETHAL, K. H.: Die Bündelnagelung. Wien: Springer 1961.
HERZOG, K.: Nagelung der Tibiaschaftbrüche mit einem starren Nagel. Dtsch. Z. Chir. **276**, 227 (1953).
— Die Technik der geschlossenen Marknagelung des Oberschenkels mit dem Rohrschlitznagel. Chirurg **31**, 465 (1960).
JUDET, R.: Luxation congénitale de la hanche. Fractures du cou-depied, rachis cervical. Actualités de chirurgie orthopédique de l'Hôpital Raymond-Poincaré. Paris: Masson 1964.
— JUDET, J.: The use of an artificial femoral head for arthroplasty of the hip joint. J. Bone Jt Surg. B **32**, 166 (1950).
KROMPECHER, S.: Die Knochenbildung. Jena: Fischer 1937.
KÜNTSCHER, G.: Die Marknagelung. Berlin-Göttingen-Heidelberg: Springer 1962.

Küntscher, G.: Praxis der Marknagelung. Stuttgart: Schattauer 1962.

Lambotte, A.: Le traitement des fractures. Paris: Masson 1907.

— Chirurgie opératoire des fractures. Paris: Masson 1913.

Letournel, E.: Les fractures du cotyle, étude d'une série de 75 cas. J. Chir. (Paris) **82**, 47 (1961).

Maisonneuve, M. J. G.: Recherches sur la fracture du péroné. Arch. gén. Méd., 2e et N. sér. **7**, 165 (1840).

McElvenny, R. T.: The treatment of non-union of femoral neck fractures. Surg. Clin. N. Amer. **37**, 251 (1957).

— The immediate treatment of intra-capsular hip fracture. Chir. orthop. **10**, 289 (1957).

Moore, A. T.: Hip joint surgery. An outline of progress made in the past forty years. 1963.

Müller, M. E.: Hüftnahe Femurosteo-tomien, 2. Aufl. Stuttgart: Thieme 1970.

— Internal fixation of fractures and for non-unions. Proc. roy. Soc. Med. **56**, 455 (1963).

— Intertrochanteric osteotomy in arthrosis of the hip-joint. Proceedings Sect. Meeting ACS in coop. w. Germ. Surg. Soc., June 26–29, 1968. Berlin-Heidelberg-New York: Springer 1969.

— Compression as an aid in orthopaedic surgery. Reprint from "Recent advances in orthopaedics", edit. by G. Apley. London: Churchill 1969.

Pauwels, F.: Der Schenkelhalsbruch, ein mechanisches Problem. Stuttgart: Enke 1935.

— Gesammelte Abhandlungen zur funktionellen Anatomie des Bewegungsapparates. Berlin-Heidelberg-New York: Springer 1965.

Perren, S. M., Allgöwer, M., Ehrsam, R., Ganz, R., Matter, P.: Clinical experience with a new compression plate "DCP". Acta orthop. scand., Suppl. **125** (1969).

— Huggler, A., Russenberger, M., Allgöwer, M., Mathys, R., Schenk, R. K., Willenegger, H., Müller, M. E.: The reaction of cortical bone to compression. Acta Orthop. Scand., Suppl. **125** (1969).

— — — Straumann, F., Müller, M. E., Allgöwer, M.: A method of measuring the change in compression applied to living cortical bone. Acta Orthop. Scand., Suppl. **125** (1969).

— Hutzschenreuter, P., Steinemann, S.: Some effects of rigidity of internal fixation on the healing pattern of osteotomies. Z. Surg. **1**, 77 (1969).

— Russenberger, M., Steinemann, S., Müller, M. E., Allgöwer, M.: A dynamic compression plate. Acta Orthop. Scand., Suppl. **125** (1969).

Riede, U., Willenegger, H., Schenk, R.: Experimenteller Beitrag zur Erklärung der sekundären Arthrose bei Frakturen des oberen Sprunggelenks. Helv. chir. Acta **36**, 343–348 (1969).

Schenk, R., Willenegger, H.: Zur Biomechanik der Frakturheilung. Acta anat. (Basel) **53** (1963).

— — Zur Histologie der primären Knochenheilung. Langenbecks Arch. klin. Chir. **308**, 440 (1964).

— — Morphological findings in primary fracture healing. Symp. Biol. Hung. **7**, 75–86 (1967).

Schenk, R. K., Müller, J., Willenegger, H.: Experimentell-histologischer Beitrag zur Entstehung und Behandlung von Pseudarthrosen. Hefte Unfallheilk. **94**, 15–24 (1968); 31. Tagg, Berlin 1967.

Schneider, R.: Die Marknagelung der Tibia. Helv. chir. Acta **28**, 207 (1961).

WATSON-JONES, R.: Fractures and Joint Injuries. Edinburgh: Livingstone 1955.

WEBER, B. G.: Die Verletzungen des oberen Sprunggelenkes. Aktuelle Probleme in der Chirurgie, Bd. 3. Bern u. Stuttgart: Huber 1966.

— Fractures of the femoral shaft in childhood. Injury **1**, 1, July (1969).

WILLENEGGER, H.: Versorgung von offenen Frakturen. Chirurg **38**, 341–347 (1967).

— Prevention and management of infection in osteosynthesis. Proceedings Sect. Meeting ACS in coop. with Germ. Surg. Soc. Munich, June 26–29, 1968.

WILLENEGGER, H.: Problems and results in the treatment of comminuted fractures of the elbow. Reconstr. Surg. Traumat. **11**, 118–127 (1969).

— GUGGENBÜHL, A.: Zur operativen Behandlung bestimmter Fälle von distalen Radiusfrakturen. Helv. chir. Acta **26**, 81 (1959).

— MÜLLER, M. E., ALLGÖWER, M.: 178. Ergebnisse der Behandlung von Mehrfachverletzungen der Gliedmaßen (einschließlich Schultergürtel und Becken). Langenbecks Arch. klin. Chir. **322** (1968) (Kongreßber.).

Subject Index

The Dynamic Compression Plate (DCP)

By M. Allgöwer, P. Matter,
S. M. Perren, T. Rüedi
26 figures
VI, 45 pages. 1973
DM 18,–; US $7.00
ISBN 3-540-06466-4
German edition available
under the title: "Die Dynamische Kompressionsplatte (DCP)"
An improved version of the
standard compression
plate for internal fixation
of fractures has been
developed, and its technical basis and potential
applications are explained
in this book. The effects
of the plate have been
studied in biomechanical
experiments and it has
been used in more than
1500 fractures.
Contents: General Aspects
of the Dynamic Compression Plate (DCP).
The Concept of Dynamic
Compression Plates
(ASIF-DCP).

M. E. Müller, M. Allgöwer,
H. Willenegger:

Technique of Internal Fixation of Fractures

With contributions by
W. Bandi, H. R. Bloch,
A. Mumenthaler, R. Schneider, S. Steinemann,
F. Straumann, B. G. Weber
Revised for the English
Edition by G. Segmüller
244 figs. XII, 272 pp. 1965
Cloth DM 88,–; US $33.90
ISBN 3-540-03374-2

M. Watanabe, S. Takeda,
H. Ikeuchi:

Atlas of Arthroscopy

Entirely revised second
edition
134 figs. in color
IX, 176 pages. 1970
Cloth DM 102,–; US $39.30
ISBN 3-540-05268-2
Published by Igaku Shoin Ltd., Tokyo.
Sole distribution rights for the USA,
Canada, and Europe (including the
United Kingdom): Springer-Verlag

R. Burkhardt:

Bone Marrow and Bone Tissue

Color Atlas of Clinical
Histopathology
Foreword by W. Stich
Translated by H. J. Hirsch
721 colored figs.
XII, 115 pages. 1971
Cloth DM 248,–; US $95.50
ISBN 3-540-05059-0
Distribution rights for Japan:
Igaku Shoin Ltd., Tokyo

Journals

Calcified Tissue Research

Editorial Committee:
B. Engfeldt, H. Fleisch,
R. M. Frank, B. A. Friedman
(Secretary), R. P. Heaney,
B. E. C. Nordin (Secretary),
F. G. E. Pautard (Secretary), C. Rich, D. B. Scott
(Secretary), K. M. Wilbur
Published in English
Approx. 4 Vols. a year
Price upon request

Medical Progress through Technology

Editorial Board:
G. O. Barnett, D. H. Bekkering, U. Gessner,
W. Giere, D. W. Hill,
B. Horisberger, R. Magnusson, O. Mayrhofer,
M. Oshima, C. D. Ray
(Editor-in-Chief).
M. Schaldach, J. Toressani,
K. Yamaguchi
Published in English
1 Vol. a year
Price upon request

Prices are subject
to change without notice

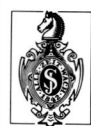

Springer-Verlag Berlin Heidelberg New York

München Johannesburg
London Madrid New Dehli
Paris Rio de Janeiro
Sydney Tokyo Utrecht
Wien

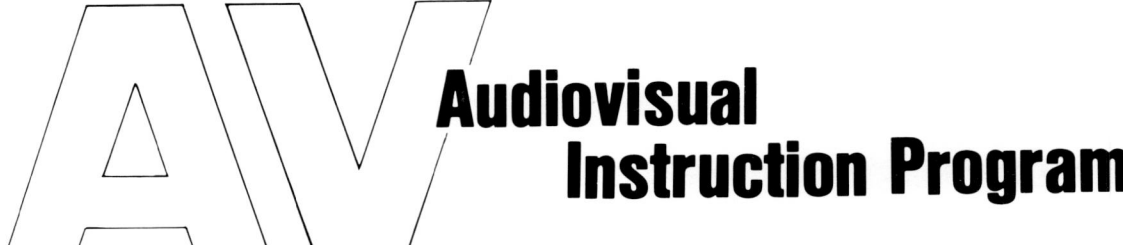

Audiovisual Instruction Program

Film Series: Internal Fixation of Fractures

**Internal Fixation
Basic Principles and Modern Means**
Medical advisors:
M. Allgöwer, Basle; S. M. Perren, Davos

Internal Fixation of Forearm Fractures
Medical advisors:
Th. Rüedi, Basle; M. Allgöwer, Basle;
A. v. Hochstetter, Basle

**Internal Fixation of Noninfected
Diaphyseal Pseudarthroses**
Medical advisors:
M. E. Müller, Bern; R. Ganz, Bern

Internal Fixation of Malleolar Fractures
Medical advisor:
B. G. Weber, St. Gall

Internal Fixation of Patella Fractures
Medical advisor:
B. G. Weber, St. Gall

Medullary Nailing
Medical advisors:
Ş. Weller, Tübingen; F. Schauwecker, Tübingen

**Internal Fixation of the Distal End
of the Humerus**
Medical advisors:
C. Burri, Ulm; A. Rüter, Ulm

Internal Fixation of Mandibular Fractures
Medical advisors:
B. Spiessl, Basle; J. Prein, Basle; B. A. Rahn, Davos

Corrective Osteotomy of the Distal Tibia
Medical advisors:
M. Allgöwer, Basle; Th. Rüedi, Basle

The Biomechanics of Internal Fixation
Medical advisors:
S. M. Perren, Davos; B. A. Rahn, Davos; J. Cordey,
Davos

Book and slides:

Manual of Internal Fixation
by M. E. Müller, Bern; M. Allgöwer, Basle;
H. Willenegger, Liestal

Films on Allo-Arthroplasty:

Total Hip Prostheses
(3 parts)
Medical advisors:
M. E. Müller, Bern; R. Ganz, Bern

Part 1: **Instruments. Operation on Model**

Part 2: **Operative Technique**

Part 3: **Complications. Special Cases**

**Elbow-Arthroplasty
with the New GSB-Prosthesis**
Medical advisors:
N. Gschwend, Zurich; H. Scheier, Zurich

Technical data:
Eastmancolor, magnetic sound, optical sound
16 mm, Super-8, EVR, VCR, TED-disc

All films available in English and German;
French versions in preparation

Sales:
Springer-Verlag, D - 1 Berlin 33, Heidelberger Platz 3

■ Please ask for special brochure

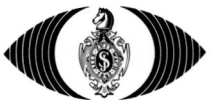

**Springer-Verlag
Berlin Heidelberg New York**
München · Johannesburg · London · New Delhi
Paris · Rio de Janeiro · Sydney · Tokyo · Wien